RDA:
Rats, Drugs and
Assumptions

Majid Ali, M.D.

**One of America's foremost spokespersons
for preventive medicine and
author of the Life Span Health Library**

Associate Professor of Pathology (Adj)
College of Physicians and Surgeons
of Columbia University, New York
Visiting Professor
Liu Hua Qiao General Hospital, Guanzhou, China
Director, Department of Pathology, Immunology and Laboratories
Holy Name Hospital, Teaneck, New Jersey
Chief Consulting Physician
Institute of Preventive Medicine, Denville, New Jersey
Fellow, Royal College of Surgeons of England
Diplomate, American Board of Environmental Medicine
Diplomate, American Board of Chelation Therapy
President, American Academy of Preventive Medicine

Library of Congress Catalog Card Number
95-77960
ISBN 1-879131-07-2

Ali, Majid
RDA: Rats, Drugs and Assumptions Majid Ali.--1st ed.

Includes bibliographical references and index

1. Empirical Medicine
2. N^2D^2 Medicine
3. Energetic-Molecular (EM) Medicine
4. RDA: Recommended Daily Allowances
5. Science and Medicine
6. Spontaneity of oxidation in Nature
7. Environment and Human Biology
8. Oxidative molecular injury
9. The Blood and Bowel Ecosystems

10 9 8 7 6 5 4 3 2 1

Published in the USA by

LIFE SPAN PRESS
95 East Main Street, Denville, New Jersey 07834
(201) 586-9191

RDA:

Rats, Drugs and Assumptions

A book that challanges most of the cherished assumptions of drug medicine. It lays bare many of the deceptions in medical statistics—most of them intended, it seems. It shows how results of valid medical research are deliberately distorted to promote long-term use of drugs of dubious value. It exposes the deep prejudice of practitioners of drug medicine against natural, nontoxic drug therapies.

This book clearly delineates the scientific basis of energetic-molecular events that cause disease, and shows how accelerated oxidative injury to human enzyme systems—comprised of energy, detoxification and digestive enzymes—is the cause of all disease processes. Furthermore, it describes how oxidative enzyme injury leads to disruptions of the bowel, blood and other body organ ecosystems.

This book marshalls evidence for the viewpoint that injured enzymes cannot be revived with drug therapies. What is required is a global restorative strategy that reduces further oxidative enzyme injury and facilitates repair of damaged enzymes by appropriate nutritional, environmental, self-regulatory and fitness approaches. It provides sound scientific basis for effective, nondrug therapies for reversing chronic degenerative, ecologic and immune disorders. Most importantly, this book defines new dimensions of preventive medicine and a promotive philosophy of health.

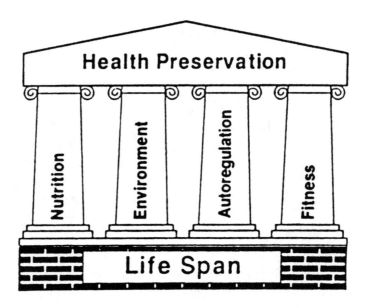

Perfection of means and confusion of goals seem—in my opinion—to characterize our age.

Albert Einstein

To all my patients, medical and nursing staffs of the Institute of Preventive Medicine, Denville, New Jersey, and my colleagues at the American Academy of Preventive Medicine.

Acknowledgments

I am most grateful to my patients whose true-to-life suffering and the recovery process gave me insights into the nature of the healing response. They were—and will always remain—my teachers.

I am indebted to my colleagues in the American Academy of Preventive Medicine, the American Academy of Environmental Medicine and the American College for Advancement in Medicine who patiently listened and critiqued my theory that, at a basic energetic-molecular level, spontaneity of oxidation in nature is the cause of all diseases. This seemed too simplistic an idea at that time. They didn't laugh me out of the conference halls during the early 1980s when I first began to present my basic theory and nondrug therapies based on it. The editors of the Syllabus of the Academy allowed me to publish my theory even when essential experimental and clinical evidence for it was lacking in some critical areas.

I thank Jerrold Finnie, M.D., Dolores Finnie, R.N., Maria Lissandrello, Lisa Rosen, Cathy Johnson and Peggy Weiner for their editorial work; Barry Weiner for his sketches for the title pages for book chapters; Ronald Rizzio and his staff at the library of Holy Name Hospital, Teaneck, for complying with my endless requests for literature searches; and the staff at Life Span Press for their unfailing support. I am especially grateful to Sister Patricia Lynch, President, Holy Name Hospital for her support of my work in preventive medicine.

Talat, my wife, is forever my best resource.

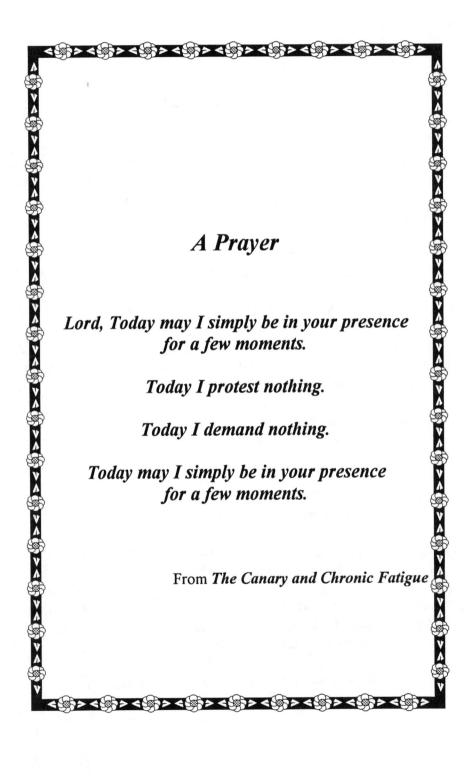

A Prayer

Lord, Today may I simply be in your presence
for a few moments.

Today I protest nothing.

Today I demand nothing.

Today may I simply be in your presence
for a few moments.

From *The Canary and Chronic Fatigue*

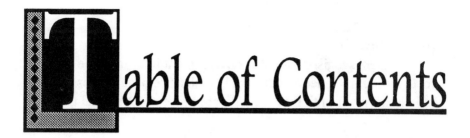

Table of Contents

PREFACE

The notion of Recommended Daily Allowances (RDA) is the most pernicious idea of 20th-century medicine.

In 1940 the Food and Nutrition Board established amounts of several nutrients that it considered sufficient to prevent some nutritional deficiency diseases. This was unequivocally the worst medical folly ever foisted on the American people by government experts. None of the "experts" who sat on the Nutrition Board proclaiming the RDA doctrine had ever practiced nutritional medicine. Notwithstanding, the RDA doctrine led to a widespread assumption among physicians that nutrients play no role in reversing chronic degenerative, ecologic and immune disorders. It led to the second and more dangerous assumption that diseases could only be treated with drugs. Little did anyone recognize that these two seemingly innocent assumptions would rob millions of Americans of untold opportunities in using nontoxic, nondrug nutrient therapies for disease prevention and treatment of chronic disorders.

The tragic error of the RDA is that it went on to spawn generations of physicians who turned their backs on the essential healing properties of nutrients, and became staunch opponents of all nondrug therapies. Ignorant in the true nature of the healing response and ill-informed about the role of nutrients in it, they declared all nutrient therapies quackery and relentlessly persecuted physician-nutritionists. Drugs and scalpels became the only acceptable tools of the trade. Laws were enacted to revoke the licenses of practitioners who practiced unconventional (meaning nondrug and nonsurgical) therapies.

HEALING IS A NATURAL STATE OF ENERGY

When life begins, it begins to end. The healing response occurs as a natural response to the aging phenomenon—beginning at the onset of life and lasting till life ends. Both the aging and healing phenomena are energy events. Injured tissues heal spontaneously. Damaged molecules, cells and tissues are programmed to generate their own healing cues. External factors may facilitate or impede the healing response, but they cannot set the wheels of healing in motion. Good medicine must be centered on this.

Injured tissues heal with nutrients—not with drugs. Vitamins, minerals, essential fatty acids and amino acids perform a myriad of metabolic functions in the body. How did it come to pass that all these nutrients were assigned metabolic roles to prevent only a few nutritional deficiency diseases? This is a simple but revealing question. Physicians are among the most highly educated, hard working and diligent individuals in any society. They see human suffering in ways no other profession does. Their whole lives are dedicated to alleviating suffering. Yet, when it comes to reversing chronic disorders, they have become impervious to the most elementary of ideas: that injured tissues heal with nutrients, and nutrients must be considered the most logical and natural therapy. I have often wondered why my colleagues in drug medicine cannot see this.

Why has the use of nutrients in clinical medicine been neglected to date? American taxpayers have paid dearly for a huge body of research in nutrition. With rare exceptions, such studies clearly demonstrate the health benefits of nutrients—drawing conclusions that, in general, are entirely predictable on teleologic grounds alone. (After all, the healing response evolved with nutrients over eons.) Why have the results of all such research been excluded from clinical medicine? Why have the healing potentials of vitamins, minerals and essential amino and fatty acids been so maligned in the U.S.? Why have nutritionist-physicians been so harassed by the disease doctors of drug medicine? The answers to all these questions have to do with the establishment of RDAs—the minute amounts of vitamins and minerals that the Nutrition Board assumes are necessary to prevent a few deficiency diseases such as scurvy (by vitamin C), beri (by thiamine), pellagra (by niacin), rickets (by vitamin D) and others.

ASSUMPTION OF IRREVERSIBILITY

The irreversibility of chronic disease is the underlying premise of drug medicine in the U.S. This assumption leads to the erroneous belief that chronic disease can only be managed by suppressing its symptoms with drugs. This assumption is not formally taught in medical school. Rather, it grows quickly in the minds of young physicians as they recognize that drugs and scalpels are the only tools of their trade—and that only quacks talk about the regenerative capacity of the body and nondrug therapies to facilitate that process.

DRUG MEDICINE: A MEDICINE OF BLOCKADE
NUTRITIONAL MEDICINE:
A MEDICINE OF FACILITATION

Chronic disease is a state of deranged physiologic processes. *Drugs are designed by chemists* to quickly relieve symptoms by blocking such processes. Even when used in the recommended doses, these drugs produce toxic effects over time with long-term usage. *Nutrients, by contrast, were designed by nature* to facilitate healing responses in a slow and sustained fashion. From extensive personal experience—as well as that of my colleagues in nutritional medicine—I know that nutrient therapies have a far greater margin of safety than drugs, even when used for decades. I cite the following examples:

Drugs block cell membrane channels that normally regulate the flow of essential minerals such as calcium, potassium and magnesium, i.e., calcium channel blocker drugs such as Calan and Cardizem. A partial list of the toxic effects of such drugs, given in the *Physicians' Desk Reference* (PDR), includes heart block, palpitations, sexual difficulties, loss of consciousness, congestive heart failure, depression, loss of memory, insomnia, tinnitus, tremors, liver injury, loss of hair and abdominal symptoms. *Magnesium is nature's calcium channel blocker.* It works slowly but never creates the adverse reactions caused by calcium channel blocking drugs. Looseness of the bowel movements is the only change with oral magnesium therapy that may be seen in a negative light—not a bad effect from a life span perspective.

Drugs block cell membrane receptors, i.e., Beta blocker drugs used for high blood pressure, such as Inderal and Lopressor. A partial list of the toxic effects of such drugs given in the PDR include congestive heart failure, a type of heart block called AV block, low blood pressure, Raynaud's type vascular insufficiency (cold hands and feet), depression, fatigue, lightheadedness, memory loss, constipation and/or diarrhea, colitis, loss of hair, lupus-like condition, impotence and bone marrow suppression. *Taurine is nature's membrane receptor stabilizer.* It is a potent antioxidant, and occurs in large amounts in almost all cells. Its clinical benefits in preventing and controlling heart rhythm disturbances have been observed by all reporting clinicians. It, of course, has none of the adverse effects of beta blocker drugs.

Drugs block essential enzymes, i.e., ACE inhibitor drugs for high blood pressure such as Capoten and Vasotec. Toxic effects of such drugs listed in the PDR include chest pain, heart palpitations, Raynaud's reaction, cough, skin eruptions, bone marrow suppression, pancreatitis, glossitis (inflammation of the tongue) and many other reactions. *Magnesium and calcium are nature's enzyme regulators.* These minerals optimize the functions of enzymes that in turn regulate the contractility of muscle cells in the vessel walls and so normalize blood pressure.

Drugs block or inactivate mediators of inflammation—the essential response in injured tissues that precedes the repair and healing phenomena. Examples: histamine-inactivating drugs such as Benadryl and Seldane. Adverse effects of such drugs include drowsiness, fatigue and concentration difficulties. *Bioflavonoids, pantothenic acid and histidine are nature's antihistaminics.*

Drugs block the various arms of the immune system. Example: steroids that suppress the immune response. Toxic effects of such drugs are far-reaching and include vulnerability to infections, poor healing responses, osteoporosis, stomach ulcers, psychosis and other conditions. *Essential amino acids and fatty acids, minerals and vitamins are nature's immune enhancers.*

Drugs block the energy and detoxification enzymes of the body even when that is not their intended goal. Example: The commonly prescribed ulcer drug Tagamet suppresses the essential detoxification enzymes included in the cytochrome P-450 system. *Vitamins are nature's energy and detoxification enzymes.* Notable among them are pantothenic acid, thiamine, niacin, pyridoxin, vitamin B^{12} and other members of B complex.

THE TRAGEDY OF RDA

Underlying the notion of RDAs are four dangerous assumptions that have had a profoundly detrimental impact on medical thinking over the last several decades.

First,

nutrients do not play any metabolic roles in the healing process, except those identified in the prevention of a handful of nutritional deficiency diseases.

Second,

because nutrients are of no value in the management of chronic degenerative, ecologic and immune disorders, such disorders can only be treated with drugs.

Third,

because drugs can only suppress symptoms of chronic degenerative, ecologic, immune, nutritional, stress-related or physical disorders, such disorders must be accepted as irreversible.

Fourth,

because drugs cannot normalize deranged cell membranes and revive damaged bowel, blood and cellular ecosystems, a sound, *working* knowledge of human ecosystems is of no relevance to clinical medicine.

EMPIRICAL MEDICINE EVOLVES INTO AN ENERGETIC-MOLECULAR (EM) MEDICINE

Since humankind began to search for ways to alleviate suffering caused by illness, medicine has been empirical—it sought to use therapies that worked and were safe. In empirical medicine, safe and effective therapies are not discarded just because it is not known how they work. This is the *core* principle of the philosophy of the great ancient healing arts of

India, China and Greece.

The empirical medicine must now evolve into an "energetic-molecular (EM)" medicine—a medicine that holds the enduring principle of empiricism of the ancient healing arts and adds to it the science and technology of energetic-molecular (EM) dynamics of health—dis-ease—disease continuum. The medicine of future—I am certain—will be this EM medicine. I devote the chapter entitled A Changing Medicine for a Changing Time to my vision of what such a medicine will be—and how it will continue to evolve. This is a medicine based on EM events that occur in molecules (and cells and tissues) before they are injured and changed. It is not based on the study of how dead and decaying cells and tissues look under the microscope *after* they have been damaged by disease.

Physicians who practice drug medicine assume that the chemistry of disease is all they need to know. Sadly, most physicians practicing drug medicine do not know even the chemistry of drug medicine in any detail—otherwise they would quickly learn the reasons why drugs cannot reverse chronic disease, and why every attempt should be made to substitute nutrients for drugs in chronic disease as soon as possible.

The new EM medicine is based on the two well-known —and fundamentally essential—facts of biology:

1.   EM injury to cells, tissues and body organs is reversible.
2.   EM healing response in injured cells, tissues and body organs occurs spontaneously and requires an ample supply of essential nutrients.

In acute illness, drugs are necessary to break the hold of

EM derangements that feed upon each other and perpetuate disease. This is irrelevant to the care of patients with chronic nutritional, ecologic, degenerative, stress-related and physical disorders.

TEXTBOOKS WILL GO OUT THE WINDOW, PATIENTS WILL STAY

I graduated from medical school in 1963. In 1968, I passed the examination and received the diploma of the Fellow of the Royal College of Surgeons of England. Four years later, after completing my pathology residence, I was certified by the American Boards of Clinical and Anatomic Pathology. In 1974, I was appointed Director of the Department of Pathology, Immunology and Laboratories at Holy Name Hospital, Teaneck, New Jersey. From 1974 to 1986, I practiced some clinical medicine but largely devoted my time to research and the practice of pathology. I estimate that I examined over 50,000 biopsies and surgical specimens during those years. During those years, I also authored and coauthored a series of twelve books written for pathologists preparing to take their board examination. Needless to say, I became well-versed with the names of diseases and the criteria for their diagnosis.

My early years of microscopic diagnostic work with biopsy and surgical specimens gave me a growing dissatisfaction with my inability to learn about the initial EM events that cause disease. I diagnosed thousands of diseases, and learned about others that I didn't see in pathology textbooks. The EM events that initiated all such diseases remained elusive. I became acutely aware of the microscope's limitation and turned my focus to the immune system. My clinical work and research in this area—in collaboration with my colleague Madhava Ramanarayanan, Ph.D., and others—led to our introduction of micro-elisa tests for the diagnosis of food incompatibilities and food allergy.

In 1986, I began to devote more time to clinical medicine in order to pursue an active investigation of how environmental agents injure human biologic systems. This investigation allowed me to test many of the theoretical concepts that evolved over years of pathology work. For several years, I had seen clinical problems only through the eyes of my colleagues in drug medicine. Now it was time to see things through the eyes of people who suffered from such disorders. I made three decisions:

First,

never to doubt the veracity of any statements made by any of my patients. Yes, it would carry the clear risk that someone vehemently opposed to empirical medicine might try to make a fool of me by feeding me deliberate lies. If so, so be it.

Second,

to limit my inquiries to two basic elements: 1) The words a patient uses to describe his suffering; and 2) The EM events that provide the basis of that suffering. Specifically, I decided to ignore the disease names that tell me nothing—but hide much—about the cause of a patient's suffering.

Third,

and most importantly, to disregard my medical textbooks whenever a patient's clinical picture does not fit an established disease name.

This seemed a reasonable personal philosophy as I began to confront the illnesses that I knew could only be caused by the impact of internal and external environments on human genetic make-up.

HEALING IS AN ENERGY FUNCTION

Healing is a person's natural state. It is not natural to be sick. In essence, life is energy, and health is an energy state. Diseases occur when the natural energetic state of tissues is burdened by elements in a person's internal and external environments. In health, the internal environment is preserved by the interplay of genes, metabolism of food and stress-related factors; the external environment is made up of some natural hazards and an increasing number of man-made toxic pollutants.

Life is created with energy. Life is sustained with energy. Life ends when energy is depleted. When molecules, cells, tissues and organs are injured, they heal with energy, and such healing is a spontaneous process. Diseases occur when there are impediments in the way of tissue healing.

An internist's drugs never heal. A surgeon's scalpel never heals. Organs, tissues and molecules have an innate ability to heal. What drugs and scalpels do well in acute diseases is to remove impediments to healing. Self-regulation with energy— "autoregulation" as I define in *The Cortical Monkey and Healing*—works exactly the same way in chronic ecologic, immune and nutritional disorders. I maintain that this is the true nature of healing.

Mind-over-body healing does not work, notwithstanding rather limited, temporary benefits of positive thinking and affirmations. An energy-over-mind approach to healing *does*. Psychosomatic and somatopsychic models of diseases are artifacts of our thinking. Diseases are burdens on biology. These burdens are imposed on our genetic make-up by our internal and external environments. The intensity of suffering caused by these burdens is profoundly influenced by a third element: the choices we make.

PREVENTIVE MEDICINE OF ECO-RELATIONSHIPS

I define some new dimensions of EM medicine in this book—and in the companion volumes *The Butterfly and Life Span Nutrition, The Ghoraa and Limbic Exercise, The Canary and Chronic Fatigue* and *The Cortical Monkey and Healing*. In *Canary*, I write about political pundits who incubate grand schemes in their clever minds to solve America's health problems with brilliant legislative strokes. The problem with such pundits is that they cannot distinguish between *front-end* medicine and *tail-end* medicine. Front-end medicine is the prevention of disease by addressing the initial EM events that separate a state of health from a state of absence of health. Tail-end medicine, by contrast, only suppresses symptoms of advanced chronic disease with drugs.

Physicians, in general, are skeptical about the prevailing concepts of preventive medicine. They recognize that they can only pay lip service to preventive measures such as balanced diet, choice of low-cholesterol foods, relaxation, loss of excess weight and physical fitness. Their offices and clinics are not set up to effectively pursue any of these measures. (Drug doctors only know how to use drugs. How does one use drugs to prevent disease?) Even when they hear experts gloat about success in the early diagnosis of cancers of the breast and cervix, they recognize *early diagnosis is not prevention.*

Genuine disease prevention calls for focus on nutrition; food incompatibilities and allergy; integrity of bowel, blood and other body ecosystems; Fourth-of-July chemistry under the skin—oxidative storms caused by stress—and physical fitness. Mainstream physicians are neither trained nor equipped to cope with any of these problems.

The medicine of the future will study ecologic relationships: how the bowel ecosystem interfaces with the ecosystems outside the body, how the blood ecosystem interfaces with the bowel ecosystem and how cellular ecosystems interface with the blood ecosystem. It will seek to preserve the integrity of such ecosystems and enhance such relationships rather than disrupt them with chemicals. Drugs, while essential for symptom suppression in acute illness, cannot revive damaged ecosystems.

The medicine of the future for enlightened individuals will

be EM medicine of health preservation and disease reversal by natural methods. It will use natural molecules that co-evolved with human ecosystems. Such substances will include minerals, vitamins, essential amino acids and fatty acids, and natural plant and animal materials contained in herbs. It will not seek to launch a chemical attack on physiological processes using synthetic drugs. It will also harness physical and energetic healing methods of proven efficacy.

Drugs will continue to save lives in acute, life-threatening illness. However, I'm afraid that drugs will also continue to treat chronic illness for limited short-term gains and serious long-term adverse consequences—simply because there will always be stakeholders in drug medicine who will forever find ingenious ways to persuade physicians to promote their drugs.

LACK OF FREEDOM OF CHOICE IN JEFFERSON'S LAND

We Americans hold precious the Jeffersonian notions of freedom of life, liberty and pursuit of happiness. Yet, people with chronic nutritional, degenerative, ecologic and immune disorders have less freedom of choice of therapies in the U.S. than in other country in the world. The dogma of drug medicine holds that all nondrug therapies are quackery and denies Americans effective and inexpensive nutritional and herbal therapies widely used in other parts of the world. The principal reason for this is that the prevailing standards of drug medicine require that all therapies be proven effective only by the double-blind cross-over methods of drug testing. This frivolous notion is utterly irrelevant to empirical medicine, in which neither the practitioner nor the patient wants to be—or can be—blinded to the true nature of therapy for extended periods of time. What we need are sound clinical outcome studies by those who understand the principles and practice of evolving EM medicine.

I hope the information I present, and the arguments I marshall to make the case for the nondrug therapies of the EM medicine, will quell some of the ignorant animus of practitioners of drug medicine against natural, nondrug therapies. I hope this information will raise some questions about the assumption of irreversibility of chronic disease that chains physicians to the prevailing model of drug medicine. I hope that sound scientific knowledge of the eco-relationships I describe will help the professional as well as the general reader attain a genuine understanding of the rationale for nondrug therapies. I also hope these materials will help my readers make informed, enlightened choices in matters of health and disease.

Majid Ali, M.D.
Teaneck, New Jersey
August 1, 1995

A Letter to the U.S. Congress

Two elements characterize medicine in the U.S. today: The cost of health care continues to escalate, and the health of Americans continues to deteriorate. If the two trends were to hold, a time can be foreseen when the nation's total resources will have to be committed to health care, and everyone will be unwell.

On December 28, 1993, the Commerce Department announced that total health care spending in the U.S. will exceed $1 trillion in 1994 (The New York Times News Service, Dec. 12, 1993). As far as the deteriorating health of Americans, consider the following:

1. Pediatricians in Baltimore County prescribed drugs to six percent of the children there for disciplinary purposes (*JAMA* 260:2256; 1988). There are communities in the U.S. in which a still larger number of children are administered Ritalin, amphetamines and other drugs to control hyperactivity/attention deficit disorders.

2. The incidence of chronic fatigue among our children and adults is pervasive—one in four Americans saw his family practitioner for chronic fatigue according to some studies (*JAMA* 260:929; 1988).

3. It is felt that as many as 44 percent of adult Americans need antianxiety drugs (*N Eng J Med* 328;1399; 1993).

4. One in four American males is considered to suffer from disordered breathing while sleeping and is thought to require a machine to assist breathing (*N Eng J Med* 328; 1230; 1993).

5. The incidence of cancers of the breast and prostate is increasing in epidemic proportions, while progress in cancer treatment during the last 35 years is considered a failure (*N Eng J Med* 314:1226; 1986).

6. Deaths and the risk of death from asthma and other respiratory disorders are increasing as are immune disorders among Americans of all ages (*N Eng J Med* 321:1517; 1989).

7. Coronary angioplasty and bypass surgery do not reverse coronary artery disease; notwithstanding, the number of these procedures is skyrocketing.

The more we spend, the sicker we get. How can this be? In my view, the two core problems of American medicine are: 1) We address the 21st-century problems of environment, nutrition and stress with 19th-century notions of disease and drugs, and 2) We have raised generations of physicians who believe all nondrug, nonscalpel therapies are quackery.

Nutrients—not drugs—heal injured tissues. Drug medicine is a medicine of blockage. Drugs—essential as they are for acute, life-threatening diseases—work by blocking essential physiologic processes, i.e., calcium channel blockers block cell membrane channels, ACE enzyme inhibitors block enzymes that are necessary for the production of certain essential hormones, beta blockers block beta receptors on cell membranes, antidepressants block the uptake of some neurotransmitters.

The fact that nutrient therapies work is suppressed today. Herbal prescriptions in experienced hands are both safe and effective for chronic disorders. Americans prefer nondrug therapies to drug regimens (*N Eng J Med* 328:246;1993), yet the leadership in mainstream medicine vehemently opposes natural, nondrug therapies. Many natural, nondrug therapies are considered effective by those who prescribe them. But why do we allow those who neither understand nor use natural therapies to dismiss them as ineffective? The U.S. Congress must answer these questions before it can change the direction of medicine in the U.S.

Medical research in the U.S. is outstanding. We outspend all other nations in new drug and technology development. Our hospitals are far better equipped than those of any other country. American physicians, by and large, are well-trained, knowledgeable, diligent and caring professionals. So why are we Americans so disappointed with the results? Why do so many Americans look to natural, nondrug and nontechnology solutions to our health problems?

Why is it that the more we spend, the sicker we get?

SCIENCE HAS NOT FAILED MEDICINE, MEDICINE HAS FAILED SCIENCE

Science in medicine is widely misunderstood. This simple fact alone can provide answers to the questions I raise in this letter. Science in medical research in the U.S. is true to the scientific tradition, but medicine is on a dangerous course when it greatly distorts real data generated by valid studies to meet the financial demands of our drug and medical technology industries. For example, the *real but meager 1.8 percent* reduction in the rate of heart attacks obtained with a drug was reported as a *bloated 44 percent* reduction in the risk (*N Eng J Med* 321: 129; 1989). In another example, a paltry 1.2 percent reduction in the mathematical rate of heart attack obtained with a another drug was reported as a robust but nonmathematical 34 percent risk reduction (*N Eng J Med* 317:1241; 1987). I cite a large number of such studies to support my contention.

Why are such data "massaged" to render the insignificant benefits of long-term drug therapies statistically significant? The answer is really simple: Americans won't take drugs for decades to reap the putative benefit of reducing the *rate* of heart attack by only one to two percent. The real data do not support the long-term use of drugs for chronic degenerative, nutritional, ecologic and stress-related disorders. Data are misrepresented to physicians who then use the distorted data to persuade patients to accept drug regimens. The same holds true for mechanical devices, such as breathing machines for persons with sleep disturbances caused by the stress of modern life.

We cannot address environmental, nutritional and stress-related problems with synthetic chemicals. All our prevailing drug therapies are based on notions of disease, based in turn on microscopic studies of tissues *after* they have been damaged by disease. The 21st century calls for medicine to address the energetic-molecular events that occur *before* cells, tissues and organs are injured. This requires a major intellectual adaptation that is unsettling for physicians trained only in drug therapies.

Preventive medicine cannot be practiced with drugs—this is self-evident. Disease prevention requires management of the environment, nutrition, stress and physical fitness. However, no real effort is made in drug medicine to address these issues. Indeed, physicians who practice nutritional and environmental medicine are aggressively persecuted by those who sit on hospital governing and state licensing boards. Americans pay an exorbitant price for this—in missed opportunities for healing with natural therapies, in escaping the toxicity of avoidable drugs, and in avoiding the high cost of unnecessary diagnostic and treatment procedures.

EMPIRICAL MEDICINE IS MALIGNED IN THE U.S.

A core problem in the U.S. today is that we have raised generations of physicians who believe that diseases can be treated only with drugs or scalpels. They dismiss as quackery all empirical therapies that have been proven effective by extensive clinical experience in the hands of physicians who practice empirical medicine, employing nondrug and nontoxic nutritional, environmental and physical therapies that *do* work. It is profoundly ironic that those who speak vehemently against empirical medicine seem to have the least understanding of how poorly prevailing medicine measures up to the standards of science in medicine. Consider the following:

Much, if not most, of contemporary medical practice still lacks scientific foundation

JAMA 269:3030; 1993

Only one in ten of the most common diagnostic or therapeutic methods has any research basis

JAMA 263:278; 1990

What can be done? I make five specific proposals to the U.S Congress:

First,

it should enact legislation that will ensure freedom of choice in health care for all U.S. citizens.

Ironically, although Americans are known to hold dear their right to the pursuit of freedom of life, liberty and happiness, people with chronic illness in this land of Jefferson have less freedom of choice when it comes to therapy than those in any other country. The dogma of drug medicine emphatically denies Americans thousands of effective and inexpensive nondrug therapies widely used elsewhere. The principal reason for this is that the prevailing standards of drug medicine hold that any therapy that cannot be double-blinded and crossed-over cannot be scientifically valid. All nondrug therapies are considered unproven, unscientific and irresponsible. This frivolous notion is utterly irrelevant to holistic medicine, in which neither the practitioner nor the patient wants to be—nor can be—blinded to the true nature of therapy for extended periods of time.

Second,

it should enact legislation that will liberate physicians who practice empirical medicine with natural, nondrug therapies from the tyranny of drug medicine.

Physicians who use the nondrug therapies of empirical medicine live in constant—and well-founded—fear of harassment and revocation of their licenses, regardless of how impeccable their credentials might be. Anyone can ascertain the legitimacy of this statement by attending conferences of the American Academy of Environmental Medicine and the American College of Advancement in Medicine, the two main groups of physicians who practice preventive medicine and use nondrug therapies.

Article II.1 of the *Declaration of Helsinki,* signed by the U.S. and adopted by the World Assembly, Helsinki, Finland, 1964, provides that "In the treatment of the sick person, the doctor must be free to use a new therapeutic measure, if in his judgment it offers hope of saving life, reestablishing health, and alleviating suffering." Most physicians refrain from natural, nondrug therapies not because such alternatives are not effective but because they are fearful of losing their licenses. The practice of medicine must be safe and effective—and physicians must be held accountable for their work. However, peer review function for the safety and efficacy of nondrug therapies must not be conducted by conventional doctors who sit on state licensing and hospital boards and—who, by their own admission, know nothing about natural, nondrug, nonsurgical alternatives to drug therapies. The licenses of most physicians who employ nondrug therapies are threatened at one time or another—and sadly too often revoked—for prescribing unconventional therapies (translation: nondrug, nonscalpel alternatives.)

The courts have consistently upheld the patient's right to make an informed decision and assume the risk of therapies outside Western allopathic medicine. However, many physicians who are prosecuted by the licensing boards for unconventional therapies do not have the resources to successfully ward off the boards' actions and defend their licenses.

Third,

> Congress should enact legislation that removes disincentives for American citizens to the use of nondrug therapies.

Nondrug nutrient and herbal therapies are much less expensive than drug therapies—people who have used both options will readily attest to this. However, studies have shown that at present only people in higher socioeconomic groups avail themselves of nondrug therapies—largely because only they can afford to pay twice for health care, once as a premium for health insurance and again as an out-of-pocket expense when insurance companies refuse to reimburse for nondrug therapies.

Fourth,

> Congress should enact legislation mandating that the safety and efficacy of all therapies for chronic disorders be evaluated via long-term clinical outcome studies.

Congress has the responsibility to ensure that all therapies paid for with public funds be safe and effective. However, nondrug therapies cannot be evaluated using the prevailing short-term, double-blind cross-over model for drug research. Drugs produce effects rapidly—and, since they are interruptive in action, eventually produce toxic effects (or lose their efficacy as tissues learn to metabolize them differently). Nutrients and herbs are enabling agents for the healing response, but exert their effects in a slow and sustained fashion. Those familiar with both the prevailing drug therapies and nondrug alternatives for chronic disorders know that nondrug therapies yield long-term clinical outcomes that are far superior to those obtained with drugs.

Fifth,

> *Congress should assert that the patient's assessment of the efficacy of therapies for chronic disorders—and not that of the treating physician—must be regarded as the centerpiece of valid clinical outcome studies.*

Who is a better judge of the efficacy of any therapy, the physician or the patient? In acute illness, clearly, the correct answer is the physician. In acute illness, the judgment of the patient is often clouded by pain, suffering, fear and uncertainty about recovery—hence, the physician is in a far better position to assess the clinical value of the therapy. Does that also hold for chronic nutritional, ecologic, immune or stress-related disorders? I do not believe so. No matter how knowledgeable and experienced the physician might be, one thing he cannot do is get under the skin of his patient and know his pain and suffering the way he does—month after month, year after year. This is an element of crucial importance. It explains why drug medicine dominates health care in the U.S. today: patients are completely excluded from the process of determining what works and what doesn't, and drugs are prescribed as the only valid therapies.

Science is the search for truth. Science is true observation. Science is accuracy and precision in measurements. Science in medicine, however, must be subordinate to one higher principle:

it must promote health and prevent disease. Drugs and medical inventions that do not serve these twin goals cannot be deemed medically desirable, no matter how scientifically valid the research data may be. (We don't use poisons in medicine just because science gives us the capability to produce them.) Medical research is *not* scientific if it causes more harm than good.

A great free society must provide freedom of choice in health care for its citizens. Congress can assure this freedom by considering the five proposals outlined in this letter.

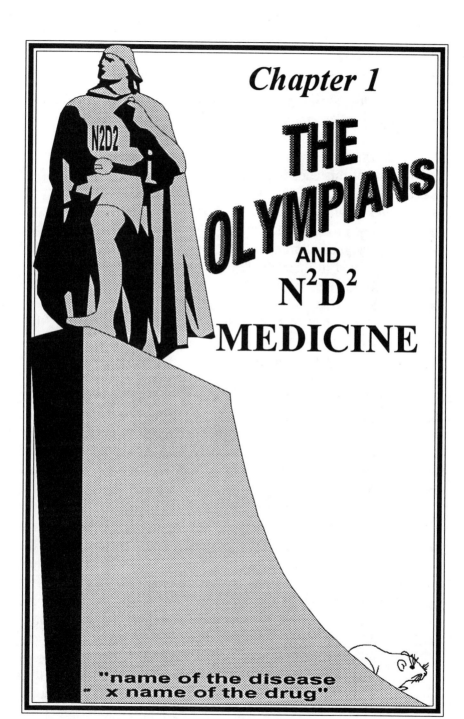

Chapter 1

THE OLYMPIANS

AND

N^2D^2

MEDICINE

"name of the disease x name of the drug"

In the beginning, as Choua tells the story, diseases descended from Mount Olympus.

Before there was anything, there was Chaos, a vast void. Then a part of this enormous emptiness condensed to give birth to Gaea, the earth, who, in turn, gave birth to Uranus, the starry sky. When Uranus grew up he became his mom's mate, and together they produced 12 Titans, the Elder Gods of Olympia. The Titans reigned supreme after Cronus, the chief Titan, started time. They lived in their abode high on Mount Olympus. Cronus grabbed power and ascended to the throne by castrating his father, Uranus. (At the behest of his mom, Cronus used a flint sickle to achieve that feat as his dad lay by his mom's side. After he forced three of her children back into her womb, Gaea grew disgusted with her husband.)

Cronus then married his sister, the goddess Rhea, and sired five sons. It was foretold that he would be banished from Mount Olympus and bound to the underworld by one of his own sons—a warning he took so seriously that he ate his five sons. The goddess Rhea was inconsolably saddened by the loss of her five sons. When her sixth son, the almighty god Zeus, was born, she had the newborn secretly carried to Crete and tricked Cronus into thinking that a stone wrapped in swaddling clothes was his new son. Cronus swallowed the stone. Zeus grew up and did exactly as had been foretold: He led his five brothers (regurgitated in error by Cronus after he swallowed them) against his father and the other Titans. The fight nearly destroyed the universe. But Zeus wrested control of Olympia, and sent Cronus and his cronies packing to the underworld.

Mortals lived happily on Gaea—the earth as it was then called—for untold ages. They were a merry and playful people who built little mud houses on the foothills of Mount Olympus and by the beaches where hills met the open sea. They ate what grew on the earth—when the earth grew it. Angels visited them at nightfall, lovingly slipping them into peaceful slumber. In the morning the sun gently nudged them from their beds to frolic among the berry bushes for breakfast. They breathed clean air and drank the pristine water of newly melted snow from the mountains. No one knew how *not* to feel well in those good times for there hadn't been any bad times.

The problems for the mortals, as Choua continues his story, began when almighty Zeus let his brother, the god Hades, take charge of the underworld. Hades was dark, austere and inexorable. He was irked by the earthlings' constant playfulness. To teach them diligence and endurance, he created maladies to afflict earthlings. Then he blew the maladies into the mists surrounding the highest peaks of Mount Olympus. The maladies floated in the mists until they ultimately descended upon the mortals.

MALADIES FROM MOUNT OLYMPUS

Some Olympian maladies gave the earthlings high fevers and black urine, while other maladies turned their eyes deep yellow and their stools clay-colored. Still other maladies caused skin sores, eye eruptions, bowel blisters and muscle tumors. Many earthlings died. Some maladies caused chronic fatigue, aching muscles, stiff joints, recurrent sore throats with swollen glands, mood swings, and problems of mood, memory and mentation. The sick earthlings cried out in anguish. Others who tended the sick saw their pain and suffering but were helpless, for they didn't know from where the afflictions had descended and had no idea how to alleviate the suffering. The mortals were frightened. There was much confusion and commotion—but no relief.

Some lesser Olympian gods often visited earth. Chief among them was the god Pan, a wonderful musician and a frequent gay companion of the woodland nymphs. Pan was a boisterous, merry god, with the head and torso of a man and horns and hindquarters of a goat. This goat god, as he was playfully called by the Olympians, was ugly, and though he was always in love with one nymph or another—his love remained unrequited. Perhaps because of this, Pan had an evil streak—sometimes he howled at night, making spine-chilling noises and spreading deep fear among the earthlings. Tormented by Olympian maladies and terrified by the god Pan's pranks, the earthlings cried out in anguish. Not knowing what to do, they made offerings to appease the Immortals on Mount Olympus and pleaded with them for deliverance.

Finally, Almighty Zeus took pity on the mortals. He asked his son, Hermes—the messenger god and the conductor of souls in the underworld who wore winged shoes and carried a Caduceus wand—to investigate why the mortals were making such a fuss.

Hermes, an inventor and a master of the art of divination, flew down to the earth and found the earthlings in total disarray— sick, disheartened and dejected. It took Hermes little time to figure out what ailed the mortals and who was behind the turmoil—his own son, Pan, and his uncle, Hades. But sickness among the mortals didn't move this Immortal. He decided not to engage in problems that held no interest for him. He flew back up to Mount Olympus to inform the Immortals about the mischief of Hades and Pan, and to tell them about the desperate strait the mortals were in.

AESCULAPIUS, SON OF APOLLO

After Hermes departed, the earthlings made more offerings to the Immortals and pleaded more fervently for mercy. Again, the Olympians felt distracted by the mortals' pleas and conferred with each other to review the situation. The Immortals never criticized other Immortals in defense of mere mortals. The council of Olympian Gods heard Hermes's report but ignored the part relating to the miscreants, Hades and Pan. In the end, they asked Aesculapius, who lived on Mount Pelion, to descend to the mortals and comfort them.

The Olympian gods knew Aesculapius had a very special reason for being sympathetic to earthlings. His mother, Coronis, was an earthling herself. No one knew who his father was. Coronis was a maiden in Thessaly. She was so stunningly beautiful that Apollo, a randy bachelor and a ladies' man of considerable repute, fell victim to her charm when he first laid eyes on her. But Coronis fell in love with a mortal and conceived Aesculapius. It remains unexplained to this day why she preferred a mere mortal over Apollo, a handsome youthful god and the deity of light. The choice was a bad mistake for poor Coronis! Enraged by the news, Apollo persuaded his sister, Artemis, Goddess of Chastity, to reach for her quiver of arrows and kill Coronis. Then the Immortals stood around the funeral pyre as the dead body of Coronis was put to flames. Watching her engulfed by the flames, and smitten by a pang of guilt, Apollo snatched unborn Aesculapius from the burning womb of his earthling mother. Apollo then took Aesculapius to Chiron, the aging but kindly Centaur who lived on Mount Pelion. (All other Centaurs were savage beasts, half-horse and half-man.) When Aesculapius grew up, Chiron taught him all about the secrets of Olympian remedies, such as cooling potions and warming salves. As a young man, Aesculapius often thought about his mother, wondered who his father might have been and how he might have looked. At times his heart would become heavy with sadness. On such occasions he would quickly turn to his consuming passion of perfecting remedies.

So it was, Choua continues, that the Olympians returned Aesculapius to the land of his mother. They knew he was skillful at making potions and concoctions with the Olympian herbs that they themselves had no use for, for they were never sick themselves. They knew Aesculapius was of kind heart and compassionate soul. The Olympians also knew something else: that in his passion to alleviate suffering and treat the sick, he would be tempted to reveal to the mortals things that only the Immortals should know.

Zeus knew something about inner conflict and turmoil, though he never let anyone else know this secret aspect of his being—perhaps because it would have detracted from his image of all-powerful, almighty Olympian. He became the supreme, All-Father God by populating the heavens and earth through promiscuous liaisons. He had a prodigious capacity for making love—and was known to woo everything that moved. A lover of all females, he had to forever disguise his appearance—turning into a swan here and a bull there to escape the suspicious eyes of his wife, the goddess Hera. While he reigned supreme over Olympia, as the God of Skies and the Father of Seasons, Wise Laws, Justice, Peace and Fate, he suffered incessantly from the compulsions of hormonal surges, forever facing the embarrassment of being caught in the beds of other gods' goddesses. Olympians didn't much care when Zeus laid with the mortal maidens and earthlings' wives. Or when he swooped down as an eagle and carried earthling boys to Mount Olympus and made them his lovers. So Zeus knew something about the pangs of guilt and conflict—and could easily see the conflict that would befall Aesculapius as he began to tend to the sick among his mother's people.

Yet, Zeus knew better than anyone else in Olympia, that Immortal matters could not be revealed to mere mortals. So, in the full Olympian court, Zeus sent thunder to warn Aesculapius that he must keep the mortals blinded to the maladies of the Immortals. Aesculapius assured the Olympians that he understood their wishes, and promised never to reveal divine things to the earthlings. He then bowed repeatedly before Zeus and his council of Olympian gods to express gratitude for being permitted to practice the art for which he had so diligently prepared.

THE BLINDED DISEASES FROM MOUNT OLYMPUS

Aesculapius was a great teacher and had a genius for organization. When he descended among the people of his mother, he was initially shocked and hurt by the sickness and suffering among them. But he soon recovered, got the Olympians to banish the god Pan from earth—though not completely—and began his healing work in earnest. He neatly classified all Olympian maladies and, realizing that the mortals had limited capacity for comprehension, simplified matters and called the maladies *diseases*. Next, he arranged all diseases into DRGs—disease-related groups—and assigned them appropriate DRG codes. To some mortals, he taught the names of diseases, always remembering to blind them from Olympian maladies, as he promised Almighty Zeus. Aesculapius called his disciples *disease doctors* and blessed them with great knowledge about the diagnosis of his diseases.

Aesculapius also knew that the earthlings were gullible and feeble-minded, and could not help but meddle with Olympian matters. Certainly, he couldn't trust that they would leave his disease names alone. He sternly told the mortals that they were going to be blinded to all Olympian maladies at all times, and that they must never pry into the matters of the Immortals. Specifically, he laid down a law that earthlings must never ask questions about Olympian diseases—about their origin, their course, and their outcome. The earthlings understood and swore their unwavering allegiance to the blinding principle of Aesculapian's teaching. The disease doctors were deeply touched by Aesculapius' kindness and devotion.

Thus, as Choua continues the story, *blinded disease doctors* came into being. And faithful to their promise, they remained so for ages—never questioning the origin, course and outcome of Olympian diseases. Indeed, to this day when young men enter medical schools, the first thing demanded of them is *blind* loyalty to Aesculapius's classification of diseases.

REMEDIES FROM MOUNT OLYMPUS:
THE BLINDED DRUGS

After teaching the earthlings about diseases, Aesculapius turned his attention to treating diseases with Olympian remedies. He flew up to the Olympian court and pleaded with the gods for permission to bring Olympian remedies to the mortals. At first, the gods vehemently rejected Aesculapius's pleas for they knew the earthlings could not be trusted.

"Meddling is minced deep in mortals' marrows," the Olympians told Aesculapius. They warned him that remedies of the Immortals could not be handed over to fickle and feeble-minded earthlings.

Aesculapius was deeply disappointed for he knew his disease doctors couldn't cure Olympian maladies without Olympian remedies. Tears of compassion welled up in his eyes as he saw distressing images of sickness, pain and anguish among his mother's folks. Apollo, who watched the proceedings in silence, saw in Aesculapius's sad eyes an ephemeral image of his mother's eyes. Moved by that memory, he interceded with other Olympians on behalf of Aesculapius. (God Apollo had a soft heart for Aesculapius and regarded him as his own son, albeit soiled by the sperm of some mortal). Olympian gods also knew of Apollo's tenderness for Aesculapius. They agreed to let Aesculapius take Olympian maladies on one condition:

"O' Aesculapius! thou must forever keep the mortals blind

to Olympian remedies," Olympians sternly warned Aesculapius a second time. "Keep them totally blinded, always and forever."

Tearfully, Aesculapius accepted the condition and, at that very moment, forgave Apollo for burning his mother alive. Aesculapius returned to the mortals with Olympian remedies and told them of his promise.

"The Immortals demand that you must always be blinded to their remedies," he addressed the mortals solemnly on his return. "You must never snoop around when I compound Olympian remedies. You must prescribe remedies only and exactly as I teach you. You must never speculate about their origin or their nature. Positively, never improvise! Never question! Never dispute! Never pry! And, never, never break my blinding code!"

The mortals realized the risk Aesculapius was taking for their salvation. They felt a crushing weight of gratitude toward him and promised repeatedly never to be disobedient, never to question.

"We'll never deviate from the truth of your teachings," they assured Aesculapius. "We'll never question your Olympian remedies—never doubt their efficacy, never look for their side effects, never wonder about the inner workings of your potions, and never search for alternatives. Above all, we'll never, ever break your blinding code."

Aesculapius felt proud and nodded with gratification. He blessed his blinded disease doctors.

BLINDED DISEASE DOCTORS
OF BLINDED DRUG MEDICINE

For a long time, the mortals never directly spoke about Olympian remedies—referring to them only with vague gestures, and in hushed tones. Such communication with gestures and whispers became cumbersome, as their practices flourished and they began to publish their blinded studies. Finally, they sent a delegate to Aesculapius and pleaded for a solution to that awkward problem of communication among themselves and their patients. Aesculapius considered their plight in silence for some moments, then smiled as he came up with a brilliant solution: he named the Olympians remedies *drugs*. (The word drugs, he thought, blended well with both divine diseases and disease doctors.)

Thus, as Choua's story proceeds, came into being the *double-blinded disease doctors of blinded drug medicine*—blinded once to the nature of Olympian diseases, and a second time, to Olympian drugs. Early disease doctors of drug medicine remained completely blinded and utterly faithful to Aesculapius. They built a massive altar of a god Aesculapius with pure gold. (They had horded enough of that metal by that time.) For worship on that altar, they wrote a code of blinded conduct that passed from generation to generation without a single word ever being changed. Such was their devotion to the god of the double blind. Indeed, to this day, their successors dutifully worship on that altar, with immeasurable gratitude and a great sense of privilege.

To this day, the successors of those early drug doctors demand that young men entering their schools pledge loyality to the Aesculapius's principle of divine double-blindedness. *To this day, they reject as unscientific all therapies that have not been approved by their Aesculapian double-blind, cross-over code.*

CENTERS OF BLINDED EXCELLENCE

The disease doctors of drug medicine built massive stone edifices on the foothills of Mount Olympus and began to practice the profession Aesculapius taught them. Thus, as Choua's story moves on, came into existence the first *centers of blinded excellence of blinded disease doctors of blinded drug medicine.* Aesculapius's disciples followed their guru's teachings to the letter and enforced them rigorously and rigidly among their trainees. They never asked any questions about Olympian diseases and drugs and never probed into divine matters as promised. Those centers of excellence were utterly devoted to Aesculapius's holy book, the *Physician's Desk Reference (PDR)*. With single-minded purpose, the disease doctors built greater and greater centers of blinded excellence. Those centers thrived, and disease doctors brought much relief from pain and suffering to the sick—and much riches upon themselves.

THE ALTAR OF THE GOD OF DOUBLE-BLIND

With time, the blinded drug doctors began to feel

awkward praying at the same altar of Aesculapius as the lay folks. Healers kneeling with the healed? The question once raised could not be put to rest except by some method of distinguishing themselves from the lay earthlings. So they called a congress of drug doctors to address the problem. The congress decided to recognize a new god, the god of the double-blinded. Diseases, they held steadfastly, were what Aesculapius said they were—maladies from Mount Olympus. They reaffirmed that they—mortals in the healing arts—had to remain blinded to Olympian diseases for their own good. Furthermore, they affirmed that drugs were cures from Mount Olympus, and they were to stay blinded to them, as this was the will of the Olympians. They vowed to keep their diseases and drugs high above their families and fortunes, and to defend them as they would their honor, even with their lives. They promised themselves never to let a mortal utter a sacrilegious word against the diseases and drugs from Mount Olympus. It seemed only natural that they build a great marble edifice to house a towering statue of their new God of the Double-Blind. And so they did that.

Soon, word of their untold wealth spread far and wide among the countries surrounding Mount Olympus. Many folks traveled long distances to try their luck. The disease doctors quickly organized themselves to keep the newcomers out of their profession. Hungry, goldless and without food stamps, most of the newcomers were disillusioned quickly and returned to their countries with sad hearts. Yet, some of them stayed on and built mud huts at some distance from the foothills of Mount Olympus, hoping not to confront the disease doctors with in-your-face competition. Disease doctors were comfortable in their stone centers and decided not to mess with the outcasts—as they were called, as long as the outcasts stayed clear of their turf on the foothills of Mount Olympus.

QUACKS AND EMPIRICAL MEDICINE

Trouble began when some of the outcasts began to experiment with alternative therapies.

The outcasts were immensely excited to observe that some of their alternative therapies worked. The sick earthlings reported rapid relief from the pain of bloated bellies, swollen joints, muscle spasms and bladder problems, and control of infections. Their wounds healed quickly. Emboldened by early successes, the outcasts tried many other therapies, holding on to what worked and discarding what didn't.

Thus, as Choua tells with a wink, began empirical medicine—a brand-new system of caring for the sick. The *core* philosophy of this medicine was that what worked—and was safe—was worth trying again. What didn't work or was toxic was to be discarded on an empirical basis. "Exciting stuff!" quacks congratulated each other when they presented case histories at their congresses. Pretty soon they had many alternative therapies, which they forever tinkered with to make them more effective. The outcasts also figured out ways to tap into the energy of their tissues, calling it the *Spirit, life force, Chi, limbic energy* and other names. They also experimented with meditation and self-regulation.

Just because an earthly therapy works and is safe is not a reason to use it, disease doctors countered peevishly. Next, they found out that the outcasts were taking liberties with disease names—turning, twisting and distorting the sacred labels handed down by the Olympians. They gave each other disturbed, furtive looks and spoke in hushed tones.

Then came the unthinkable: The outcasts began to openly defy the gods of Mount Olympus and loudly proclaim that the diseases of the earthlings had earthly origins. Disease doctors were stunned by this heretical notion. What diseases didn't descend from Mount Olympus? They cringed as they asked each other the question. Did Aesculapius mislead us? Or worse, is he a liar? They felt sharp pangs as they contemplated the unthinkable.

"O' Aesculapius! Where art thou?" they cried as they threw dirt on each other's hair in mourning. Aesculapius was not heard from. As days passed, disease doctors were inconsolable. Dark days were followed by darker nights, but Aesculapius didn't show. And, as if that wasn't enough, the outcasts propounded an even more preposterous theory that diseases could be treated with earthly remedies—cooling potions, heating salves and cleansing concoctions made from the earthly weeds, leaves and roots. What an abomination! they cried with unspeakable anguish. Earthly remedies for Olympian maladies! How could that be?

"Blasphemy!" screamed the disease doctors in agony. "May death visit upon the outcasts before the Immortals discover their intransigence," they prayed convulsively. But the outcasts didn't die. They didn't even get sick. Instead, they became emboldened as days passed and Aesculapius didn't show up to chastise them. "Oh, Olympian gods! Smite the non-believers with your wrath," the drug doctors pleaded with the Immortals directly when they gave up hope of seeing Aesculapius soon. "Heretical notions must not be tolerated in the healing arts! The outcasts—the doubters, the nonbelievers in divine diseases—must be destroyed forever."

The outcasts were not intimidated by the curses of disease doctors. They shrieked back in harsh, raspy, ducklike voices.

The Olympians were amused by the raucous earthlings. They liked the loud quacking of the outcasts among the mortals and dubbed them *quacks*. So, as Choua's story advances, quacks came into being, a title bestowed upon the outcasts by the Olympian gods themselves.

MOUNT FUDGE

As the anguish of the disease doctors grew, so did the excitement among quacks. They became increasingly belligerent, shouting in ever louder voices their blasphemous notions that diseases didn't descend from Mount Olympus. To pour fuel on the fire, the quacks even desecrated Mount Olympus and called it Mount Fudge—the high mountain where maladies are blinded and the drug data are fudged. The disease doctors convulsed with rage as they saw their most sacred beliefs so reviled. They feverishly prayed to the Olympians for early signs of an impending quack annihilation.

Strangely, the Olympian gods were not irked. When they looked down at the earthlings, they smiled knowingly at the mortals' follies.

The disease doctors called a convention to deal with the spreading cancer of heretical notions of diseases and drugs among quacks. Some spoke with much vitriol against quacks, while others talked somberly of some safe and sure strategy for success. Finally, everyone agreed on one common goal: the total destruction of quacks and their empirical medicine.

The disease doctors then organized an association of drug doctors, established disciplinary boards to govern the practice of their craft, and appointed to their boards only those who they knew couldn't think for themselves. They first licensed themselves and then censored quacks for professional misconduct.

THE GREAT WAR OF N²D² AND EMPIRICAL MEDICINES

And, so it was, as Choua continues his story, that the disease doctors of drug medicine ferociously fought quacks and their empirical medicine for a thousand years. They vowed to wage war and subdue everything that threatened their double-blinded medicine. They pledged to burn all quack manuscripts describing theories of earthly causes of heavenly diseases. They proposed bills and had them passed them into laws banning all discussions about the nature of their sacred diseases from Mount Olympus (to which they were most gratefully blinded) and against all attempts to replace their divine drugs (to which they were equally and gratefully blinded) by the accursed, earthly alternative therapies.

At their annual congress of the blinded disease doctors of

blinded drug medicine, a wise delegate proposed a brilliant solution. He first emphasized the absolute need for a rallying cry that could bring all of them together, then he proposed the following slogan:

N^2D^2 medicine =
name of disease X name of drug

The entire congress instantaneously fell in love with the slogan. They unanimously adopted a resolution that declared N^2D^2 medicine the official name of their profession. The resolution was later proclaimed at an official ceremony.

"We shall ordain that whenever a disease doctor treats a sick man," the wise delegate proclaimed during the annual banquet that evening, "he shall begin his work with the name of a disease and end it with the name of a drug. *And between the name of the disease and the name of the drug, there will be nothing, positively and categorically.* Each disease doctor will swear allegiance to N^2D^2 medicine."

"By Almighty Zeus!" the whole conference resonated in unison, "each of us will take the oath of N^2D^2 medicine! So be it! So be it."

"Praise thee, O' Olympian gods!" the wise man continued. "None of us will ever betray our lord, Aesculapius! In N^2D^2 medicine, there shall never be any question about our Olympian diseases. Of course, all diseases descended from Mount Olympus! I know it! You know it!"

"You know it! We all know it!" the N^2D^2 doctors chanted, trembling with excitement.

"We have been—and we will always be—blinded to our Olympian drugs! I know it! You know it!"

"You know it! We all know it!" the audience screamed in chorus.

"In N^2D^2 medicine, we shall never permit any discussion of Olympian matters," the wise delegate led the conference. "Of course, all diseases and drugs descended from the high abode of the Immortals. We have been—and always will be—blinded to Olympian maladies and Olympian remedies! I know it! You know it!"

"You know it! We all know it!" the crowd exulted.

QUACKS FIGHT BACK

The quacks were not intimidated by the show of solidarity among N^2D^2 practitioners. They organized a congress of empirical medicine to respond to N^2D^2 medicine. There was much inflammatory rhetoric. Some of the speakers made wild pronouncements that mortals are made sick by earthly substances. "Hilariously funny stuff," someone in the audience soberly observed. Other speakers—their judgment clouded by the passion of argument—lost all reason and logic and muttered strange things in incoherent sentences. The congress soon degenerated into shouting matches of outlandish ideas.

Some quacks spoke like lunatics, proclaiming that diseases actually arose from within individual body organs. Some others, carried by the flight of misbegotten ideas, proposed yet more outlandish causes of disease.

"Ho! Ho! Ho! The bowel bloats and billows and blisters!" A quack bellowed.

"Far out! Far out!" many quacks shrieked in a frenzy of feeding on ludicrous ideas.

"Hey! Hey! Hey! The heart putters, palpitates and plummets," Another quack howled.

"Hurray! Hurray!" the quack audience shouted.

"Bullay! Bullay! Bullay! The brain bickers, burns and boils over!" A quack burped loudly and the whole quack congress bursts into laughter.

Many quacks presented similarly stupid ideas about diseases beginning in the liver, kidneys, adrenals and other body organs. Some of them even talked about injury to body ecosystems, such as the battered bowel ecosystem and the blood ecosystem invaded by viruses and yeasts. In the quack congress were some spy N^2D^2 docs who concluded that the quack ideas of diseases were too crazy to be taken seriously. So they later reported their findings to the high council of N^2D^2 docs.

FBA:
THE MOUNT FUDGE-BLINDED ASSOCIATION

There was yet more to come in the quack congress. Some speakers who followed stoked the fires of hatred against the N^2D^2 doctors. They openly ridiculed the dogma of N^2D^2 medicine. The claims of cures from Mount Olympus, they cried out defiantly, were phony. They jeered disease doctors and declared their data fudged.

Then came the ultimate insult—one of the quacks viciously declared that Olympian drugs were without any value, and that the N²D² docs shamelessly used them to bilk the sick of whatever gold they had. Furthermore, they shouted that drug doctors were brazenly blinding the gullible sick.

And, then as if all that wasn't enough, one quack rose to pour yet more venom. He contemptuously called the association of drug doctors FBA—Mount Fudge-Blinded Association. The Mount Fudge-blinded, he fumed, were not only blinded to diseases and drugs, they were also blinded to common sense. He then rebelliously dared the FBA commissioner to take action against quacks. He proclaimed that natural remedies made from flowers, leaves and roots of earthly plants were there to stay. No one, he angrily hissed, could keep quacks from using their natural remedies.

Little did the quack know that, years later, his challenge would be accepted by the FBA commissioner. The FBA agents would assault a quack clinic with drawn spears to confiscate all the plant remedies there. That quack would be quite well-known for fomenting trouble among other quacks. The FBA commissioner would swear that he would ruthlessly enforce his drug rules on all quacks—and that he certainly had the legal authority and means to do that. The geek among the drug doctors—quack-busters as they called themselves—gleefully celebrated the occasion with wild chants.

The Olympian gods watched the territorial turf strife among the mortals in healing arts with amusement. Some of them put wagers on who would come out the winner, the N²D² doctors or the quacks? Nothing humored the Olympians more than when they heard disease doctors call themselves *healers*. The Immortals were hilarious when they heard drug doctors tout their work as *quality care* rendered with the highest possible *scientific* standards.

HEALERS AND THEIR QUALITY CARE

There were other things that amused the Immortals. When drug doctors talked to their politicians, they always emphasized that they kept the *patient's best interest above the financial interests of N^2D^2 doctors*. The Immortals preferred high quality humor. The disease doctors' unending reference to the *patient's best interest* provided them with much comic relief. And so it was, Choua says, that the Olympians found drug doctors to be more endearing than quacks. *Drug doctors were more proficient at making things up, and the Olympians liked that.*

The lay mortals were also much amused by the squabbles among their health care professionals. Drug doctors had more gold, so they were more visible and influential among politicians. Quacks appeared largely to attract the poor, and that fact was often used by drug doctors to strengthen their case: "If the poor were not stupid, they would know better than to go to quacks," N^2D^2 doctors spoke scornfully. "And, of course, if they were not stupid, they would have more gold to afford us." Still, many poor mortals continued to see quacks.

The mortals continued to honor Aesculapius as no other mortal. They recognized him as a great benefactor. The sick, maimed and dying came in herds to be healed and cured by the great Aesculapius. When cured, they built temples of glistening marble to glorify him. As time passed, they built statues of Aesculapius and deified him. That raised a few eyebrows among the Olympians. Aesculapius was after all the son of a mortal. Still, the Immortals, in deference to Apollo, didn't take any action.

AESCULAPIUS SLAIN: DARK DAYS FOR EMPIRICAL MEDICINE

It is said that the worship of the idolaters went into Aesculapius's head and he committed the cardinal sin against which he had been repeatedly warned. In a fit of passion to heal, he brought a dead mortal back to life. A mortal bringing a dead mortal back to life! The Immortals were incensed. The mortals must not be trusted, they complained loudly to Almighty Zeus. The mortals must be kept in their place, they demanded furiously. Almighty Zeus himself had warned Aesculapius harshly against that unpardonable sin. To appease the infuriated Immortals, and to teach all mortals an unforgettable lesson, he struck Aesculapius with his thunderbolt and slew him. All Immortals except Apollo were pleased with Zeus's action.

(Merry and playful on most occasions, the Olympian deities were vile, vituperative and vindictive when they saw their honor in jeopardy. Zeus was sometimes irked by the praise other Immortals heaped on Apollo—the handsome, youthful God of Music, Prophecy and Healing. He knew Apollo's had a soft heart for Aesculapius. The murder of Aesculapius was a shrewd political move on Zeus's part: It dealt a severe blow to Apollo's

pride, and at the same time, it ingratiated all other Olympians to
Zeus. Apollo—also God of Truth and Light—was nobody's fool.
He understood Zeus's trickery. To avenge the death of his son,
Apollo killed Zeus's armorers, the Cyclopes.)

The news of the slaying of Aesculapius spread like wild
fire among N^2D^2 practitioners, striking fear in their hearts in a
way they had never known before. "With Aesculapius gone, how
will we ever know the will of the Immortals?" they mourned.
Then they called another congress, then biggest ever, and bowed
their heads in total silence, seeking enlightenment. But nothing
happened. Finally, exhausted with hunger and dehydration, one
by one, without uttering a word, they slowly and sadly walked
back to their centers of excellence. The congress simply died.

The effects of the news of Aesculapius's death on quacks
was quite different. Shaken to their cores—and morbidly afraid of
the Immortals—the quacks went underground. And, to this day,
as Choua's story goes, the quacks remain underground.

"Time heals all wounds as it wounds all heels. N^2D^2
doctors consoled each other when the initial shock at
Aesculapius's death subsided. Seasons changed, and they
eventually settled back into their richly rewarding work as
healers. For days, then months, they expected the quacks to
surface again with their obnoxious notions of earthly causes of
heavenly diseases. But the quacks remained underground. And,
with passing years, they realized that they had the healing arenas
all to themselves.

In their hearts, N^2D^2 practitioners continued to worship
Aesculapius. But, in public, they always prayed to Almighty Zeus
and invoked his mercy before they cut into people with their

scalpels and poured Olympian remedies down the throats of the sick. They did the same when they opened their N^2D^2 congresses. Verily, they were grateful to Zeus for one thing: His slaying of Aesculapius had driven quacks underground and out of their hair. "Almighty Zeus, thou be praised!" they chanted fervently whenever they thought of quacks.

BLESSINGS OF N^2D^2 MEDICINE

"Let me count the blessings of N^2D^2 medicine," the president of a national congress of N^2D^2 doctors addressed the membership one day, many centuries later. "First and foremost, it saves us from the effort of thinking. Thinking is hard for everyone, and we N^2D^2 doctors are no exceptions. Our lives are hard to begin with, and need not be made any harder by the requirement of thinking every time we put an ill person on our drugs. Besides, Aesculapius told us not to think. He warned us that if we ever thought about Olympian diseases and drugs, we would go astray. Just look at quacks! Where did their thinking take them? Underground!"

"Blessed are the blinded," the audience resonated with great excitement.

"Life is comfortable when everything is black and white. Shades of gray are hard on everyone and..."

"And we N^2D^2 doctors don't like shades of gray either," the audience completed the president's sentence with loud clapping.

"There is not much point in pushing shades of gray in a doctors's work," intoned the president wisely. "Our patients pay us for disease names that are crisp and clear. They don't like shades of gray anymore than we do. N^2D^2 medicine abhors shades of gray—it likes its drug names crisp and clear—none of that nonsense of immune enhancement that quacks talk about."

"And what happens if the clinical situation is not black and white?" someone in the crowd said, raising his voice.

"Nay! Nay!" the president retorted, "The clinical situation in N^2D^2 medicine is never *not* black and white. We are the blinded! No! We are the double-blinded—once, when we were blinded to Olympian maladies, and again when we were blinded to Olympian remedies."

"Praise the Olympians!" the crowd shouted in unison. "It is never *not* black and white in N^2D^2 medicine."

"We'll build great centers of blinded excellence where everything will be blinded. Everything! All diseases! All drugs! Cancer, heart diseases, arthritis and immune problems," the leader proclaimed jubilantly.

"And Epstein-Barr syndrome, *Candida*-related complex and *C. difficile* colitis," the crowd roared joyously.

"And shirker's syndrome, Yuppie syndrome and all-in-the-head syndrome," the president thundered. "Our scientists at the Centers for Disease Control have deftly—and scientifically—established criteria for chronic fatigue syndrome. They have decreed that chronic fatigue syndrome must never be diagnosed when the patient has any known organic or psychiatric cause for fatigue. Now isn't that a brilliant stroke? A dazzling tribute to Aesculapius? Utterly faithful to his admonition that we shall never think about the cause of disease? An astounding feat of N^2D^2 medicine?" The president fired a volley of questions at his flock.

"Chronic fatigue syndrome descends from Mount Olympus," the crowd chanted.

"If N^2D^2 geniuses at the CDC weren't so brilliant," the president yowled, "every fool would look for the cause of chronic fatigue in organic or psychiatric diseases, wouldn't he?"

"He would! He would!" the crowd intoned.

"Quacks would search for the cause of chronic fatigue syndrome in their foolish ideas of food allergy, wouldn't they? They would look for the cause of chronic fatigue in their frivolous notions of the multiple chemical sensitivity syndrome, wouldn't they? They would find the cause of chronic fatigue syndrome in their stupid theories of battered bowel ecosystem and violated blood ecosystem, wouldn't they? Can you imagine intestinal parasites and prolonged bowel transit time causing chronic fatigue syndrome?" the leader grimaced.

"Blessed are the blinded! For they shall never search for the cause of the divine chronic fatigue syndrome in earthly things," the followers chanted.

"The greatest blessing of N^2D^2 medicine is the rich variety of tongue-twisting disease names that no patient can ever decipher. It gives us, the champions of N^2D^2 medicine, the aura of knowledge and respectability that we desperately need to use the billing codes for maximal remuneration."

"Billing codes! Billing codes!" The crowd bellowed with deafening noise.

WEEPING NOSES, BLOATING BELLIES, CRAMPING MUSCLES

"Without our N^2D^2 disease names, how would we have treated noses that weep, bellies that bloat and limbs that ache?" the leader bellowed.

"Indeed, how would we have?" the crowd responded.

"N^2D^2 diagnoses are Olympian gifts that we'll forever

cherish," the president spoke slowly, weighing each word with a deep sense of gratitude. "Do you realize how inconvenient it would be for our neurologists if they didn't have the diagnosis of chronic headache—and the CPT reimbursement code to go along with it—for those who complain of their head hurting all the time?" the president asked the congress.

"By goddess Athena!" the neurologists in the crowd responded with zest. "It would be most difficult. And, without the CPT code, how would we bill for our services?"

The president's question about headache reminded the neurologists of Athena, Goddess of Wisdom and Arts, who sprang fully armed from Zeus's skull when he suffered a severe headache. Zeus swallowed his first wife, Titaness Metis, just before she delivered her first born, Athena, because he was told his second child would overthrow him. Pretty clever! Zeus ate up his wife so she couldn't bear him another child. Then he developed a headache—presumably because Metis wasn't very digestible—and had his forehead cleaved open for relief. Out of the opened skull emerged Athena.

"And how embarrassing would it be if our gynecologists didn't have the diagnosis of PMS and its CPT code for women who are always suffering from PMS?" The president asked solemnly.

"By goddess Hera!" the N^2D^2 gynecologists shouted with one voice. "It would be most embarrassing. And what would have we done without the PMS CPT code?"

The gynecologists in the hall knew that Hera, the jealous wife of Almighty Zeus, *always* acted *PMS-y*—even when she was not premenstrual. It's hard to imagine any female not acting PMS-y with a philandering husband like Zeus, alternately thundering and decoying, they mused.

"And how unseemly it would be for our sleep specialists to lack the diagnoses of sleep-disordered breathing for those who sleep fitfully and breathe unevenly," the leader led the followers.

"By Selene, the mood goddess!" the sleep specialists followed with zest. "It would be most unseemly without the proper CPT billing code."

The sleep specialists adored Selene who once saw a youth of indescribable beauty in a cave on Mount Latmus. She couldn't help but lay beside him and kiss his eyes. The youth slumbers in that cave to this day.

"And how awkward if our rheumatologists didn't have the diagnosis of chronic backache to use for those who complain of pain in the back all the time?" the voice from the podium trailed off in a groan.

"By god Hephaestus!" the N^2D^2 rheumatologists in the crowd replied in shrill voices. "It would be most awkward! Most awkward without the CPT code! How else would we have coped with chronic pain in the back to those whose backs ache all the time?"

The N^2D^2 rheumatologists knew that Hephaestus suffered from chronic backache. There were several reasons for that. To begin with, he was lame but worked hard at his crafts, creating uneven strain on his sacroiliac joints due to the uneven length of his legs. Once when his dad, Zeus, brutally attacked his mom, Hera, he stumbled to defend his mom. Zeus, enraged by the sight of his own son rising against him, abruptly lifted lame Hephaestus and slammed his back hard against rocks. Hephaestus's back hurt much after that period of misunderstanding in the first family of Olympia.

There were other causes for Hephaestus's backache. He was ugly and Zeus—it seems to spite Aphrodite, his daughter of surpassing beauty—gave her in marriage to him. (Olympians preferred to marry their sons to their daughters—arguably to hold the threads of Olympian DNA tightly together.)

The goddess Aphrodite, it turned out, was her daddy's girl—forever craving lovers of all descriptions. She wasn't very discreet about her illicit liaisons and caused poor Hephaestus much embarrassment and aggravated his chronic back condition. Finally, Hephaestus trapped virile Ares, the God of War, in bed with his wife with a thin but resilient net hung over Aphrodite's bed. The gods Apollo and Hermes poured salt on his wounds, jesting about how they themselves wouldn't mind being caught with a damsel of Aphrodite's beauty. Hephaestus wouldn't free Ares until the captive promised to compensate the captor for the dowry he paid Zeus for Aphrodite. (Clever businessman, Zeus! He collected the dowry even when he married his daughters to one of his own sons.) Ares agreed but, once freed, refused to keep his word, causing Hephaestus yet more backache.

Poor Hephaestus! His wife always hopped in and out of other gods' beds—and the pads of mortals when gods were not readily available. His back always hurt.

"And wouldn't it be clumsy if our internists weren't able to fall back on the diagnoses of anxiety state and panic attacks for those who are always anxious and panicky?" the president spoke in a mock panicky tone.

"By god Pan!" the N^2D^2 internists also responded in mock panic as they recalled the mischievous nocturnal howling of the god Pan. "It would be most clumsy."

"And how inept we would look if our jaw surgeons were without the TMJ diagnosis for those who keep their jaw muscles clenched till their heads hurt."

"By goddess Demeter!" the N^2D^2 jaw surgeons trolled. "We would seem incompetent." They recalled how tight-jawed with anguish the goddess Demeter, full sister and lover of Almighty Zeus, looked when her daughter, the goddess Peresphone, was abducted by the god Hades, her brother and her daughter's own uncle. Demeter's TMJ was caused by being deeply dismayed at her brother's conduct and her daughter's plight.

"No wonder the goddess Demeter suffered from TMJ," Choua broke his story to comment. "My jaws tighten up just thinking about the family tree of Olympians and keeping straight in my mind who married their sisters, made love to their daughters, abducted their nieces and, disguised as eagles, carried little boys from earth and make them their lovers."

"Yeah, and how do you think your listeners feel when your story turns and twists like that?" I teased Choua.

Choua looked puzzled for a fleeting moment, then recovered, grinned and proceeded with his tale.

"And do you know how discomfiting it would be for our gastroenterologists if the Olympians hadn't blessed them with the diagnosis of irritable bowel syndrome for those whose bowels are always irritated, bloated and cramped?" the president continued his learned discourse.

"By trumpeter god Triton of Sea!" the fellowship of gastroenterologists affirmed. "It would be most discomfiting. What would we have done without the *blessed* irritable bowel syndrome?" The N^2D^2 gastroenterologists loved it when Triton blew his concha shell. It always reminded them of the loud gurgling they heard with their stethoscopes in the bowel of patients who suffered from irritable bowel syndrome.

"And can you imagine how silly our cardiologists would look if they didn't have the diagnosis of coronary artery disease?" the president went on.

"By the goddess Atropos!" the N^2D^2 cardiologist followed, "We would look silly."

The Fates were three powerful goddesses who determined man's life span. The first one, Clotho, wove the thread of life—created *your* oxidative spark to usher life in, Choua winked again. The second, goddess Lachesis, measured out Clotho's yarn—you might say decided the length of DNA strands that encode for antioxidant enzyme systems that dampen the oxidative flames. The third, goddess Atropos, did the next important thing: She determined the length of stay for humans on planet earth. The N^2D^2 cardiologist were awed by the whimsical Atropos. She held the scissors of death, ready to clip the coronary arteries at the slightest provocation. The cardiologists and cardiac surgeons built great edifices to glorify their goddess Atropos and decorated them with blurping, beeping and buzzing Star Wars electronic gizmos. Then they called those edifices coronary care units. The earthlings came from far and away to make offerings to goddess Atropos. The N^2D^2 cardiologists benefited handsomely.

"Tell us, our revered president," the N^2D^2 congress asked, "Tell us about radiologists. How true are they to our lord Aesculapius?"

"Our radiologist friends," the president became somber, "they weasel words like no one else does—or can. Don't they? They are masters of writing fiction, aren't they? Their radiology reports keep us—and our patients—in the drak, and well-blinded. We refer our patients to them with two or three possible diagnoses. They return them back to us with four, five and sometimes as many as seven possibilities. Do you know how disturbing it would be if they didn't add to their reports the blessed words *'to be clinically correlated?'* We all know what that means, don't we?" the president grinned broadly.

"What does that mean?" the crowd asked excitedly. "What does *'to be clinically correlated'* mean?"

"It means: *'Silly, don't ask me. I don't know!'*"

"By Tantalus, the monster of deprivation!" the radiologists in the crowd exclaimed, "It means *I don't know. We are—and will always remain—true to our lord Aesculapius.*"

"And the pathologist!" the N²D² congress asked their president lovingly. "Tell us about the pathologist."

"Ah, the pathologist," the president sighed. *"When the pathologist has nothing to say, he says it so elegantly.* Do you know how utterly futile it would be if he didn't have all those topsy-turvy, tongue-twisting words to fill up the pages of his reports—words that not even we disease doctors, let alone our patients, can understand? How very scholarly! How scientific?"

"By god Proteus!" the N²D² pathologists in the congress cheered. "It would be utterly futile!" They revered Proteus, who changed his shape at will when things didn't go his way. "Proteus sustains us. He is the one who taught us how to vacillate this way and that way until no one knows where we stand. And don't we do that so well?"

"You do! You do!" the president applauded the pathologists. "Truth be told, you pathologists dazzle the sick more eloquently than anyone else. Aren't your pathology reports longer the less you pathologists know about maladies from Mount Olympus?"

"Do you know when a pathologist should move to another town?" Choua asked again, breaking the story line again.

"When?" I asked.

"When tumors he diagnosed as benign begin to metastasize," Choua replied churlishly. "And, do you know the story of a one-armed pathologist?"

"No," I replied.

"Once upon a time a pathologist lost an arm in an accident and lost his job during his recovery period. Many months later, he saw an advertisement for a one-armed pathologist that puzzled him, but he applied anyway. The search committee liked him and offered him the position. After thanking them for their confidence, he asked the committee chairman, a surgeon, why they had advertised for a one-armed pathologist. The surgeon smiled and replied, 'Oh, that's simple. You see, we are fed up with pathologists who look at our tumor biopsies and say, "On the one hand, the tumor has microscopic features of a benign neoplasm, but on the other hand it could be malignant. So, now we insist that our pathologist have only one hand." Choua finished his story within the story, smiled at me, and, finding me unamused, continued.

"Now, our dearest president," the N^2D^2 congress pleaded with their president, "would you enlighten us about the psychiatrist."

"Aha! The psychiatrist!" the president's eyes lit up. "The psychiatrist is the truest among us—truest to our lord, Aesculapius. Truest to the promise he made to the Olympians! Never to think about the nature of Olympian remedies! He never indulges in silly thoughts about the possible cause of psychiatric diseases, and he is committed to the belief that the cause of all psychiatric illness is *unknowable—totally, completely, utterly.* Some of us sometimes err and read underground writings of quacks and their quackish notions of foods and chemicals being the cause of our heavenly diseases. But not the psychiatrist! No sir! Not him. He is above all that. He never looks for the cause of illness in nutrition, nor does he ever reflect on the role environment might play in any illness. He dutifully sits—and does so at hourly rates—as his patients spill their guts. True professional that he is, he never lets anything come between him and the clock that announces the next patient so that the first one can be politely showed to the door. Yes Sir! The psychiatrist among us, he is the purest! The pristine! Never troubled by silly thoughts about causes of human suffering."

"How did that come to pass?" disease doctors asked, their mouths gaping with awe. "How did the psychiatrist become so enlightened?"

"Not easy! Not easy at all!" the president drawled. "They go through many years of training before they lose all ability to think about the cause of disease. Not easy at all! It requires a lot of caffeine and, of course, other drugs help as well. Also, I think, because they always remind each other what happened to the goddess Psyche when she failed to abolish her thoughts about the nature of Olympian matters," the president explained.

Psyche was firmly and clearly told by her lover, Cupid, to completely abandon all thoughts and suppress her curiosity about him. Gods were not to be seen by the mortals they made love to. Cupid told Psyche never to open her eyes to see him when he visited her in the darkness of night and made love to her.

Cupid put Psyche in a great palace with colorful fountains and running streams. He filled the air with music even though no musicians could be seen. He provided her with all earthly comforts. Alas! Psyche disobeyed Cupid and great tragedies befell her. Psyche had two vile sisters who visited her in the palace and were smitten with jealousy. They persuaded Psyche to check out whether Cupid was really a handsome god or a loathsome monster. Poor Psyche! She fell for the trap. She used the lamp given to her by her sisters to look at the naked body of her lover, Cupid, as he lay by her side, spilling some oil and burning him. Cupid was revealed as the God of Love who could never live where trust was lacking. Poor Psyche was abandoned and wandered around in the wilderness doing menial jobs for years before Cupid healed his burns, found her in the wilderness and persuaded Zeus to make her immortal and let him marry her.

"And then they lived happily ever after," the crowd cheered wildly. "And the psychiatrists learned their lesson from the story of Psyche: Never look into the nature of matters! Right?"

"Right!" the president nodded his head excitedly in approval. Then he became solemn again. "There are yet other blessings of N^2D^2 medicine." The president seemed to be coming close to the end of his dissertation. "It is hard work to figure out what foods cause adverse reactions. It is harder still to know what chemicals do to human biology. How can anyone figure out which one of 70,000 odd chemicals that we eat, drink and breathe causes reactions?"

"How does N^2D^2 medicine help?" the audience asked, even though they knew the answer to the question.

"Simple!" the president grinned. "N^2D^2 medicine has declared that food allergy is an all-in-the-head problem and has pronounced chemical sensitivity to be obsessional psychopathology. See how neatly N^2D^2 medicine resolves messy problems that get in the way of treating diseases with drugs of choice?"

"Blessed are the blinded! Blessed are the double-blinded!" the audience chanted joyously, enthusiastic about the new insights into the workings of N^{2}D^2 medicine.

"And if those are not enough blessings for you?" the president continued, "N^{2}D^2 medicine has also solved the problem of nutritional medicine created by quacks. It has denounced all ideas of nutritional disorders as a pathologic belief system. How clever? If a patient believes some foods give him colitis, isn't that the clearest proof of his distorted belief system against drug therapies. I tell you, I love N^{2}D^2 medicine."

"We all love N^{2}D^2 medicine," the audience chanted in chorus.

Quacks' Foibles

Quacks, Choua continued his story, were terrified when Zeus slew Aesculapius and went underground. But their foibles continued.

Quacks were as inquisitive as they were disputative. They could never control their curiosity about the nature of earthlings' maladies. They could never stop arguing among themselves about the theories and hypotheses they were obsessed with at any given time. They spun all kinds of stories about how factors in earthlings' internal and external environments made them sick. The bowel fascinated them to no end. The bowel lining, they postulated, separated the human body from whatever surrounds it, a kind of interface between it and the life around it. They fabricated exotic theories about death beginning in colon and suggested that disorders like headache and skin eruptions could be treated with bowel remedies. N^2D^2 docs were stunned by such preposterous propositions.

And when quacks were not engaged in silly speculation about the role of the bowel, they talked about the kidney being a waste organ. They propounded yet more asinine theories of the lymphatic system being an immune defense system and about lymph dumping waste into the blood and the kidney excreting toxins with the urine. Then they imagined that when the free flow of toxins in lymph and urine was blocked, earthlings became sick. "What nonsense?" N^2D^2 docs cried out when they heard such crazy ideas. The geek among them—the quack busters as they called themselves—wrote articles ridiculing quack theories about toxins and declared that quacks themselves were toxic with silly ideas of body toxins.

Quacks were not distracted. They spun a different yarn about the liver. They imagined that the toxins in the body were detoxified in the liver. They claimed that when earthlings were sick and didn't want to eat, it was because the liver was under stress—only quacks could have dreamed up a quackish idea like that. They also believed there were herbs that strengthened the liver.

PROMETHEUS, THE LIVER AND REGENERATION

A quack notion that tormented N^2D^2 docs most was the quack claim that the injured body tissues were capable of regenerating. This seemingly innocent idea struck at the heart of the core notion of irreversibility of tissue injury of N^2D^2 medicine. Quacks went on to proclaim that earthly remedies facilitated that regeneration and repair process, and that Olympian drugs were really not necessary—a sacrilegious idea that distressed N^2D^2 docs much.

Another quack notion that picqued N^2D^2 docs was the concept of dis-ease—a reversible, pre-disease state of absence of health. Quacks claimed that if that state of dis-ease could be identified early, disease could be prevented. To put that crazy idea to test, quacks proposed a unique program for disposal of human excreta. They called it hygiene. "What is disease prevention?" N^2D^2 docs asked each other, baffled and suspicious of new troubles. "What does drinking water have to do with disease? How can diverting the flow of fecal matter protect mortals from the Olympian diseases?"

The response of some N^2D^2 docs to quack notions of regeneration and healing was totally unexpected. "By god Prometheus! There is hope yet for the quacks," they exclaimed. Actually that was not the first time N^2D^2 docs had tried to co-opt the quacks. Divisiveness—the senior among them said—was not good for business. If quacks couldn't be killed outright, perhaps they can be absorbed as second-class citizens in the Olympian hierarchy. If tissue regeneration seemed to fascinate the quacks, it must have something to do with the god Prometheus, they reasoned. Perhaps there was some hope for them—hope of their coming to their senses and returning to the Olympian gods.

The clever Titan Prometheus and his scatterbrained brother Epimetheus stayed neutral in the war between their nephews, Zeus and their Titan brothers. For this reason they were spared imprisonment in Tartarus. Yet, Prometheus had little love for Zeus and the Olympians who had incarcerated their Titan brothers in the underworld.

Prometheus shaped man out of mud and was much intrigued by his own creation. When the time came to distribute characteristics among man and animals, he made the mistake of permitting his brother, Epimetheus, to dispense various elements to the creation. Epimetheus foolishly gave away all the good ones—courage, cunning, speed and the like—to animals. Nothing was left for man. Prometheus was dismayed when he discovered there was nothing left for his favorite creation. He thought hard and, to distinguish man from animals, gave earthlings an upright posture—like Olympian gods. That didn't go over big with the

Immortals, but they decided not take action against Prometheus. Still, Prometheus wasn't satisfied. He thought of ways to embellish his favorite creature, man, even further. And, then the unimaginable happened. Prometheus, in direct defiance of Zeus, flew up, lit up his torch from the sun, brought it back to the earth and gave it to the earthlings. Fire, he thought, would give man an advantage over all other creatures. Zeus had never been angrier. He chained Prometheus to a rock in the Caucasus and sent an eagle every day to lunch on his liver. And everyday the liver grew back the missing piece.

The N^2D^2 docs were awed by the way Prometheus's liver grew back each day. They suspected Prometheus's hand in the quack notion of regeneration. Many of them hoped that some day common sense might grow in the quacks' heads just as the liver grew in Prometheus's body. They remained hopeful that one day they would co-opt quacks if they couldn't destroy them.

QUACKS AND ATTENTION DEFICIT DISORDER

N^2D^2 docs knew that quacks suffered from hyperactivity and attention deficit disorders, Choua continued.

"You *know* that as a fact, or are you just guessing?" I asked, surprised.
"It seems most likely. In fact, I'm pretty sure of that," Choua rubbed his temple in hesitation, as if wondering whether his story was losing credibility with me.
"I know Olympians were hyperactive and often showed signs of attention deficit disorder, but you haven't told me

anything yet about the earthlings that might indicate that too," I countered, encouraged by Choua's hesitation.

"Only hyperactivity and attention deficit disorder could have led quacks so far astray," Choua recovered quickly. "How else could they have developed preposterous theories linking Olympian diseases with earthly causes. Do you know they actually believed that sugar was bad for children and that it made them hyperactive? Another quack foible held that sugar caused glucose-insulin-adrenaline roller coasters that triggered attacks of anxiety, heart palpitations, jitteryness and lightheadedness. Quacks were not to be believed! Some of them actually believed that cupcakes and chocolate caused learning problems in schools. Amazing stuff!"

"How did N^2D^2 doctors counter that?" I asked.

"They hired professors from the great centers of blinded excellence to come and lecture mothers about the benefits of sugar as a safe source of energy. They also used choice language to ridicule quacks and reported them to licensing boards."

"What else did quacks talk about?" I asked.

"Quacks invented many new diseases. One of their favorites was environmental illness. Bizarre stuff! They said that innocent chemicals such as formaldehyde could cause headaches. And that safe chemicals such as tetrachloroethylene, which dry cleaners used, could cause brain fog. Imagine, cleaning solutions causing brain fog! Quacks were crazy. Then they babbled against household cleaners and pesticides. Do you know why they talked about brain fog so often?" Choua asked.

"Why?"

"Because they were fogged out most of the time themselves. How else would they think that electromagnetic fields from power lines could cause cancer in children. Very imaginative, those rascal ecologists!" Choua muttered. "Those quacks were something else," Choua mused. "They didn't stay with the same idea for too long. Hyperactive, attention-deficited rogues, those quacks!"

"What came next?" I asked.

"Many delusional ideas. One outrageous idea was the notion that earthlings were made up of energy, and that diseases developed when energy patterns were blocked. Some of the quacks hallucinated and dreamed of energy meridians in the body. Some thought-reality-dissociated quacks looked at such meridians and began to play around with them, ultimately spreading lies among themselves that diseases could be treated by pressing or putting needles into points along those meridians or simply by pressing those points—accupressure as they called it. Imagine that!"

"What did N²D² doctors think of that?" I asked.

"You forget Aesculapius had forbidden thinking among them. They ridiculed the whole scheme as shameless quackery. But the quacks didn't let up. They meditated, experimented with breathing techniques and claimed to develop *energy treatments*. Hyperactive as they were, one thing followed another and pretty soon they had many schools of energy medicine."

"Schools of energy medicine? Wow!" I couldn't control my excitement.

"Yes. They taught their students how to diagnose all their invented diseases by looking into the iris of the eye, pinna of the ear and into points on the foot—I think they called that reflexology."

"Did those therapies really work?"

"Many sick claimed the therapies had worked for them. You know how the power of suggestion works, don't you? The gullible always fall for such quackery. But N²D² docs were safe from such charlatans—for Aesculapius had forbidden thinking, and, truth be told, after a while they couldn't have thought even if they tried. Old habits die hard."

"Fascinating stuff, Choua. Tell me more," I urged.

"There were crazier things," Choua replied churlishly.

"Oh, no! What could be crazier than that?"

"Some of them propounded a strange law of the similars. It theorized a weak solution of the substance that causes illness can cure it."

"They were an imaginative lot, weren't they?" I mused. "What did N^2D^2 doctors do about that?"

"Hyperactive quacks were too hyperactive for N^2D^2 docs. Before they could react to the quacks' new ideas, quacks came up with yet newer ones. One of them said diseases could be caused by bugs. Now *that* caused a riot among N^2D^2 docs," Choua chirped.

"Who was that quack?" I asked.

"And that's not where he stopped," Choua ignored my question. "He then proposed the preposterous idea that he could prevent infections by preparing vaccines against the bacteria that caused them. Now, that really riled the N^2D^2 docs. 'How dare a quack dream up vaccines to prevent Olympian infections? How dare he make his vaccine from earthly bugs?' they fumed. Then there was another quack, crazier than the other."

"What did he say?" I asked.

"That nut said you can prevent childbirth fever simply by washing hands before delivering babies," Choua winked.

"How did the mainstream physicians take that one?"

"N^2D^2 docs put that rebellion out fast. They drove him to an asylum. He was followed by a nut who was a surgeon, and he claimed that his scalpels and other surgical instruments could be sterilized with some earthly potions that killed the bugs. Some fool! He thought he could prevent surgical wound infections by such stupid steps. You see, quacks fed upon each other's ideas. Soon, a quack claimed he had discovered a potion—the silver bullet that killed the bugs but left the sick earthling unharmed."

"What happened to that nut?" I asked. "Did they incarcerate him in an asylum as well?"

"No! A strange thing happened," Choua rubbed his eyes, then continued. "Iris, the messenger goddess, told the president of the N²D² congress that the potion, the silver bullet, was actually an Olympian remedy. The Olympians had hidden it in a mold and later sent a flaming flamingo to reveal it to the mortals. The N²D² doctors fell in love with that potion and fed the baby earthlings with tons of that stuff."

"Did that silver bullet work?" I asked. "Did it really kill the bugs and left the body organs of the sick babies unharmed?"

"Unharmed, my foot!" Choua erupted. "What kills one form of life kills another! It's that simple."

"Did N²D² doctors understand that?"

"To understand such things, you have to think first. Didn't I tell you N²D² docs were forbidden to think by Aesculapius. They fed the sick babies the flamingo potion for sore throat, and when that didn't work, they took out their tonsils. When the babies developed yet more infections, N²D² docs prescribed yet more flamingo potions, then removed their adenoids. Next the tiny ear tubes of the babies became blocked by allergies. N²D² docs poured yet more flamingo potions into their little bodies. When that didn't work, they operated on their ears and inserted plastic tubes."

"Did that solve the problems of the little babies?"

"How could it?" Choua retorted. "Those babies grew into teenagers who had much trouble with acne for which N²D² dermatologists prescribed broad-spectrum flamingo potions. That therapy cleared the pimples for some months but wrecked their delicate bowel ecosystems. Many of the young women developed yeast infections. Years later, many of these young people developed autoimmune disorders such as colitis, asthma, vasculitis, underactive thyroid glands, lupus and multiple sclerosis."

"What did quacks think of Olympian diseases?" I asked.
"For example what did they think of the various types of
arthritis—rheumatoid arthritis, rheumatic arthritis, juvenile
arthritis, lupus arthritis, Lyme arthritis, psoriatic arthritis,
Reiter's arthritis, migratory arthritis, polyarthritis and God-
knows-what-else arthritis?"

"And Zeus-knows-what-else arthritis! That's how quacks
ridiculed N^2D^2 doctors," Choua grinned impishly.

"Explain that, Choua! I'm not sure I understand that."
"You see, quacks sometimes played moles and tricked disease
doctors into thinking they were sick. They asked them questions
about what caused rheumatoid arthritis and juvenile arthritis. And
about how lupus arthritis and psoriatic arthritis might begin. Of
course, the N^2D^2 doctors always looked up to Mount Olympus
and told them that those were Olympian diseases and that what
they might be and how they might begin weren't destined to be
revealed to them. Quacks listened to N^2D^2 doctors on such
occasions politely and later laughed hysterically among
themselves. How stupid can you get? they asked each other. Why
have so many different types of arthritis if you don't know the
cause of any of them and if all you prescribe for them are
Olympian steroids and immunosuppressant ambrosia? They
derided N^2D^2 doctors."

"And how about colitis?" I asked. "Aren't there many
types of colitis? There are ulcerative colitis, Crohn's colitis,
microscopic colitis, collagenous colitis, spastic colitis, channel
colitis, ischemic colitis, stercoral colitis and, of course, there is
the all-time popular inflammatory bowel disease. What did quacks
say about that?"

"Quacks had more fun with colitis than they did with
arthritis. They thrived on ridiculing N^2D^2 doctors for colitis

classification. They knew that all disease doctors could do about all those types of colitis was to look up to Mount Olympus. They knew it wasn't destined for them to know the causes of Olympian colitis. The treatment, of course, was Olympian steroids and immunosuppressants. Sometimes they preferred anti-inflammatory nectars from Olympia," Choua chuckled.

"And how about skin disorders? Hives and atopic dermatitis? Acne vulgaris and acne rosacea, psoriasis, pemphigus and others?"

"No difference there either!" Choua laughed lightly. "N²D² doctors always looked up to Mount Olympus when they were asked such questions. Then they went on to prescribe Olympian steroids and skin creams that hid the skin lesions but nothing else. Nothing was ever cured, but the repeat business for N²D² dermatologists was lucrative. Quacks knew all that and complained incessantly among themselves about the deception of such drug therapies."

"How did they know it was deception?" I asked. "Did they have any earthly remedies that worked for those skin disorders?"

"That was the thing! Quacks by that time had learned enough about the altered states of bowel ecology and knew that skin disorders respond well when bowel ecology is restored and protected from flamingo potions."

"And how about other types of autoimmune disorders?" I changed the subject rather than challenge Choua's narration. "How about multiple sclerosis, lupus, under- and overactive thyroid states, myasthenia gravis, and vasculitis?"

"Why should those be any different?" Choua groused. "The cause was always up there on Mount Olympus and the treatment always Olympian steroids. Fortunately for N²D² doctors, Olympian steroids came in so many different shapes and colors that the sick earthlings rarely knew that their immune systems were being suppressed with the same Olympian remedy. Quacks had much fun with those diseases as well."

"How about degeneratory disorders? Coronary artery disease. What did N^2D^2 doctors think caused that problem?"

"A plumbing problem! That's what they thought it was. The disease came from Mount Olympus. Some of them became quite adept at the plumbing job—you know the roto-rooter stuff, zapping the plaques with lasers. When that didn't work, they bypassed the plaques."

"Did that work?" I asked.

"How could it? Plaques form due to metabolic problems which N^2D^2 doctors were not allowed to think about."

"Why didn't the pathologists challenge the heart surgeons? Even when you talk about double, triple or quadruple bypasses, you knew that plaque formations affect all parts of coronary arteries. So, why didn't the pathologists speak up?"

"Pathologists speak up against surgeons? Are you crazy or stupid?" Choua scowled. "Surgeons have too much power. Remember, they appoint the pathologists. Besides, surgeons feed the pathologist with their biopsies. The pathologists were not that stupid! They wouldn't bite the hands that fed them."

The Wrath of Zeus

The Olympians watched the squabbles among the earthlings with amusement. They were humored by the defiant attitude of quacks. Earthlings! they shrugged. Little beasts! they smiled. Miserable little worms intellectualizing about our affairs!! they shook their heads. But time wears everything down. And so it was, Choua's story continued, that Olympians lost interest in N^2D^2 docs and quacks.

The god Poseidon, Zeus's brother and God of Sea, had a violent, volcanic temper. He had an unhappy marriage with Amphitrite, a sea nymph—mostly because, like his brother, he had a roving eye. He was irked by the fact that Zeus on Olympia had a wider range of striking for beautiful damsels while he was restricted to mostly slimy, slithering sea creatures. Every now and them, Poseidon succumbed to sibling rivalry. Zeus's frequent heavyhandedness, of course didn't help matters much.

On one occasion, at Hera's provocation, Poseidon joined Apollo in a plot to dethrone Zeus. They captured and bound Zeus to a couch, and threatened to kill him. Fortunately for Zeus, the nymph Thetis—who had spurned Poseidon on several occasions—happened to learn of this. She brought Briareus, the 50-headed monster, to guard Zeus, effectively squashing the rebellion. In revenge, Zeus hung Hera by her heels from Olympus and sent Apollo and Poseidon to servitude in a distant penal colony. He, himself, stood on Mount Olympus, brooding.

It was then that a quack, while presenting a research paper to a quack congress, had the audacity to insult the Olympian remedies. Zeus was besides himself. "Those pitiful rogues! Those miserable ants!! Those abominable creatures!!" Zeus thundered. It was then when he decided to put an end to all quackery.

"What did he do? Kill them all with his thunderbolt?" I felt a chill.

"No. As angry as Zeus was then, he had just escaped death himself. His anger wouldn't have dissipated with the simple death of quacks." Choua shuddered as he continued. "At that moment Zeus decided on a cruel revenge that the mortals would forever remember. Sudden death by a thunderbolt, he thought, would kill quacks before they would know what hit them. He wanted to inflict pain slowly, inexorably, for a long time. He wanted them to hurt and bleed while he watched. To this purpose, he decided to use N^2D^2 docs as the agents of mass destruction of quacks. He knew N^2D^2 docs would cherish the role, getting even after suffering insult at the hands of quacks for centuries."

"What did he do?" I asked nervously.

"Zeus was mean-spirited then. He disguised himself as the FBA commissioner. He scheduled a global health congress—the likes of which had never been seen before—and called in all the assistant commissioners of FBA, all heads of licensing boards, all bigwigs of the Joint Commission of $N2D^2$ Hospitals, all honchos of state N^2D^2 societies, all chairmen of professional ethics committees, all executive officers of drug companies, all chiefs of medical boards of insurance companies and all prosecutors in the departments of professional misconduct. During the cocktail party the evening before the conference opened, he put a special blend of ambrosia and nectar in their drinks and so seeded in their hearts an inquenchable thirst for the blood of quacks. He then..."

"What happened," I interrupted Choua, unable to contain myself.

"What happened next was entirely predictable. Zeus's special blend had its intended effect. Everyone attending the congress woke up in the morning as thirsty as a bloodhound, with an inquenchable desire for quacks' blood. They fumed with rage in the congress hall and swore that they—each in his own way—were going to kill every last one of the quacks. The congress unanimously decided to strictly ban all quack therapies. All nutritional therapies were outlawed. All herbal remedies were disallowed. All physical methods of relieving pain were declared illegal. All methods of self-regulation, meditation and stress reduction were denounced as sorcery. All clinical ecology methods of diagnosis and treatment were forbidden. Trigger point injections with glucose were proscribed. (Olympian steroid injections were allowed.) Bio-oxidative therapies were terminated. Joint manipulation, kinesiology, reflexology, hydrotherapy, massage therapy—all those alternative therapies were condemned."

"How did they do all that?" I asked.

"Zeus, wearing the robe of the FBA commissioner hauled in all quacks. He ordered his nymphs to drag out all their books and sacred manuscripts and burned them in the presence of quacks. He then sent his Cyclopes to raid their clinics and confiscate and destroy all earthly remedies. He first suspended their admitting privileges, then revoked their licenses.

"Still, Zeus's anger was not mitigated. He had all the assets of the quacks impounded—their bank accounts seized. Then Zeus moved on to their families. First, he planted seeds of discontent in the hearts of their wives which soon matured into flaming disgust. Many quack wives deserted their husbands.

Zeus's wrath didn't even spare the children of quacks. He made other children at school hate them and jeer at them, shouting, 'Hey, hey, little quackling, your quack dad is cracking.'

"Some ecologists tried to escape into Mexico and some nutritionists took boats to China and India. But all that was to no avail. Zeus had the NAFTA law passed and that brought Mexico under control."

"And India?" I asked. "Didn't India stick up for its own? Indians are a proud people. They have very old traditions of using natural Ayurvedic and other therapies for thousands of years. Why didn't the Indians tell the FBA commissioner to go fly a kite? Why didn't they protest the FBA's heavyhandedness?"

"Those Ayuvedics? Naw! They were no match for the *scientists* from the office of the FBA commissioner. None of them had any double-blinded studies with which to defend their natural therapies. Besides, they were too poor and disheartened to fight back. The Indian N^2D^2 docs, by contrast, were rich and well connected to their politicians. Zeus made the Indian N^2D^2 docs first dismiss the quack theories as stupid old wives tales, then defrocked and destroyed all quacks. Of course, the Indian drug companies celebrated the events by throwing elegant yacht parties for N^2D^2 docs."

"I didn't know Indians had so many yachts." I said surprised. "Tell me about China? The Chinese love to defy Potomac city. Didn't they tell the FBA commissioner to go jump in some lake?"

On a visit to Beijing, some Chinese physician-friends proudly spoke about traditional Chinese medicine. There were simply too many Chinese—a billion and half by the year 2025—to be treated with N^2D^2 Star Wars technology, they explained. The Japanese couldn't build enough electron microscopes and the

Americans enough MRI scans for them. The Chinese remedies, my hosts asserted, were there to stay. But on the other hand when I visited an emergency room in a Jinan hospital later in that trip, all IV drips administered for heatstroke contained antibiotics. I was surprised that the Chinese were using antibiotics to manage cases of heatstroke. My companion, a perceptive young Chinese physician, smiled and said, "These young Chinese only know Western medicine. If they didn't put antibiotics in IV drips, they wouldn't know what else to do."

"China?" Choua rolled his eyes at me when I returned from my thoughts of my China trip. "Many years earlier, some Chinese businessmen had implored the FBA commissioner to let them import their herbs into the N^2D^2 country. The FBA commissioner had insolently rejected their pleas. When Zeus, impersonating the FBA commissioner, first approached the Chinese, they laughed out loud at him, then arrogantly dismissed him as a fool who knew nothing about Chinese heritage and pride. Zeus was not amused. Transforming himself into the chief delegate from Potomac city, Zeus appeared in the Great Hall of People by sprawling Tiennamen Square. And standing below a huge picture of Mao, he sternly warned the Chinese of dire consequences if they didn't abolish completely *Ti Chi* and *Chi Gong*, their herbal and food remedies, and if they were not totally subservient to the dictates of the Chinese N^2D^2 docs. He informed them that the powerful people of Potomac city would revoke the most favored trade status of China if they didn't desist from all quackery. Finally, he warned them to either publish double-blinded N^2D^2 drug studies or perish. The Chinese decided not to perish and accepted the FBA terms—just as they had a hundred years earlier, when the British forced them to accept their poppy flower gifts after the Chinese lost the Opium War in the Pearl River delta."

"And the Russians?" I asked.

"Poor Russians! They had nothing, not even clean syringes. They degenerated into experimenting with light therapy, which they could afford. That brought much amusement to the folks at the FBA."

"And the Germans?" I asked. "The Germans are well-known for their ingenuity in using natural therapies such as neural therapy. The Germans also had little respect for the FBA. What did they do? Didn't they fight back?"

"You forget Germany was also the mecca of the N^2D^2 drug industry. Too many Dueche marks! Although it is true that the German people had little respect for the FBA, that didn't hold for the German drug agency. They had close ties with the office of the FBA. As things went by in Potomac city, so did they go in the city by the Rhine."

"And the French?" I persisted. "The French loved their homeopaths. At one time, more than one-third of the French preferred homeopathy to N^2D^2 medicine, didn't they?"

"Too many N^2D^2 Eurodollars there! The Common Market did them in. Zeus had no difficulty in persuading the French to kill off all quacks who practiced homeopathy."

"And the African countries! What happened to their indigenous remedies?" I persisted.

"You're a funny man, Mr. Pathologist!" Choua sneered. "You think the naked, starving Africans would be a threat to the FBA commissioner and his swarming hordes?"

"So, what is the point of your story?" I asked, flustered.

"None!" Choua replied churlishly. "Every story doesn't have to have a point."

I stretched and closed my eyes to rub them. When I opened my eyes, Choua was gone.

Chapter 2

Prince Chaullah and Science in Medicine

Choua came over one day. I was at my microscope.

"What is science in medicine?" he asked without greeting me. That's not unusual for him.

"Science in medicine is the same as it is outside medicine," I replied.

"What is science?" Choua asked, moving closer to the window in my office and looking out.

"Science is measurements," I answered.

"And?" Choua prodded, without turning to look at me.

"Reproducibility."

"And?"

"Accuracy."

"And?"

"Precision."

"And?"

"What is on your mind, Choua?" I asked. "Where is this leading us?"

"So you think science is measurement, reproducibility, accuracy and precision, is that it?" Choua went on without acknowledging my inquiry.

"Yes! That's about it."

"What about observation?"

"Yes! That too," I agreed, realizing that as usual Choua was much closer to the subject than I.

"Which one of those is most important?"

"I would say measurement. Reproducibility is obviously important but it comes after measurement. But I don't know which one of them is most important."

"What if they clash with each other?"

"What do you mean?"

"I mean if they are inconsistent or incompatible."

"Give me an example of how measurement and reproducibility clash with each other, Choua, and I'll see if I can come up with the answer *you* want," I said, irritated.

"What I want is simple. I want to know what you *doctors* think science is." Choua spoke sharply, as he suddenly turned to face me and then moved away from the window and closer to my desk.

"Well, tell me how measurements and reproducibility clash with each other?" I repeated.

"Suppose you observe something once. Now suppose someone else fails to make that observation. That would be a problem, wouldn't it?"

"Yes," I agreed, not knowing where Choua was leading. "Actually, Choua, this is exactly the reason why we Americans insist on reproducibility before we accept medical statistics as scientifically valid."

"I know *that*," Choua brushed my point aside. "Suppose a friend sees a mouse scurry away to a dimly-lit corner of a room. You don't see the mouse. Now, would you say your friend's observation is not true—scientifically invalid—just because you didn't make the same observation?"

"Not really," I replied.

"Not really?" Choua raised his eyebrows. "Would you say it was a scientifically valid observation even if your friend made it but you didn't?"

"Don't be ridiculous, Choua," I chided. "There is no science in seeing or not seeing a mouse. Many times people think they see mice in dark rooms when in reality they mistake shadows for rodents."

"Think about what you are saying," Choua's voice rose. "Your friend saw the mouse so he knows it was there. You didn't see it. Yet, you're so ready to cast doubt on the validity of your friend's observation."

"Choua, you're confused. Valid scientific observations must be reproducible."

"Oh, is that so?" Choua frowned. "If your friend couldn't persuade the mouse to put up a repeat performance, you would reject his observation."

"Choua, you are confusing science with..."

"With what?" he snapped. "We are talking about observation, aren't we? Your friend saw the mouse. You didn't. Was it there or not?"

"Yes, it was there," I yielded.

"So his observation was correct even if you couldn't confirm it, even if he couldn't reproduce it. Right?" Choua was in a combative mood.

"Right! But what does that have to do with science?" I asked, frustrated.

"Science is observation. *It's that simple!*"

"Yes, but the observation has to be valid," I asserted.

"Who decides what is scientifically valid and what isn't?" Choua narrowed his eyes. "What are you saying? Is your friend's sighting scientifically valid or is your failure to see the mouse scientifically valid?"

"I'm not saying anything about your frivolous proposition. That's all." I saw the logic in Choua's argument, but he still irritated me.

Choua stared at me blankly for a few moments, then turned, walked to the window and looked out again. I watched him in silence, wondering what it was that he wanted to tell me and why he wouldn't speak plainly. Choua can be direct and succinct in arguing his case, or he can wear me down with his circuitous reasoning. Science in medicine! That's simple enough. But why did he have to bring a mouse into this discussion? I wondered.

"How often do patients respond well to a drug initially only to have the drug lose its efficacy over time?" Choua asked softly, seemingly lost on the distant horizon.

"Often," I replied.

"How often?"

"I don't know how often, but it is not uncommon. What's your point?"

"The point is that you doctors have distorted ideas of what science is and what it isn't. Tell me what you would consider unscientific, the initial effectiveness of the drug or its inefficacy later on?"

"Now you're distorting things," I rebuked him. "There are valid scientific reasons that explain why people develop drug resistance after using drugs for some time," I challenged.

"Do all people develop drug resistance? Does such resistance develop at the same rate in all cases?"

"No! But that's obvious. No two patients are exactly the same."

"*Aha! No two patients are exactly the same*!" Choua chuckled. "I was hoping you would say that. Tell me why does that happen?"

"Because people are different. There is this matter of biochemical individuality—people metabolize different drugs differently. That's old hat. I don't know why you are getting excited about that."

"So a physician needs to know if a given patient responds to a given drug. Right?" Choua winked.

"Yes," I agreed.

"And that holds regardless of how many double-blind cross-over studies have been done with that drug. Right?"

"Right!"

"How does a doctor find out whether a drug will work for a given patient or not? And if it does work, how does he know how long its efficacy will last?"

"By clinical experience."

"So it's the clinical observation—the empirical experience—of what does or doesn't work that matters. Right, Mr. Clinician?" Choua taunted.

"Clinical experience is based on what works and what doesn't," I ignored his tone.

"And that holds whether there are or aren't any double-blind cross-over studies for a given therapy," Choua snapped.

"Choua, you are utterly irrational when it comes to double-blind cross-over studies. I don't know why you are so rabid about this drug research model," I scolded him.

"Because that's where the trouble begins. That is the wellspring of poisonous thinking for young medical students," Choua replied belligerently.

"Without blinded and controlled studies, how does one find out what works and what doesn't?" I asked.

"By careful observation."

"How does one know that a given observation is accurate, and that the benefit attributed to one therapy actually didn't accrue from another?" I persisted.

"That's what being an astute clinician is all about, isn't it?"

"You can't practice medicine without controlled studies, Choua. Understand that, will you?" I said, exasperated.

"Why not? What's wrong with simply observing what works and what doesn't? Isn't that what great Greek physicians of the past did before the *geek* doctors of today took over?"

"You miss the whole point," I said, suppressing a smile at his play on words. "If those great Greek physicians of the past had the technology and the statistical methods of the geek doctors of today, they would have used them as well. They would also have used the double-blind cross-over method."

"You *really* think your methods of drug research are perfect, don't you?" Choua frowned.

"Nothing is perfect in medicine but it is a good model," I

replied uncompromisingly.

"Good model, eh!" Choua rubbed his forehead with his hand, looked around, moved over to a pile of journals in the corner and pulled one of them out. "Listen to this:

We found that 36 percent of 815 consecutive patients on a general medical service of a university hospital had an iatrogenic illness. In 9 percent of all persons admitted, the incident was considered major in that it threatened life or produced considerable disability.

N Eng J Med 304:638; 1981

This is the truth behind your pseudoscience of drugs," Choua spoke contemptuously. "Iatrogenic illness—diseases caused by your ill-advised therapies—is hurting millions of people."

"That is a real problem," I agreed.

"Don't you ever reflect on what your wonderful therapies do to people *after* they have been proven safe and effective by your blessed double-blind cross-over science?" Choua asked sternly. "You ride your high horses of pseudoscience of drug medicine and push those chemicals on gullible people, never thinking about what the long-term consequences of poisoning human biology with chemicals might be."

As medical students, we were never troubled by such questions. Life was simple then. We accepted as scientifically valid whatever we were taught by our professors. Why wouldn't we?

Our professors had all the knowledge, statistics, graphs and illustrations. We were regularly cautioned against unscientific nonsense that passes for herbal and nutritional medicines and were rigorously warned against charlatans, quacks and other miscreants involved in health fraud. Drugs and scalpels were the only valid therapies. I don't remember any professor putting it in exactly those words, but the message was always clear.

In the two major ancient civilizations—China and India—healing arts are entirely based on empirical observations made over centuries. And so it was in the healing arts that prevailed in ancient Egypt, Assyria, Babylon, Greece and Rome. Medicine was based on trial and error—whatever worked was accepted and what didn't was rejected. There were no controlled studies. Of course, this evolved slowly over centuries. But, in Pakistan then, and in the United States now, empiricism is not held in high esteem in medicine.

HERBALISTS AND DRUG DOCTORS

"Let's assume that three herbalists make an observation about the healing effects of an herb on three patients," Choua posited. "Would you accept those as valid observations?"

"Yes." I felt relieved at his sudden composure.

"Now, suppose three drug doctors try to repeat the same observation in three different patients and fail to observe the beneficial effects of that herb. Do the drug doctors invalidate the observations of the herbalists?"

"It does call into question the validity of the first set of observations, doesn't it?"

"That's the crux of the problem!" Choua became excited again. "The observations of the drug doctors do not invalidate the observations of the herbalists anymore than the observations of the herbalists invalidate those of the drug doctors. Actually, the only valid conclusion that can be drawn from this is that the herb worked in the hands of the experienced herbalists but didn't in the hands of the drug doctors. There is nothing wrong with that at all. Herbalists have learned to make their herbs work for them while drug doctors haven't."

"It's not that simple, Mr. Logic," I teased. "If the herb has any effects, drug doctors should be able to demonstrate them as well."

"Drug doctors do not have the patience to wait for the slow, sustained effects of herbs. They want their results quick and..."

"And dirty?" I poked.

"I wasn't going to put it that way," Choua grinned. "But you have the gist of it. Drugs are potent chemicals and do produce closely reproducible *short-term* results. Herbs and nutrients work slowly—and safely, without any of the toxicity caused by drugs. It's that simple! But you doctors can't see any of that, can you?"

"If observations about herbs and drugs are made carefully enough and under controlled conditions, they really cannot conflict with other observations," I refused to yield the argument.

"Of course, it can," Choua said emphatically. "If what you claim to be true is really true, your *proven* safe and effective drugs wouldn't be sending people to hospitals by the millions, would they?"

"You can't help it. Exaggeration is in your marrow." I showed my frustration.

"Exaggerate, eh! Remember what the *Journal* said: One of three Americans admitted to a hospital has a disease caused by doctors. You drug doctors don't like to talk about such things, do you?"

"Your cyclopean eye sees things only one way," I scolded him.

"You keep writing about changes in human biology," Choua went on, ignoring my comment. "You say when we change something in biology in one way, we change everything in biology in some way. But I don't think your disease doctors of drug medicine understand any of that—how synthetic chemicals damage human ecosystems."

"We have to have concrete information—hard data obtained with blinded and controlled studies—when we care for the acutely ill. You cannot be whimsical in matters of life and death. There is no room for error there," I persisted.

"Aha! So you think that you must have suitable control subjects when you treat patients with acute, life-threatening illnesses. Is that the point? Tell me, where do you go looking for such controls? And, if the illness were *really* acute and life-threatening, wouldn't the controls die if you gave them mere placebo starch pills?"

"Controls for acute illnesses can be..."

"Why would you want to blind an acutely ill patient anyway?" Choua interrupted me tartly. "What possible clinical advantages can there be in that? Why do you have to blind his physician? What conceivable benefits can there be if the physician doesn't know what therapy he is administering to an acutely ill patient? How can you ever rationalize that on a scientific basis? How can you ever justify that on moral grounds? You really don't see how preposterous your logic is, do you?" Choua scowled.

"What's your point, Choua?" I asked, exasperated. "The whole point of double-blind cross-over studies is to separate specific effects of drugs from nonspecific results—to determine what drugs work consistently and what do not."

"Don't sidestep the issue," Choua spoke sharply. "We are

talking about what science is and what it isn't. Consistency of results is a matter of empirical observations. Drug use today is as empirical as the use of herbs was in ancient China and India. Science is only accurate observation—nothing more, nothing less. Repeated accurate observations give us our empirical sense of what does and doesn't work." Choua waved his hand disdainfully.

"Being an astute clinician doesn't mean that we ignore all the benefits of modern controlled studies." I held my ground.

"Uh! Controlled studies again. You do have blinders on, don't you? You can't breathe without your *blessed* controlled studies, can you? Don't you understand why sick people see their physicians? To alleviate their suffering! Relieve pain! Reverse the disease process! Don't you understand any of it?"

"Yes, yes, I do! But without blinded study we cannot..."

"Clinical outcome, Dr. Blindfold," Choua rudely interrupted me. "Clinical outcome! That's the only thing that matters. Why do sick people see their doctors?"

"To get well."

"That's right! That's what people want when they are sick and when they wish to stay well. And that's what you should be looking for as well—not some frivolous, made-up numbers. A patient is his only valid control. There is no one quite like him. He knows how he felt before he got sick. Regaining his health is the only *control* he cares for. If you can alleviate his suffering and reverse his disease, then he knows you have succeeded, and so do you. It matters little if there were or were not any double-blind cross-over studies to prove anything. Can't you see any of this?" Choua's tone was outright insulting.

"You are entitled to your opinion, Choua," I countered gently. "But modern medicine cannot progress with such a simplistic approach—without controlled studies."

"Oh God! Controlled studies again!" Choua bellowed with palpable anger.

Then suddenly he was calm. He squeezed his lower lip between his teeth, whistled in a subdued tone and smiled. I have seen him go through such sudden mood swings a thousand times. Still, it amazes me how quickly his anger dissipates and his face lights up.

"I want to tell you a story," Choua grinned mischievously. "Go ahead, Choua. I'm ready for another story," I replied.

PRINCE CHAULLAH'S STORY

Once upon a time there was a king. He was strong, wise and kind. He was at peace with the kings of neighboring realms who bestowed much respect and honor upon him.

His kingdom was a peaceful one. He was a just king and ruled his subjects with fairness and compassion. His subjects revered him. People were prosperous. Everyone had enough to eat. There were only a few miscreants, and the king's soldiers were quick to apprehend them and present them to judges who dispensed justice swiftly and decisively in open forum. People liked that.

The king was enlightened. He loved literature, sculpture and architecture just as he did martial arts and athletics. After the harvest, week-long festivals were held throughout the kingdom, with food, games and prizes. The king presided over the ceremonies held in the capital that always included music, art shows and readings of the works of great writers and poets.

Those were good times.

The king had a son named Chaullah. Prince Chaullah was the apple of his father's eye and the pride of his mother, the queen. The king wanted his prince to be the greatest of all kings, strong and capable in body, quick in mind, wise, just and compassionate. To that end, the king sent messages out to all parts of his kingdom and to other kingdoms as well, announcing that he was searching for tutors for his prince and promised great rewards. There was a great response from places far and wide. Hordes of tutors arrived for the great honor. There were mathematicians and historians, poets and scholars, artists and architects. The king appointed a committee of his courtiers to select the best among great tutors for his prince. And so it was done.

Prince Chaullah studied many subjects under the able tutelage of his many gifted teachers. He received instructions in all disciplines befitting his status as the heir to the throne. Months passed and then years. The king awaited anxiously for the day that the tutors would declare their work done and present Prince Chaullah to the king for some tests. Then, the great day arrived.

Prince Chaullah appeared in full court wearing a flowing crimson silk robe, with a glittering bejeweled crown on his head. He walked erect and with solemn dignity. He was followed dutifully by his many tutors, walking side by side in two rows, wearing robes of many colors. Everyone in the court stood up to greet the procession. The king motioned his courtiers to take their places and asked his prince to walk closer to the throne that he shared proudly with his queen. Prince Chaullah obediently approached his parents and bowed low in submission. His tutors stayed behind. The king then looked at the tutors and graciously asked them to take their seats close to the throne.

"Are you ready for a test?" the king asked them with a gentle smile.

"Yes we are, our Lord!" they crowed in unison with excitement.

"Have you chosen a test for the prince?" the king demanded.

"We beg our Lord to choose the test," they replied with one voice.

"Very well then, we shall choose the test," the king smiled again and reached deep within his royal robe to pull something out. His fist was clenched as his hand emerged from the robe. He waved his hand from side to side to let the full court witness how tightly his fist clenched the object in his hand and that what it held couldn't be seen by anyone. Then he extended his closed fist to Prince Chaullah and asked,

"Tell us, my Prince Chaullah, what do I hold in my fist, hidden from your eyes?"

Prince Chaullah looked at the closed fist and then toward his tutors. The tutors shook their heads and nodded him on. The prince then returned to his father's closed fist and gazed at it intently for some moments. Then he closed his eyes, as if meditating on the fist. More moments passed. Nothing but silence prevailed in the court. Yet excitement rose among the royal audience until it was palpable.

"It is a stone!" Prince Chaullah exclaimed as he opened his eyes.

"Oh my God, blessed are we all!" the king shouted jubilantly. "You're right! You're right, our prince."

There was a rush of loud mumbling throughout the court.

The tutors breathed sighs of relief and lowered their heads in gratitude.

"Tell us now, our Prince, what is it?" the king asked as the noise in the court subsided.

Prince Chaullah craned his neck to get closer to the king's closed fist, stared at it for a while, moved his head back a little and then closed his eyes again. A hushed silence spread over the court again as everyone waited for the moment of revelation. Within moments, Prince Chaullah's frame began to sway to and fro; his face contorted slightly; his eyes still closed. Anticipation surged in the silent court. All eyes fixed on the Prince.

"It has a hole in the middle!" Prince Chaullah cried out, his eyes still closed. "It is made of stone and it has a hole in the middle," he smiled as he opened his eyes.
"God be praised! God be praised!" the king stood up with exhilaration. "You're absolutely right, our Prince Challah."
"God be praised!" Prince Challah rejoined. Then he looked at his tutors who all nodded approvingly.
"Now, tell us what is it?" the king asked.

The king's question seemed to baffle the prince, but he recovered quickly. Looking at the king's outstretched arm and tight fist, the prince closed his eyes and slipped into another trance. Silence befell the court again. The prince was quiet much longer this time. The courtiers remained motionless as the king and queen studied their prince's intense face.

"It's rounded! It's rounded!" Prince Chaullah suddenly erupted.
"So it is! So it is!" the king roared.

"It's made of stone. It has a hole in it. It is rounded," the prince repeated.

"Right! Our great prince. Right!" The king rose, bent forward and kissed the prince on his forehead. "Now tell us, my son, what is it that I hold in my clenched fist?"

For the fourth time, Prince Chaullah scrutinized his father's fist for some moments and then slowly closed his eyes. Soon his body began to sway, first gently then with sharp jerky movements. His lips were tight now, his teeth clenched. Then he began to tremble. The queen, who sat quietly all this time, could no longer calmly witness the proceedings. She stood up abruptly in evident discomfort, sending a wave of shock through the court. The king also rose and warmly held his queen's hand with reassuring affection. They both then sat down to wait for their son to emerge from his trance and reveal the identity of the object hidden in the king's fist. Then it happened.

"It's a millstone! A millstone," Prince Chaullah screamed. "It's made of stone. It has a hole in the middle. It is round. Yes, that's what it is! It's a millstone!"

"Wha...at?" the king suddenly stood up, jolted by the prince's answer. "A millstone in my fist?" His voice cracked.

"Yes! A millstone!" the prince responded amiably.

"Think, Prince Chaullah, think again! A millstone in my clenched fist?" The king thundered, shook his head violently and looked at the tutors. His whole body trembled with rage. The tutors quivered in terror. The courtiers froze in their places.

Prince Chaullah was stunned by the king's response to his answer. He trembled a little and then murmured, "It's a round stone with a hole in the middle. It's a millstone. What else could it be?"

The king angrily motioned all the tutors to follow him to the back chambers and stormed out of the court.

"How could it have happened?" he thundered and waved his arms.

The tutors stood before the king, their eyes downcast, their bodies shaking beneath their robes. Moments passed.

"I demand to know!" the king thundered again. "How could it be? How can anyone smart enough to deduce that an object hidden in a clenched fist is a round stone with a hole not know that a clenched fist cannot hold a millstone?"

"If our lives be spared, we..."

"Answer!" the king shouted in rage. "Your lives are spared."

"Our Lord, we taught him everything we knew," they answered with one voice.

"How could it be?"

"We taught the prince all we could," they spoke again. "He recognized it was a round stone with a hole in it."

"How could he not know that a round stone with a hole clenched in my hand could only be a pearl and not a windmill stone?" the king roared on.

"Our Lord, we taught Prince Chaullah all we could. But there are things that can't be taught," they murmured softly and lowered their heads.

Choua finished his story, looked at me for a few moments, then was gone.

A SHOOTING STAR IN HOPATCONG

"Suppose it is a clear summer night at Lake Hopatcong," Choua spoke as he stood in the door the next day. "Some people sitting by the water see a shooting star."

"Yes!" I knew right away that it was going to be a continuation of the tirade of the previous day.

"Would you say that is a valid observation?"

"Yes, I would."

"Now suppose it is cloudy in Cambridge, New Haven and Bethesda."

"Okay!"

"The clouds blinded the folks in Cambridge, New Haven and Bethesda."

"Go on, Choua." I began to see his line of reasoning.

"The folks blinded by clouds don't see the shooting star."

"Yes."

"Now tell me, is the observation of people in Hopatcong scientifically valid or not? I mean is it scientifically correct to say that indeed there was a visible shooting star in Hopatcong?"

"Yes," I agreed, amused by the trial lawyer's oblique questioning.

"But the folks in Cambridge, New Haven and Bethesda failed to see the shooting star. They could not confirm the observation made by the folks at Hopatcong."

"Go on."

"Now, suppose the folks in Cambridge, Bethesda and New Haven proclaim that what the people in Hopatcong claim they saw wasn't really there. The Cambridge, New Haven and Bethesda folks assert they are specialists in sighting shooting stars, and, further declare there is really no way that lay people at Hopatcong could have seen what the specialists didn't with their high-tech tools. So they believe the Hopatcong people simply imagined the whole thing."

"I don't know where it is leading us, Choua," I complained, concealing my amusement at his logic.

"Was there a shooting star or not?" he asked.

"Yes, there was."

"How do you know?" Choua squinted impishly.

"Because the people in Hopatcong saw it."

"Even if the specialists at Cambridge, Bethesda and New Haven insist it wasn't there?" Choua pressed.

"Didn't you just say they were blinded by clouds?" I asked.

"So we can agree that the folks at Cambridge, Bethesda and New Haven didn't see it because they were blinded. Can we?"

"Yes!"

"Now tell me, what would have happened if the night was clear also at Cambridge, Bethesda and New Haven, but the specialists there decided to wear blindfolds. Could Hopatcong folks have seen the shooting star?"

"Yes, of course. You just said that," I answered with irritation.

"Could the specialists at Cambridge, Bethesda and New Haven have seen the star through their blindfolds?" Choua pressed on.

"Not if their blindfolds were any good. But what's the point of all this, Choua?" I asked angrily.

"The point, Dr. Gullible, is that it's not the fault of Hopatcong people that specialists at Cambridge, Bethesda and New Haven wore blindfolds. If the specialists choose to blindfold themselves and cannot see what everyone else can see, it is not a matter of science, is it? Don't you get it? That's exactly what *your* high priests of science are doing to nutritional and environmental medicines. First, these champions of N^2D^2 medicine flatly reject the idea that nutrients and herbs can work. Next, they refuse to see what is so obvious—nondrug therapies do work. They spurn the clinical experience of ecologists and nutritionists. They dismiss the statements of patients who get better with nondrug therapies. Then they wear blindfolds and claim to be scientists. Science is observation. If an observation cannot be reproduced, it does not mean the observed phenomenon didn't take place. What matters is whether the observation was correct."

"It's not that simple!"

"Not that simple, eh?" Choua growled. "How many Chinese and Indian herbs do you use in your practice?"

"Many."

"Do they work?"

"Why would I use them if they didn't work?" I asked with annoyance.

"Did the Chinese or Indians ever prove the efficacy of their herbs using a blessed double-blind cross-over?"

"No," I answered with a smile. "They based their methods on empirical knowledge."

"What is empirical?" Choua frowned.

"What works! It is knowledge of things that work by common observation. Isn't that what you told me yesterday?"

"Aha! What works. So you don't care whether the specialists at Cambridge, Bethesda and New Haven are blinded to the value of nutrients and herbs or not. You use them because they work."

"Yes, but it is not that simple with drugs. We don't have thousands of years to determine the efficacy of new drugs. So we must have valid statistics," I said firmly.

"Oh yeah! Statistics. You do need them, don't you?" Choua asked sarcastically. "And your statistics have to be blinded and crossed-over, don't they?"

"We need hard data."

"Yes, you do. I have no problem with that. The real issue is whether the data has to be gathered by specialists who choose to blind themselves or whether they can be gathered by astute clinicians who do not wish to work blindfolded?"

"Choua, I know you have problem with double-blind cross-over drug studies, but seriously, how can you introduce newly synthesized drugs without some safety studies?"

"Why do you have to blind anyone to find out how toxic a chemical is?" Choua shot back.

"How can you assess drug toxicity without statistics?" I demanded.

"Why not? How do you assess drug toxicity anyway? Drug toxicity causes symptoms that patients tell you about. Drug toxicity shows up in abnormal laboratory tests. Why do you need to blind yourself to make such simple observations?"

"I told you why! For objectivity and statistical validity!" I replied contentiously.

"Statistical validity again!" Choua shook his head in disgust.

"Yes! For statistical validity," I repeated belligerently.

Choua looked at me with piercing eyes and then with a vacant expression—as if to determine whether I was earnest in my argument or playing devil's advocate. I looked back at him impassively.

"How do good clinicians practice their art?" he asked after some minutes.

"What do you mean?" I asked.

"How often do they follow their own intuitive senses about the nature of their patients' suffering? How often do they go to libraries to check statistics?"

"Actually that happens all the time." I sensed an obvious weakness in his argument.

"Oh!" Choua murmured softly and raised his chin with his hand. "So they subordinate their clinical senses to medical statistics. Is that what *good* clinicians do?" Choua emphasized the word *good*. "How often do you use statistics to make your clinical judgment calls for your patients?"

"You miss the point. I may not use statistics to choose therapies for individual patients, but I rely on statistics that give me a sense of what to expect in terms of clinical outcome."

"I doubt that! I doubt that very much," Choua spoke churlishly.

"That's funny. You claim to know my clinical work more than I do," I mocked him.

"You go by what does or doesn't work!" Choua responded calmly. "You establish in your mind what does or doesn't work by repeated empirical observation. When you put together outcome statistics to publish your studies, your data statistically validates what you already learned by your empirical observation. Isn't that so?"

"In a way, you..."

"You confuse clinical observations made with sick people with physical observations made with laboratory technology," Choua interrupted me, very gently this time. "Think back, Mr. Pathologist, all your unexpected research observations were about physical phenomena revealed by laboratory studies, whether made with your microscope or with analytical chemistry methods. All your clinical observations were always empirical."

Choua fell silent and stood impassively for several moments, looking at the floor. Then he slowly walked out. An hour or so later, he returned with a thick pile of journals and read aloud:

Doctors' Ignorance of Statistics

Many of us faced with someone who quotes statistics find it difficult to distinguish whether any consequent conclusion is correct or whether we have been bamboozled.

British Medical Journal
294:856; 1987

Choua finished reading and looked up.

"I know there are problems with statistics," I capitulated.
"There are problems then there are *problems*. When it comes to medical statistics, you doctors have mega problems. Let me read some more:

Wulff and colleagues sent a questionnaire to 250 Danish doctors (of whom 148 responded) to assess their knowledge of elementary statistical expressions...From nine multiple choice questions, respondents produced a median correct response of 1.4.

Do you know the best part of this story?" Choua asked when he finished reading the journal.

"What?" I asked.

"An average of only one correct answer out of six was the best achievement by those doctors who dared to respond to the questionnaire. I wonder what would have happened if the 102 doctors, who didn't respond, had taken the test."

"We are physicians, Choua, not mathematicians," I said in defense of my colleagues.

"Then why do you pretend to be scientists?" Choua snarled. "If you do not know the ABCs of statistics, why do you claim to practice the scientific method? Why do you always quote statistics when you push drugs? If you do not understand the elementary statistics—the tools of science—why do you insult others when they refuse to pump drugs into people based on medical statistics they do not understand? Don't you see what your high priests of drug medicine do? Every time they kill a holistic physician—by yanking his license—they accuse him of being unscientific. Do they ever question the efficacy of their own methods of science?" Choua nearly screamed.

"Take it easy, Choua!" I said sharply. "That's just one study."

"Just one study, eh?" Choua snapped. "Let me read some more. I quote:

...Danish doctors who replied clearly knew little (and the 102 who did not reply may have known less). Are doctors in other countries more knowledgeable? The evidence suggests not.

British Medical Journal 294:856; 1987

The statistics of drug companies bamboozle you every day," Choua continued, "with their cholesterol-lowering drug studies, with their chemotherapy drugs, with their high blood pressure drugs and with their antibiotic studies. It's not just one study. It happens every day, my dear Dr. Gullible," Choua taunted.

"As usual, you exaggerate," I replied testily.

"I exaggerate!" Choua pouted. Then his eyes lit up and he grinned broadly. "I want to tell you something about the magic of medical statistics."

"Magic of medical statistics?" I asked, puzzled.

The Magic of Medical Statistics:
Now You See It, Now You Don't

"There is great magic in medical statistics," Choua announced when he returned the next day, carrying another thick pile of medical journals. "Listen!" he began sifting through a pile of journals. "I'm going to read some magical stuff from these medical journals:

VITAMIN C IS GOOD FOR A COLD;
VITAMIN C IS NOT GOOD FOR A COLD

...there were 26 percent fewer symptomatic days observed in younger vitamin C groups, and 33 percent fewer in older girls on vitamin C...Significantly more children on vitamin C had no sick days observed in the periodic survey.

N Eng J Med 290:6; 1974

Great news for physician-nutritionists!" Choua chirped. "Now they can prescribe vitamin C freely. But, wait! Let's read some more:

Vitamin C does not seem to be an effective prophylactic or therapeutic agent for upper respiratory illness.

N. Eng J Med 295:973; 1976

Does not seem effective! What happened? Why did the *Journal* changed its mind?" Choua frowned.

> **COFFEE IS BAD FOR THE HEART;**
> **COFFEE IS GOOD FOR THE HEART**

These findings support an independent, dose-responsive association of coffee consumption with clinically evident coronary heart disease, which is consistent with a twofold to threefold elevation in risk among heavy coffee drinkers.

N Eng J Med 315:977; 1986

Twofold to threefold elevation in risk! Coffee is not good for the heart. What better proof do we need?" Choua grinned and then grimaces, "But wait! Listen to this:

These findings do not support the hypothesis that coffee or caffeine consumption increases the risk of coronary heart disease or stroke.

N Eng J Med 323:1026; 1990

Coffee, after all, isn't bad for the heart," Choua chuckled.

VITAMIN E IS GOOD FOR THE HEART; VITAMIN E ISN'T GOOD ENOUGH

(There is) evidence of an association between a high intake of vitamin E and a lower risk of coronary artery disease...these findings, together with similar findings in women, support the hypothesis that supplemental vitamin E may reduce the risk of coronary disease.

N Eng J Med 328:1450; 1993

Vitamin E may reduce the risk of coronary disease! Good news for nutritionists!" Choua shook his head excitedly, "Or is it? Let's see if the *Journal* changes its mind again:

> *Public policy recommendations with regard to the use of vitamin E supplements should await the results of additional studies.*

> N Eng J Med 328:1450; 1993.

Should await additional studies! How lucky you didn't jump at *Journal's* and start prescribing vitamin E for your patients. You must wait and see which the *Journal* next." Choua rubbed his temple gravely. "Do you realize you could have prescribed vitamin E in doses larger than the RDA amount if you had believed only part of the *Journal's* story. Tricky stuff! So easy to misread the *Journal's* mind, isn't it?"

DIOXIN IS A CARCINOGEN; DIOXIN SHOULD BE OF NO CONCERN

> *Dioxin is an extremely potent carcinogen and general toxin in rodents, perhaps the most potent yet tested.*

> N Eng J Med 324:260; 1991

Perhaps the most potent carcinogen! The *Journal* is so concerned about our environment," Choua said somberly. "It warns us so clearly against the hazards of dioxins. But then again:

> *This study of mortality among workers with occupational exposure to TCDD (dioxin) does not confirm the high relative risks reported for many cancers in previous studies.*
>
> *N Eng J Med* 324:212; 1991

Risk not confirmed! Oops, false alarm. Dioxins after all do not increase the risk of cancer. Everyone can sleep better now that the *Journal* has declared dioxin harmless!" Choua mocked. "Then again, may be we should wait. Listen to this:

> *Higher incidence in birth defects among Air Force personnel involved with spraying Agent Orange (dioxin) than in control group.*
>
> *Air Force Health Study*
> Project Ranch Hand II USAF School
> of Aerospace Medicine, 1984
> (parenthesis added)

See how some people sensationalize! Such irresponsible behaviour.

Blaming birth defects on dioxins? Awful, isn't it?" Choua groused.

> *Thus, the present exposure of the general population to environmental TCDD and related compounds should not be of concern.*
>
> *J Tox and Env Health* 30:261; 1990

By Zeus, some people have the good sense to squash bad rumors about chemicals!" Choua raised his arms in mock gratitude. "Some people have such irrational fears of chemicals. Thank God there are those who know about the safety of dioxins," Choua raised his arm in mock gratitude.

The Physicians' Health Study is a randomized, double-blind, placebo-controlled trial designed to determine whether low-dose aspirin (325 mg every other day) decreases cardiovascular mortality...There was a 44 percent reduction in the risk of myocardial infarction in the aspirin group.

N Eng J Med 321:129; 1989

Wow! A 44 percent reduction in the risk of heart attack. It doesn't get better than that, does it?" Choua crowed. "Now let's see what else the *Journal* has for us:

...254.8 (heart attacks) per 100,000 per year as compared with 439.7 in the placebo...

N Eng J Med 321: 129; 1989
(Parenthesis added)

The difference between the actual rates of heart attacks between the drug and the placebo groups fizzles down to 1.85 percent. Oops! What happened to this elegant Harvard study?" Choua winked mischievously. "A robust risk reduction of 44 percent turns into a paltry 1.85 percent reduction in rate reduction!"

"Explain it to me, Choua," I asked. "How did you turn the 44 percent reduction in risk reported by the *Journal* to 1.85 per cent reduction in heart attacks?"

"*Magic of medical statistics!* It's really quite simple. 254.8 per 100,000 comes to 2.54 percent, and 439.7 per 100,000 is 4.39 percent," Choua computed and then grinned broadly. The *Journal* ignored the sample size. I didn't. I used the raw data reported by the *Journal* and calculated the *true* mathematical reduction in the rate of heart attacks obtained with the drug. The *Journal* computed the risk reduction by ignoring the total number of people included in the study—such a risk reduction number obviously is not a *true* mathematical number. Do you see the magic of medical statistics now?" Choua made a circle in the air with his thumb and shook his head.

"I still don't understand it," I complained.

"Well, then, I'll try again. Listen to this:

No reduction in mortality from all cardiovascular causes was associated with aspirin.

N Eng J Med 321:129; 1989

No reduction in mortality! See the magic of statistics of N^2D^2 medicine. The 44 percent reduction evaporates into thin air. We're left with *no reduction.*" Choua sneered.

"Choua, you're playing games by taking one excerpt from here and one from there to make your befuddled case," I complained.

"Befuddled case! Okay, if that's befuddled, how about the world-renowned Helsinki study. Listen to this:

In a randomized, double-blind five-year trial, we tested the efficacy of simultaneously elevating serum levels of high-density lipoprotein (HDL) cholesterol and lowering levels of non-HDL cholesterol with gemfibrozil in reducing the risk of coronary artery disease...a reduction of 34.0 percent in the incidence of coronary heart disease...

N Eng J Med 317:1237; 1987

Reduction of 34 percent! Impressive isn't it? The risk of heart disease pummels down with the drug gemfibrozil, commonly known as Lopid!"

"Yeah, but I'm sure you've figured out a way to rub that number down too," I chided Choua.

"I don't need to rub anything down. The *Journal* did that! Here are the raw data before the *Journal* massaged them to build up its 34 percent risk reduction:

There were 45 deaths (rate, 21.9 per 1000) in the gemfibrozil (Lopid) group and 42 deaths (rate, 20.7 per 1000) in the control group. This difference was not statistically significant.

N Eng J Med 317:1241; 1987

See how 34 percent risk reduction fizzles down to nothing—to little over one-tenth of one percent reduction in the *actual rate* reduction. *And the difference favors the placebo control group. Less people taking the placebo pill died than those who took the drug! Amazing, isn't it?"*

"Thirty four percent down to about one-tenth of one percent—and that is in favor of the starch pill? There has to be a catch somewhere, Choua. I simply don't believe *that*," I shook my head in disbelief.

"Magic! My friend, the magic of Olympian N^2D^2 statistics! I quote the *Journal* word for word. There is no catch there. You can calculate the death rate for yourself: 21.9 per 1,000 comes to 2.19 percent and 20.7 per 1,000 to 2.07 percent. And the difference between the two actual rates is 0.14 percent. On second thought, there is a catch," Choua laughed churlishly.

"Wha...t?"

"The *Journal* put the 34 percent reduction in risk—calculated by rates of cardiac end-points on the front page of its article where everyone read it. Then it hid the actual data for deaths on the fifth page where it knew few doctors will ever discover it. You see I don't play games, the *Journal* does that,"

Choua chuckled.

"I don't understand how all that could happen. I mean how could that slip by the *Journal's* editors," I said, perplexed. "*How could they report 34 percent reduction in heart disease with drug when actually more people taking the drug died?*"

"What's there to understand? This is elementary arithmetic."

"If it is so elementary, why didn't the folks at the *Journal* pick up on it?" I persisted.

"Because it would have embarrassed them to report a lower death rate with the placebo than with the drug. Remember, they blew millions of dollars of taxpayers' money to do the study. How do they justify such an expense with such shameful outcome? Now, 34 per cent is a robust number, isn't it? It's not a real number, but who has the courage to go up against the *Journal*?" Choua whimpered.

"Okay, let's assume the authors of the report massaged the data and presented it in a misleading way. Why hasn't anyone spoken out against it so far? Over the years, we have had hundreds of speakers talk about heart disease at our hospital. They almost always refer to the Harvard aspirin and Helsinki Lopid studies. None of them ever made a distinction between risk reduction and rate reduction numbers. Why?"

"That's simple too," Choua laughed. "How many of those speakers were paid by drug makers? No! Was *anyone* of them not paid by drug companies? Why would a drug company spend money to fly its experts around the country teaching them how not to use drugs?"

"You're such a cynic," I admonished him.

"I'm a cynic?" Choua frowned. "Don't you see there were more deaths in the Lopid group than in the placebo group in this study?" Choua said with a smirk.

"But they had to do the study to find that number, didn't

they?" I offered the usual defense for such studies.

"Chickensh..." Choua stopped in midsentence.

"Don't chickensh...me, Choua," I said angrily. "How else do you evaluate the efficacy of drugs."

"The problem is not in doing such drug studies," Choua snapped. "The problem is truth in reporting the data—honesty in presenting the real data the way they emerge. No matter which they looked at the data," Choua chirped, "the true numbers for the drug are dismal. So they doctored the data, inconspicuously putting the higher death rate with the drug in the middle of the article and spashing the spurious 34 percent risk reduction on the front page—the way tabloids do it. They knew they could never promote the drug with the real data. Who would buy that silly number? That's the blunt truth about the Prince Chaullahs of N^2D^2 medicine. It's not a question of science at all. It's about selling drugs. It's about drug dollars, Dr. Gullible," Choua angrily threw the *Journal* down.

"There has to be an explanation for that, Choua. Give me the journal, and I'll read those quotes myself," I picked up the copy of the *Journal* and read.

The cumulative rate of cardiac end points at five years was 27.3 per 1,000 in the gemfibrozil group and 41.4 per 1,000 in the placebo group—a reduction of 34.0 percent in the incidence of coronary heart disease...

N Eng J Med 317:1237; 1987

Aha! Caught you, didn't I?" I said excitedly. "You used an incomplete quote. The *Journal* is right! The difference between 41.4 percent and 27.3 percent does come to 34 percent. I knew the *New England Journal of Medicine could never make such a mistake.* You distorted the case by selective quotes. The *Journal* is after all right! *There was a reduction in the incidence of coronary artery disease.* Shame on you!" I felt good about my reprimand. It's not often that I catch Choua with such glaring inaccuracy.

"Oh God! You are so thick-headed," Choua spoke sternly, then shook his head in disgust.

We looked at each other in silence. I was both irritated and baffled by his insult—baffled because on the one hand the *Journal* was so clearly right and on the other Choua was so adamant about ridiculing the *Journal* and, now, rediculing me. "What am I missing?" I wondered. Choua is not given to frivolous criticism to matters that he doesn't know well. That added to my confusion. After several moments he opened his mouth to say something, but seemingly changed his mind, and walked to the window instead. He looked out and was lost in his thoughts. I looked at the back of his head, as I had many times before, wondering what unexpected turns Choua's argument would take.

"Aren't you going to explain yourself?" I asked after a while.

"What's there to explain," Choua spoke softly this time, without turning to look at me. "Sick people go to their physicians so they can feel better, have their maladies treated, become healthy and live longer. Drug doctors doing that study fed 2,051 men a drug for a mean period of over five years. They gave placebo pills to another 2030 men. At the end of the study, more people died in the drug group than in the placebo group. More than 11 percent of the men taking the drug suffered 'moderate to severe upper gastrointestinal symptoms.' The paper withholds raw data concerning other adverse effects of the drug, so we don't know how many patients were hurt that way. About one-third of the men in the drug group dropped out—presumably they recognized the sheer stupidity of the study. Despite all that, the *Journal* had the gall to talk about a 34 percent reduction in cardiac end points.

"Tell me, do people go to their physicians so they can live longer in good health?" Choua continued. "Or do they go so that their doctors can write landmark papers about the reduction of their blessed end points while the patients get sick with drug toxicity and die sooner than the control group who had the good fortune to be in the group given the placebo pills?" Choua asked, brimming with sarcasm.

"I...I don't...I mean, I don't..." I stammered in my response.

"Suppose, a Chinese immigrant child dies in New York city," Choua turned sharply to face me, as he interrupted my flustered reply to his question.

THE DECEPTION IN RISK REDUCTION

"Suppose the cause of the death is suspected to be a toxin," Choua continued.

"What toxin?" I asked.

"Next year two Chinese children die in New York city of similar illness," Choua ignored my question. "The pediatricians are puzzled by the two cases. Then someone speculates that the children were poisoned by a fungal toxin brought into the city as a contaminant of a Chinese herb. The story leaks out that two

Chinese children have died of an fungal toxin, a toxin that was brought into the country by Chinese importers. There is concern that other children in the city may also be affected by that unknown toxin. Many parents and politicians get involved. The media feeds the frenzy. Pretty soon, someone calls for an immediate end to importation of all Chinese herbs to New York city. The folks at a major New York newspaper also get involved and run a front-page story titled:

Risk of Death in Chinese Children from a Fungal Toxin Increases 100 Percent in New York City.

The newspaper story strengthens the case for banning the entry of all Chinese herbs into the city. When criticized for its outrageous story, the newspaper uses the risk calculation method, commonly used by the *New England Journal of Medicine,* to defend its abominable position: One child died of a suspected fungal toxin the first year; two died the following year. That increases the risk of death from the malady 100 percent. Right?" Choua asked seriously.

"Well, purely on a statistical basis, that would be the case, but..."

"But it is too stupid to imagine," Choua interrupted me again. "Suppose there are 300,000 Chinese children in New York city. One in 300,000 gives us the rate of chemical injury of 0.0003 percent; two in 300,000 children gives a rate of 0.0006 percent, and the difference between the two rates comes to 0.0003 percent—that is, of course, one in 300,000 children. See how you can distort the data. People are amuse when cheap tabloids create such thrills. It would be different if a major New York paper ran the story. And yet, the *New England Journal of Medicine* gets away with such distortions of medical data regularly and with impunity. Why?"

"Why?" I asked.

"Because the *Journal* is published with drug ad money. Just pick any issue and count the ad pages."

"You're a rascal!" I chided Choua.

"More magic in medical statistics!" Choua smirked, as he picked an other journal and read:

1.6 PERCENT
IS STATISTICALLY SIGNIFICANT;
44 PERCENT
IS NOT STATISTICALLY SIGNIFICANT

The cholestyramine group experienced a 19% reduction in risk of the primary end point (heart disease events)...The benefits that could be expected from cholestyramine are considerable.

Journal of American Medical Association 251:360; 1984 (Parenthesis added)

Nineteen percent reduction in risk of primary end point!" Choua beamed.

"Let's see how you give it your Choua treatment," I said, amused.

"Not difficult at all!" Choua laughed. "We'll read some more from the same paper:

> *The cumulative seven-year incidence of the primary end point was 7% in the cholestyramine group vs 8.6% in the placebo group.*
>
> *Journal of American Medical Association*
> 251:360; 1984

Do you see the magic in medical statistics now?" Choua looked up from the *Journal*. "A *meager 1.6 perecent decrease* after a 7 to 10 year drug therapy is blown up to a *contrived number of 19 percent risk reduction*. And, that's not where the magic ends in this elegant report. Watch the flip side of this coin:

> *A few more hospitalized participants in the cholestyramine group had, as their main diagnosis, gallstones (16 vs 11) and more cholestyramine-treated participants had an operation involving the gallbladder (36 vs 25), but the differences were not significant.*

Fascinating! A dismal 1.6 percent reduction in the heart disease is considered highly significant, but a 44 percent increase in drug toxicity requiring surgery is dismissed as insignificant?"

"Why doesn't anyone expose such fallacies?"

"Why would drug makers pay a doctor to expose fallacies in drug statistics?"

"Okay, drug makers have no reason to do so. But, why don't other doctors do so?"

"Because doctors are ignorant about statistics! Haven't we established that? I mean hasn't the *British Medical Journal* established that?" Choua jeered.

"That is sad!"

"The magic continues. These drug researchers first drugged thousands of innocent, unsuspecting people. Many of them developed drug toxicities, and several required surgery. But the drug researchers promptly dismissed the toxic effects of the drugs, proclaiming that *"The benefits that could be expected from cholestyramine are considerable."* Now, readers can be expected to be impressed with the *Journal's* enthusiasm. Right?"

"Not really."

"How many of the readers of the *Journal* have the courage to ask the simple question: Since heart attacks are caused by stress and many other factors, how can anyone say whether that 1.6 percent reduction was actually due to the use of the drug or whether it was caused by lifestyle changes that people involved in such studies usually make?"

Choua finished reading the journal excerpts, his rage spent. He shook his head and walked over to the window, as if to escape the misery of the statistics that he inflicted upon himself. I looked at him in silence for some minutes and said,

"Science moves like that, Choua. By trial and error, it is self-correcting as it goes along."

"Science, my foot!" Choua turned to face me directly and erupted. "It has nothing to with science. Don't you see that?"

"How else does science in medicine advance?" I asked calmly.

"Get it through your thick head for once, for God's sake," he scowled. "It's not about science. It's about drugs. It's about drug money. Do you think the disease doctors of drug medicine, who wrote that report, didn't know the truth?" Choua was livid now.

"What proof do you have that the authors of the study knew all that?" I asked hesitantly.

"Listen to this, Mr. Drug Attorney," Choua pouted as he leaped to the pile of journals on the floor and snatched one of them. He excitedly shuffled through the journal and read:

...it is acknowledged that it is unlikely that a conclusive study of dietary-induced cholesterol lowering for the prevention of CHD can be designed or implemented.

Journal of American Medical Association
251:360; 1984

This is a direct quote from the same report of the *Journal of American Medical Association* that preaches its readers to push toxic drugs for cholesterol. Don't you see it?"

"Are you saying researchers knew their studies couldn't be conclusive?"

"I'm not saying anything. The *Journal* said that. Before

those drug doctors administered drugs to conduct that *scientific* study, they acknowledged that a conclusive study for the prevention of heart disease could not be designed. They were not stupid about the real issues. More heart attacks are caused by anger and stress than by clogged arteries. You should know that. How many times have you seen open, unclogged coronary arteries at autopsy in people who died of heart attacks?" Choua asked acidly.

"It happens!" I conceded. "To tell the truth, the majority of patients who reach the autopsy table within six hours of dying of heart attacks do not show blood clots in the coronary arteries."

"The *Journal* study had nothing to do with science. Those were N^2D^2 dollars at their best—programming the N^2D^2 doctors with nonsensical statistics to push their drugs. Don't you see it?"

Lies, Damned Lies and Statistics

"Mark Twain had the right idea. He saw through statistics." Choua began again.

"He was a humorous man, wasn't he?" I said.

"Humorous and perceptive. He would have seen through your cholesterol lies if he had been alive."

"My cholesterol lies?" I felt a twinge in my neck.

"Yes, lies with which drug companies program drug doctors to push drugs on their unsuspecting patients," Choua snarled.

"Oh, now you're being Choua! Vintage Choua! How do drug companies do all that?" I prodded.

"Take the example of cholesterol-lowering drugs! The drug makers fund the cholesterol studies and hire disease doctors to conduct them. Then, the cholesterol cats program their hired guns to extol the virtues of their drugs with bloated..."

"What are cholesterol cats?" I interrupted.

"Bloated numbers and distorted statistics!" Choua leered, not answering my question. "And doctors who prescribe the drugs simply do not understand the statistics."

"What are cholesterol cats, and how do they distort numbers?" I persisted.

"The cats! The money men of medicine! The masters of statistical lies. They program their hired guns to hide the real data—the numbers that indicate the dismally poor efficacy of the drug and use numbers that give a false indication of the drug's effectiveness of the drug."

"Can't you talk plainly for once, Choua?" I asked, bewildered.

"It's really quite simple," Choua grinned. The data showing the real reduction in the *rate* of heart attacks is hidden while they brag about bloated numbers of *risk* reduction."

"Explain, Choua, explain!" I complained.

"Risk factor is not a true mathematical number and makes the cholesterol story look good," Choua continued, ignoring my interruption. "The incidence rates—or ratios, if you prefer—are true mathematical numbers that expose the fraud in this story."

"How do they make the risk factor number look good when the real rate number isn't?"

"Simple! Very simple!" Choua grinned broadly. "Suppose there were 1,000 people over 65 years old in a city. One year, the winter was mild and ten people died of heart attacks. The following year, it was a bitter cold winter. The cold weather caused pneumonia in many people, and 20 persons died of heart attacks that were brought on by the added stress of pneumonia. Now, there are three ways you can play with these data. First, you can say that very cold weather increased the risk of death from heart attack by 100 percent—from 10 deaths during the mild-winter year to 20 deaths during the following bitterly cold winter year. Right?"

"Right!" I agreed.

"The second way you can play with these data is to say that the risk of death from heart attacks could be reduced by 50 percent if people were well protected from bitter cold—20 down to 10 deaths. Right?" Choua smiled impishly.

"Right! Go on, Choua." I acknowledged.

"The third way of reporting these data would be a truthful statement saying that the rate of heart attack could be reduced by one percent if people were well protected from bitter cold—20 deaths in 1,000 people gives us a death rate of two percent, while ten deaths produce a death rate of one percent. Right?" Choua suddenly turned solemn.

"Right." I confessed. "I know statistics can be manipulated to support any conclusion. But how did cholesterol cats convince physicians that the use of the cholesterol-lowering drugs could save patients from heart attack?"

"The risk factor for heart attack is not a real number because it does not take into account the total population studied," Choua began to elaborate the concept. "Ten heart attacks could occur in one thousand people or in one million. Yet the risk factor does not distinguish between the two numbers. The incidence rate of heart attack, by contrast, is a true number. For example, ten in one thousand people means one out of hundred, or one percent. Ten in one million would give us a ratio of one in one hundred thousand. That's simple, right!"

"Right! That's simple enough," I agreed.

"Now let's take the case of the relationship between the blood cholesterol number and heart attacks. Suppose, there are one thousand people with blood cholesterol levels of 280 milligram per deciliter (mg/dl) and 20 of them have a heart attack one year. Now we lower the cholesterol level to 220 mg/dl with our *wondrous* cholesterol-lowering drugs. The next year, ten people suffer heart attacks. These numbers are exactly the same as those we used to discuss the relationship between cold weather and heart attack. The risk reduction for heart attacks in this example would be one hundred or fifty percent, depending on what type of game we decided to play. Right?" Choua asked with a smile.

"Right!" I agreed.

"Now both of those numbers are quite impressive. Agreed?"

"Yes!"

"Now let's look at the *true* reduction in the *true* rate of heart attacks—the real benefit that may be attributed to cholesterol drugs. Again, it comes to a mere one percent—quite unimpressive by any criteria, right!"

"Right!"

"Now, do you see the problem?" Choua chuckled.

"There are lies, damned lies and statistics! Isn't that what Mark Twain said about statistics?" I asked.

"Something like that," Choua replied. "Let's see what damned lies and statistics can do. Who wouldn't be scared into accepting cholesterol drugs for decades when told they reduce the risk of heart attack by fifty percent? On the other hand, who would agree to take drugs for decades—with all the hazards of drug toxicity—just to reduce the incidence rate of heart attack by less than one percent?"

"Especially when most heart attacks appear to be precipitated by stress anyway," I repeated what I said earlier.

"Quite right!" Choua went on. "Now do you see the way cholesterol cats program their N^2D^2 researchers to churn out the numbers that they want?"

"Why don't physicians see through all this?"

"Physicians are busy caring for the sick. They trust the leaders in cholesterol research to provide guidance. The problem is that the leaders in cholesterol research are funded by cholesterol fat cats who program them to massage the data, and report it in ways that grossly exaggerate the potential benefit of drugs. This keeps the true-to-life incidence of heart attacks hidden, and conceals how ineffective cholesterol-lowering drugs really are."   "That's hard to accept," I ignored the insolence in choua's comments.

"The hired guns of the cholesterol cats use the risk-reduction values of 17%, 34% and 44% for the Lipid Research Clinics, the Helsinki and the Physician's Aspirin studies respectively. The actual numbers for rates of incidence reductions in these three studies were 1.16%, 1.30% and 0.93% respectively. Now do you see the problem?"

"But, Choua, are those numbers really correct?" I expressed my doubt. "I mean if those numbers are true, why didn't anyone expose the tricks of the cholesterol cats?"

"There is no problem with those numbers," Choua shot back. "Anyone can check the references."*

"I can't believe that no one challenged such blatant distortions, if indeed those were distortions," I expressed doubt again.

"Some do," Choua smiled. "But you know how that is. The challenges get buried in the fine print because the cholesterol cats have the money to keep distorted data flashed on the screens in the conference rooms of the nation's hospitals. Here, I'll read something interesting:

In the Helsinki Heart Study...no statistically significant difference in overall mortality was noted. The cholesterol-lowering trial that has been most widely cited is the Lipid Research Clinics-Coronary Primary Prevention Trial (LRC-CPPT), in which patients were treated with cholestyramine or placebo. The difference between the study groups in overall mortality was negligible.

N Eng J Med 323:946; 1990

No statistically significant difference in overall mortality! How

---

Journal of American Medical Association 352: 351; 1984; *New England Journal of Medicine* 317: 1237, 1987; and 321: 129; 1989.

many doctors do you think ever think of such data? How often do you think they are reminded of such data by the hired guns of cholesterol fat cats?" Choua snarled.

"I agree there is a problem when all the cholesterol speakers are paid by drug makers," I conceded.

"The Lipid Research Clinics study was published in 1984. Remember this is the same study I quoted earlier that pronounced *'The benefits that could be expected from cholestyramine are considerable.'* The Helsinki Heart Study was published in 1987. It took some folks three years to point out the distortion. How far do you think they went with it? Tell me, what subjects are discussed most frequently by the visiting speakers at your hospital?"

"Cholesterol, heart disease, hypertension, arthritis..."

"Why is that so?" Choua interrupted.

"Because funding by drug makers is most readily available for those subjects?" I ventured a guess.

"The cholesterol speakers robotically regurgitate the bloated risk-reduction data. How often have you seen anyone in an audience expose their ignorance—or worse, exhibit deliberate deceit? The cholesterol fat cats keep getting fatter. There are many other similarly absurd numbers that cholesterol cats use to program their hired guns—to throw around and to deceive the uninformed."

"For example?"

"Well, one commonly made statement by cholesterol doctors is that a one per cent difference in serum cholesterol is associated with a 2.6 per cent difference in the risk of heart disease. There were other deceptions in the cholesterol story."

"Why doesn't anyone catch such glaring errors? Why doesn't anyone write articles exposing the blatant deception in such statistics?"

"You're so gullible! Cholesterol cats don't let something

like that be published in their journals. Such articles are promptly rejected."

"That's not true," I challenged him. "The *British Medical Journal* had published a paper against the cholesterol story."

"What did it say?" he asked.

"It documented a systematic bias in the cholesterol literature. The studies that supported the prevailing cholesterol story were included in the citations six times as frequently as those that opposed it," I explained.

"So, I stand corrected," Choua jeered. "How did that report escape the guardian angels of cholesterol drugs?"

"Perhaps it will change."

"Science has not failed medicine, the Prince Challahs of N²D² medicine have failed science."

PUNISHING 99 TO FAVOR ONE

"You trivialize the cholesterol issue and you demonize cholesterol-lowering drugs," I chastised Choua. "You *do* know that government and medical groups have set national goals to reduce the blood cholesterol levels and prevent heart disease, don't you? And those goals are based on the studies you cite."

"Yeah! Yeah!," Choua drawled belligerently. "I also know who sets those national goals—the same N²D² docs whose cholesterol research is funded by drug makers."

"High blood cholesterol level is a risk factor, your preachy sermons against risk reduction numbers notwithstanding," I said, annoyed by his recalcitrance. "If the population has elevated cholesterol level, then the use of risk factor is valid. Isn't it?"

"No, it isn't," Choua said impatiently.

"One of the two people who had a heart attack in your example was saved by lowering his blood cholesterol level. That's worth it, isn't it," I asked.

"It depends upon how you look at it," Choua answered indifferently. "You think of one person who will benefit from drugs and I think of the remaining 99, whose fat metabolism will be disrupted by the drugs for decades, who will develop chronic fatigue, myopathy, liver injury and bone marrow suppression. You don't realize the mischief in your risk reduction numbers, do you?"

"What mischief?" I asked, uncertain of his point.

"The mischief of make-believe numbers that reduce the risk of heart disease for one or two percent while you drug or operate on the innocent 98 or 99 percent who do not use your great medical advances. Why not offer safe nutritional therapies to all and teach them self-regulation for reducing stress?"

GUT-TWISTING SURGERY
FOR LOWERING CHOLESTEROL

"Here is another very interesting intem," Choua resumed.

The Program on the Surgical Control of Hyperlipidemia (POSCH), a randomized clinical trial, was designed to test whether

> *cholesterol-lowering induced by the partial*
> *ileal bypass operation would favorably*
> *affect overall mortality or morbidity due to*
> *coronary heart disease...These results*
> *provide strong evidence supporting the*
> *beneficial effects of lipid modification in*
> *the reduction of atherosclerosis*
> *progression.*

N Eng J Med 323:946; 1990

Beneficial effects! For whom? The surgeons who made out well with fees or the poor patients who get their guts twisted with ileal bypass operation?" Choua groused.

"Hold it!" I nearly screamed at Choua. "That's outrageous! In that study, they treated patients who survived a first heart attack. They wanted to investigate exactly what they described: Whether or not fatal outcomes from heart attacks could be favorably influenced by modifying the lipid profile of patients with surgery. Choua, I don't think you have any idea how science in medicine progresses. They tested surgical approach for patients with a potentially fatal disease. All research is inescapably risky and such research probably carries greater risks. But, the whole purpose of research is to test new ideas and benefit millions of people when research proves the clinical efficacy of a surgical procedure. As for surgical fees, many of those surgeons probably didn't get a penny for performing the operation. You talk like a rabid man. No one is immune to your vituperation, and the pale of your venom has no bottom," I severely scolded Choua.

Choua seemed shaken by my sudden outburst. He stood still for several moments, looking at the floor to evade my angry eyes. Then he slowly moved back from my desk toward the window. "Go get lost in your clouds," I wanted to scream but didn't.

"Did the operation work?" Choua asked calmly after a while.

"Yes! Isn't that what the paper said?" I shot back. "Didn't they write about strong evidence supporting the beneficial effects?"

"Would you let anyone bypass your gut if you had a heart attack?" Choua asked timidly.

"Yes! No!" I flustered, then quickly recovered. "Well, no, I wouldn't."

"I didn't think you would," Choua added gravely.

"But, you miss the whole point of the study, Choua," I spoke in a conciliatory tone. "How would anyone know whether or not bowel surgery can prevent heart disease until someone conducts such a study?"

" "I'll read you some more," Choua's face lit up a bit. "Listen to this:

Overall mortality and mortality due to coronary heart disease were reduced but not significantly so (deaths overall control vs. surgery, 62 vs. 49.

N Eng J Med 323:946; 1990

Let me compute some rate numbers for you," Choua offered. "There were 417 patients in the control group and 421 in the surgery group. So the difference in the rate of heart attack comes to 3 percent. A far cry from their pronouncement of *strong evidence supporting the beneficial effects!"*

"At least there was some difference," I tried to save a lost cause.

"Three percent difference at what cost!" Choua continued. "I'll read some more:

At 1,5,7 and 10 years of follow-up, 5.3, 16.4, 25.1 and 31.5 percent of the control-group patients were taking at least one cholesterol-lowering medication. In the surgery group, the corresponding figures were 0.5, 3.0, 6.2 and 3.7 percent... Twenty-three patients underwent reversal of the bypass because of diarrhea...

N Eng J Med 323:946; 1990

That's the problem with this study. They compared apples and oranges—one group with twisted guts and the other drugged for cholesterol. Twenty-three patients had to have their guts untwisted. Interesting! Isn't it?" Choua smiled.

"Still, the surgery has some benefit," I struggled for an answer.

"Of the 421 patients assigned to surgery in that study, 22 refused the operation. I wonder what draconian measures they took to coerce the remaining 401 persons to have their guts twisted. What can be more irrational than bypassing the gut to prevent heart disease? Don't you see the utter stupidity of it? You write about the battered bowel ecosystem and about the gut lining being the true interface between man and his environment. What do you think bypassing the bowel does to its delicate ecosystem? Isn't the bowel the seat of digestive-absorptive functions that determine the long-term health of the individual? You write about the bowel being the arena where all immune battles are fought—and won and lost! About the bowel being the shield that protects the liver! About the integrity of the bowel ecosystem being the primary defense of man against degenerative disease! Will you explain to me how anyone in his right mind could ever dream up gut-twisting surgery to prevent degenerative disease in the heart?" Choua gored.

"You can't help yourself, Choua," I said, exasperated.

"There was something else quite neat about this report that I don't think you picked up on." Choua grinned.

"What?" I asked, a trifle put off.

"The authors deftly sidestepped the embarrassment of their conclusions. Note that they didn't make an outright recommendation that patients who suffer heart attacks should have bowel-twisting surgery. They seem to have come to their senses—a bit lit late for the unfortunate 421 who were used as guinea pigs—and recognized the sheer stupidity of twisting the bowel for a metabolic problem. Their conclusion addressed the beneficial effects of lipid modification, omitting any mention of bowel bypass surgery. *Science in medicine! Huh!*" Choua waved one hand contemptuously and walked out.

FAVORING 100 TO FAVOR ONE

"Why do you have to punish 99 to favor one when you can favor all one hundred?" Choua asked when he returned the next day.

"We don't want to punish anyone! Would you get this through your head for once?" I felt some of yesterday's bitterness return.

"Teach all 100 meditation—some of your limbic stuff—and tell them about right choices in the kitchen. Something about limbic exercise! And tell them EDTA chelation clears plaques in the heart arteries, improves collateral circulation, prevents premature aging of heart cell enzymes, reduces body burden of toxic metals, and provides a strong antioxidant defense against oxidative stress. If people did all that, then no one has to have his gut twisted or liver injured by drugs. No one *has* to live with a chemical blockade of his physiologic processes by drugs. You know, people intuitively know that chemical drugs are not good for them even, when if do not know all the chemistry that you do. Isn't that true?"

"You live in a world of your own, Choua," I said testily. "You don't face the clinical problems we face—the problems of noncompliance, of patients wanting quick fixes, of hearts that won't quit palpitating, of sugar roller coasters that won't go away, of stress, anxiety and panic attacks! Everything is black and white to you. Real life is not that simple!"

"So, what's the answer?" Choua growled. "Drug 'em! Twist their guts! Violate their heart arteries! The truth...you know what the truth..."

"No, no! I don't want to know what the truth is," I yelled. Choua looked sternly at me , then briskly walked out.

ALICE IN WONDERLAND

"Alice in Wonderland! Isn't it?" Choua asked contemptuously as he thumbed through my pile of journals the next morning.

"Yeah! But I'm not ready for another tirade," I replied tersely.

"There are a lot of Prince Chaullahs on the payrolls of drug makers," Choua ignored the irritation in my voice. "They thrive on blinded studies. Then their payers massage the data to present negative data on drug efficacy as significant and positive data on drug toxicities as insignificant. Insignificant for whom? The makers of the drugs or the victims of drug toxicity?"

"You exaggerate, Choua." I tried to reason with him.

"All in the name of science!" Choua ignored my comment. "People outside medicine would scoff at such pieces of medical literature—or shall I call it medical *illiterature*. If only they could see through the lies of drug makers and the drug doctors on their payrolls."

"What's eating you today?" I asked.

"No one outside medicine would believe the works of medicine's Prince Chaullahs, the deception of their drug masters! Why would they? They trust their doctors. Little do they realize that their doctors simply cannot tell true research from pseudo research. They do not know how to interpret raw data correctly, so they simply accept the conclusions drawn by the drug masters," Choua pressed on, "But the drug makers have the money for buying TV time to peddle their chemicals—and to hire their guns in white coats to extol the virtues of their wonder drugs. Who has..."

"We need drugs, Choua. We need good drugs!" I broke in.

"Who has the courage to go up against all that?" Choua brushed aside my objection. "The handful of physicians who see through their clever schemes are no match for them. They can always get the drug doctors on state licensing boards to threaten—and, when deemed necessary—revoke their licenses to teach expensive lessons to them and others with similar antidrug, antisurgery notions."

The Sacred Deception

"Who dreamed up the double-blind cross-over method for drug research?" Choua asked me one day.

"I don't know, but it probably was someone at some drug company," I replied.

"Why is it called double-blind?"

"Because both the patient and the physician are blinded to the use of placebo and the drug given at different times."

"Why do they blind the sick?"

"So that the patient does not know whether he is taking a drug or a placebo starch pill."

"Why is that important?"

"For obvious reasons! So that the drug researcher can tell whether there is any difference between the effects of the drug and the placebo."

"Huh! Why do they blind the doctor?"

"So that the physician doesn't know whether the patient is taking the drug or the placebo."

"Why should that be important?"

"So that the physician cannot influence the outcome of the study."

"So you think that both the patient and the physician must be excluded from the process."

"Yes, to assure objectivity in results."

"Objectivity!" Choua uttered the word slowly, as if mulling over its meaning. "Why do they do the cross-over step?" he continued.

"For additional proof. To add further strength to the

argument for drug efficacy obtained with the first step. It is to
see if reversing the order of administration of the placebo and the
drug further validates the results of the first part of the test
protocol."

"How long has the double-blind cross-over method been
used?"

"I'm not sure. Maybe since the early part of this century."

"How many drugs have been tested with this method?"

"I don't know the exact number, but..."

"But it must be in the thousands, right?" Choua
interrupted me. "Probably more. The FDA has been using this
method for approving drugs for decades. So we can conclude that
the methods have been well-tested and proven to be completely
objective and reliable. Do you agree?"

"Yes!" I replied.

"And one can say with complete confidence that..."

Choua didn't complete his sentence. He scratched his ear,
moved closer to the window, and looked out. It is not uncommon
for Choua to interrupt himself in mid-sentence like that. I looked
at the back of his head and kept quiet, anticipating Choua's return
to the subject. He always does so, though sometimes it is after
long periods of silence. Some minutes passed. Choua seemed lost
somewhere in the distant horizon. I returned to my microscope.

"Does it work?" Choua muttered, barely loud enough for
me to hear.

"What?" I looked up from my microscope.

"The double-blind cross-over! Does it work?"

"Of course, it does! Everyone knows that. That's
elementary stuff, Choua. Why do you ask?"

"Because it *cannot*!" Choua turned sharply, his eyes
intense and chilling.

I was startled. By now, I am used to Choua's contrarian pronouncements. He has a way of distorting things—or, more accurately, of looking at things through the squint of his mind that distorts what he sees. I am usually not unnerved by his iconoclastic tirades. Rather, I have come to expect such things from him—and, in general, I am amused by them. Notwithstanding, there he stood categorically rejecting double-blind cross-over—the gold standard in drug research, clearly one of the most zealously guarded precepts of American medicine.

"Now, how did you arrive at such a conclusion?" I asked, recovering.

"The double-blind cross-over model is a pious falsehood. It is the sacred deception of drug medicine," he growled.

"Wow! You are taking on the whole world, aren't you?" I tried to humor him.

"It is a deception perpetrated by the drug industry in collusion with the drug doctors on their payroll. And together they buy FDA approval," Choua continued angrily.

"Strong words, Choua," I tried to soften him. "Don't you think that is going too far? I mean, don't you think that stretches credibility?"

"A deception is a deception," he replied acidly. "It matters little how many people participate in this fraud. It matters little how prestigious are the institutions who hide behind this phony cloak of respectability. It matters little how much money there is to perpetuate this deception." Choua's anger surged with each sentence.

"You have your..."

"The FDA doesn't allow anyone to make any healthful claims for nutrients and herbs that have stood the test of time. Yet those drugs are peddled freely on TV under the cloak of scientific validity. How do they prove such validity except with that sacred double-blind cross-over deception?"

"Why do you call it a sacred deception?"

"Because it is one of the two deities of drug medicine—one of its two most sacred cows." Choua's face brightened a little for the first time.

"What's the other?" I suppressed a smile.

"The RDA deity. Drug medicine sacrifices hundreds of millions of people every year on the altar of its two deities," Choua smiled back. "The RDA deity prohibits doctors from using nutrients to reverse chronic diseases, and the double-blind cross-over deity promotes the use of toxic drugs." Choua stretched his back.

FIRST,
THE ONLY WAY DOUBLE-BLIND CROSS-OVER CAN WORK IS IF THE PATIENT IS A ROBOT

"Do you realize the only way your *blessed* double-blind cross-over can work is if the patient has neither any curiosity nor any intellect—if he is a robot," Choua continued.

"How is that?" I suppressed a laugh.

"Why do you use drugs?"

"For their chemical effects."

"Aha! So drugs have chemical effects," Choua chirped cheerily.

"Of course they do. Have you lost your mind, Choua? What kind of a question is that?"

"Well, if drugs have any chemical effects, won't those effects be felt by the patient—sooner or later?"

"Yes, so?"

"So, Mr. Objectivity, if the patient feels any of the chemical effects of the drug, wouldn't he know he is taking a chemical? Wouldn't the drug effects reveal to him that he is taking a drug?"

"But wouldn't the placebo effect make him feel as if he were taking some drug?" I countered.

"Do starch pills really have any chemical effects?" Choua gave me a dig. "The deception of the placebo might throw him off for a few days, but that's about it."

"Well..."

"Well, what? How can anyone take a chemical week after week—month after month—feel its chemical effects and not wonder about what he is putting into his body? Don't you see the utter stupidity of anyone thinking that a person can be blinded to the chemical effects of a drug that he *himself* senses?"

"It's not that simple," I argued. "Almost all studies show significant placebo effects. We need to separate the effects of the placebo from those of the drug," I explained.

"Aha! Starch pills have effects, do they? If that is really true, Mr. Objectivity, why don't you simply treat diseases with placebo starch pills? Certainly starch is much cheaper than drugs and is not toxic."

"Your mind is warped. You distort everything," I rebuked him.

"Don't you worry about my warped mind! I asked you a simple question. If the placebo starch pill really has sufficient healing power, why don't you dispense starch pills for all diseases? I think it is a valid question," Choua chuckled.

"You don't understand. Any pill can have a placebo effect—the effect of a positive suggestion and a possible healing image. The placebo effect must be separated from the specific chemical effects of drugs. That's the key element—that is the whole point of using a controlled study with a placebo."

"So, what you're really saying is that the placebo effect soon wears out while the chemical effects of the drug do not. Is that it?" Choua was relentless.

"Yes," I confessed.

"What you're really saying—though you don't seem to understand it—is that the patient cannot tell the difference between the temporary effects of the placebo and the permanent effects of the drug, while the drug company can."

"No! Yes, but it's not that..."

"It's not that simple!" Choua completed my sentence mockingly. "Do you know what I find most funny about you doctors?"

"What?" I asked, embarrassed by my incoherence.

"You doctors cannot accept simple things. I guess it is because you cannot maintain your aura of prescient status with simple things. You must complicate things so that you can keep the sick ignorant about the real issues. Let's do a simple test."

"What?" I sighed.

"Let's go searching for a person who participated in a double-blind cross-over study and who couldn't tell the difference between the effects of suggestibility with the placebo and the chemical effects of the drug. Maybe, just maybe, we'll find one single such individual who will make a liar out of me and will save the day for your blessed double-blind cross-over. Shall we?" Choua laughed out loud. "Here, let me read you something:

...were enrolled in a double-blind, placebo-controlled, randomized study comparing the effects of an exercise regimen, exercise plus dietary calcium supplementation, and exercise plus continuous replacement of estrogen and progesterone...four (10 percent) women in the (hormone) group withdrew because of this (breast) symptom.

N Eng J Med 325:1193; 1991
(parenthesis added)

So much for the double-blinded, placebo-controlled model! Ten percent of the women bailed out because of symptoms. Still, the authors of the study kept the facade of double-blind. How else do you publish studies?" Choua chuckled.

**SECOND,
THE ONLY WAY DOUBLE-BLIND CROSS-OVER
CAN WORK IS IF THE DOCTOR IS A ROBOT**

"Do you realize the only way double-blind cross-over can work," Choua continued, "is if the doctor administering the drug has neither any curiosity nor any intellect—if he is a robot."

"Because if the drug has any chemical effects, it will

be..."

"Don't these doctors who agree to be blinded feel stupid about maintaining this facade?" Choua didn't let me finish.

"It's not stupid to try to be objective," I repeated my defense.

"There is nothing wrong with being objective, Mr. Objectivity," Choua ridiculed me again. "What's wrong here is the facade of objectivity. What's wrong is open deception. How can a doctor give a drug for weeks and months and not have enough curiosity or intelligence to look for the chemical effects of the drug in his patient? Does that seem logical to you? I thought the thing that they insist on most in medical schools is that students learn to observe their patients' clinical states and listen to them carefully. Doesn't that hold anymore?"

"Yes, yes!" I groaned.

"So why wouldn't a doctor fail to see the obvious?" Choua was unrelenting.

"I give up. Leave me alone, Choua," I said in exasperation.

Choua studied my face for a few moments and broke out laughing. "It's all in fun and games, isn't it? Here, listen to this:

Altogether 52 percent of the 30 women who had not undergone a hysterectomy in the exercise-estrogen group had vaginal bleeding at some point during the study.

N Eng J Med 325:1193; 1991

Interesting! Isn't it? The Prince Chaullahs who conducted the study were really blind, weren't they? I mean the researchers maintained the facade of double-blind even when more than half of the postmenopausal women in the blinded study reported that they had vaginal bleeding. Funny stuff!"

"You do have a point, Choua," I conceded.

THIRD,
THE ONLY WAY DOUBLE-BLIND CROSS-OVER CAN WORK IS IF THE DRUG DOES NOT CHANGE LABORATORY TEST RESULTS

"Do drug doctors order laboratory tests for their patients entered in their double-blind cross-over studies?" Choua asked.

"Yes," I responded.

"Why?"

"To monitor the drug use."

"Are you telling me that drugs affect the laboratory test results?"

"Yes, they do."

"How does that happen?"

"Don't ask me silly questions," I whined.

"I'm so sorry. I didn't mean to offend you. Does the placebo starch pill affect laboratory test results?"

"I don't know!" I answered, frustrated by Choua's onslaught.

"*You* don't know? You are a pathologist. How can you not know that?" Choua was relentless.

"No! Placebos don't alter the laboratory test results," I acquiesced.

"Now, if the drugs change the laboratory test results and

the placebo doesn't, both the patient and the doctor must also be
blinded to the laboratory test results. Are they?"

"Usually not."

"Oh, so they see the changes in the laboratory test results
but they do not let that information register in their minds. They
realize that if those test result changes entered their cognitive
fields, the double-blind will be double-blind no more." Choua
eyed me impishly. "Why don't the champions of N^2D^2 medicine
ever talk about this problem?"

"Go on, Choua. Pour it on!" I said with resignation.

FOURTH, THE ONLY WAY DOUBLE-BLIND CROSS-OVER CAN WORK IS IF PATIENTS FOLLOW ONLY DRUG PROTOCOLS

"Do your patients with chronic illnesses consult other
professionals?" Choua asked.

"Yes, they do."

"Why?"

"Because they often have multiple problems and require
care by professionals in different disciplines."

"When a patient begins to feel better, how do you tell
whether he is responding to your therapies or to someone else's?"

"That's a real problem."

"So the only way double-blind cross-over can work is if
the patient mindlessly does only what the drug researchers tell
him to do. This, of course, seldom happens."

"Why not?" I asked.

"Drug doctors establish all their blessed double-blind

cross-over studies with great attention to detail. They try to blind both the patient and his physician to the nature of the treatment so that they cannot in any way influence the results. They try hard to systematically strip the patient of all control over his treatment. Do you realize that the patient is essentially excluded from playing any role in his own recovery? Now, do you really think that ever happens?"

"Why not?"

"Because no chronically ill patient is ever willing to completely put himself at the mercy of his drug doctor. They do not simply suffer in silence. They do other things—in areas of nutrition, home environment, stress and fitness. Do you think there is ever a single patient who does not think of ways to alleviate his suffering in other ways—who mindlessly does, month after month, only what the drug researchers tell him to do? You see the sheer stupidity of all this, do you?"

"I don't know if..."

"No patient does that," Choua didn't let me finish my sentence. "Why don't you find me any such research subjects? We will ask them questions together. Okay?"

"Go on, Choua," I yielded.

FIFTH, DRUG RESEARCH PROTOCOLS ARE NOT TRUE TO LIFE

D^3 medicine is another of Choua's favorite terms that he uses to ridicule the prevailing drug medicine in the U.S. D^3 medicine, according to him, holds that a physician search for one disease in a patient, make one diagnosis, then treat that disease with one drug. Sir William Osler, often given the title of the father of modern medicine in the U.S. and Canada, was the most forceful proponent of the idea. He believed that all clinical data for a given patient must be evaluated carefully to fit into a single diagnostic category so that the treatment of that single disease can be undertaken with the most effective available agent—the drug of choice.

"The only way double-blind cross-over can work is if the drug research protocol was true to life," Choua shifted restlessly, "In D3 medicine, you believe your diseases, diagnoses and drugs are immutable—etched in marble. You must search for a single disease, make a single diagnosis and then use a single drug of choice."

"The Oslerian notion of one-disease-one-diagnosis-one-drug-of-choice does have considerable merit," I challenged.

"You know Sir Osler died a long time ago. The times have changed. The environment is different today. Your nutrition is different today. The stress of life is different today."

"Oslerian philosophy still has a valid place in clinical medicine," I persisted.

"Nonsense!" Choua exploded. "If Sir Osler were alive today, he would have been an ecologist and a nutritionist. Where do you think those single diseases come from anyway? Mount Pocono? Or is it Olympus?"

I suppressed a smile. In the passion of argument, Choua sometimes throws my own words back at me—seemingly forgetful of the fact that I wrote them. Choua was back on his favorite theme. I decided not to provoke him any further.

SIXTH, DRUG RESEARCH PROTOCOLS LAST FOR MONTHS, THE THERAPIES BASED ON THEM FOR DECADES

"Double-blind cross-over drug studies are done for some months," Choua resumed, "and you use the conclusions, based upon such limited studies, for recommending therapies that last for years and decades. Now does that make any sense?"

"How else do you propose we proceed?" I asked.

"You know that human metabolism makes adjustments when it is assaulted with drugs, chemicals that are foreign to it. Don't you?" Choua ignored my question. "The efficacy of the drug—as determined by the *blessed* double-blind cross-over drug research—has little relationship to the clinical value of that drug when used for long periods of time. Drugs often fail utterly when put into clinical use *after* they have been unequivocally proven effective by the double-blind cross-over studies. How do we explain such failures?" Choua asked.

SEVENTH, DRUGS ARE EVALUATED AS SINGLE AGENTS; THEY ARE USED IN THREES, FOURS OR FIVES

"Of all the things you drug doctors do," Choua spoke without making any attempt to soften his blows, "the most amusing is this: Drug companies spend enormous sums of money to test the efficacy of single drugs with your blessed double-blind cross-over. They present their data to their friends at the FDA and obtain approval for marketing the drug. What happens when the drug hits the market?" Choua sneered.

"You tell me, Choua. It's your monologue," I taunted.

"How often do you drug doctors use single drugs for your patients—I mean just one drug at a time?"

"I don't know?"

"It must be quite unusual. When you prescribe drugs, you prescribe them for individual symptoms. The more the merrier! Right!"

"Go on."

"How often do you use two drugs at the same time? How often do you know what the combined effects of those drugs might be? How often do you use three drugs at a time? How often do you know the combined effects of three concurrently used drugs?"

"Pharmacists try to warn physicians..."

"How often do you use six drugs concurrently? And eight drugs concurrently?" Choua interrupted me again.

"Why do you ask me questions if you do not have the patience to hear my answers?" I grunted.

"Do drug companies ever do double-blind cross-over drug research with the concurrent use of two drugs? Or concurrent use of three drugs? Or concurrent use of six or seven or eight drugs?"

"No! They don't!" I shook my head. "But you..."

"But what?" Choua frowned.

"Nothing. Never mind!" I leaned back on my chair.

DRUGS ARE COMPARED ONLY WITH PLACEBOS, NEVER WITH NONDRUG THERAPIES

"If this is all true, why don't mainstream doctors see the farce in double-blind cross-over research?" I asked after several moments.

"What choice do N^2D^2 docs have?" Choua shrugged. They are required by their licensing boards to practice medicine within the usual and customary standards of care—that is, within the prevailing dogma of drug medicine. If that is so, why don't the doctors who sit on licensing boards see the folly of such drug research? But, then, what can these doctors do? They have to use some scientific criteria. Where do they get their criteria? From drug companies! Where else? That is the only science they can consider acceptable. If that is so, why don't the drug companies see the absurdity in such drug research? Why do they continue to pour billions of dollars into such research? But, then, what can the drug companies do? What choice do the drug companies have? How do they get past the FDA? They have to have marketing approvals from the FDA. If that is so, why don't the folks at the FDA see this? But what choice do the folks at the FDA have? They have to use some *scientific* criteria. Where do they get their science from? From the editors of our prestigious medical journals! Where else? Now if that is so, why don't these editors see the farce in such science? Because they are drug doctors and they have to have faith in the tools of their trade. So this circus goes on and on. Who pays the price? The patient, of course!"

THE PLACEBO GAMES

"N^2D^2 docs love to play placebo games with their double-blind studies," Choua resumed.

"What are placebo games?" I asked.

"Clever stuff indeed!" Choua chuckled. "This is how the placebo games are played: The N^2D^2 docs decide before they start the study which way they want to move the placebo effect to suit their purpose."

"Move the placebo value?" I was taken aback. "What do you mean by moving the placebo value?"

"Yes sir! The game is about moving the placebo value to tout the drug that is compared with, or to put down a therapy used by holistic physicians. That's how the placebo game is played.

"Preposterous!" I yelled. "Utterly preposterous! I've never heard such nonsense. Where do you get such crazy ideas from anyway?"

"Don't lose your temper at me," Choua responded calmly. "If you want to yell at someone, yell at N^2D^2 docs who play such brazen tricks."

"I don't believe such nonsense for a moment!" I challenged. "Show me some hard evidence for it."

"I don't know why that offends you so," Choua said solemnly. "In the first part of the game, N^2D^2 docs make the clinical outcome with the placebo look very bad so that the outcome with drug looks very good by comparison. Clever! Isn't it?"

"Oh, c'mon, Choua, that's rediculous! Give me an

example. How can you make the results obtained with the placebo look bad. After all, the placebo pill is supposed not to have any effect. Indeed, if the placebo has an effect, by definition, it isn't a placebo anymore." I countered.

"You always underestimate the ingenuity of N^2D^2 docs.

"Fine! I'll cite a specific example," Choua jeered. "Watch how N^2D^2 docs make the unhappenable happen! You know that multiple sclerosis is an autoimmune disorder in which the injured immune system is so confused that it makes antibodies against the insulating sheats of nerves called myelin sheaths."

"Yes, yes! I know that," I said impatiently. "I want to know can anyone make the placebo outcome worse."

"Some N^2D^2 geniuses decided to treat multiple sclerosis with cladribine, a chemotherapy drug used for leukemia and lymphoma when other drugs do not work. Cladribine is an efficient killer T-helper immune cells."

"Patients with immune disorder need more not less immune cells. Why would anyone kill helper immune cells in a patient who suffers from a severe immune injury to his myelin nerve sheath?" I asked, incredulously. "Are you making it up, Choua?"

"Don't ask me why N^2D^2 docs use chemotherapy drugs for patients who suffer from noncancer disorders caused by injury to the immune system," Choua frowned. "N^2D^2 docs destroy the immune system rather regularly with steroids and other immunosuppressant drugs. Why does that surprise you?"

"Okay! Go on. Tell me about the placebo trick," I prodded.

"Well, the drug docs in the Cladribine study reported that the patients in their placebo group deteriorated at six times the rate at which patients on placebos did in aother reported studies."

"How could that be?" I asked.

"Magic of medical statistics!" Choua chugged along.

"Here, listen to this:

> *...since 1 control improved by at least one point and 15 remained within 1 point of baseline, the 7 patients who deteriorated by 1 point or more, must have accounted for a mean EDSS (Expanded Disability Status Scale) of at least 2.36 points...These changes are strikingly different from those in placebo group of other trials. In the Canadian trial...the mean EDSS deterioration in the placebo group was 0.39...*

Lancet 344:537; 1994

See how cleverly these N^2D^2 docs turned an expected value of detrioration from 0.39 to 2.36 points—an increase of about six hundred percent! Clever fellows, these N^2D^2 docs, aren't they?"

"That's unbelievable! How did the author explain such discrepancy?"

"They didn't. What I will now quote to you is from the letter someone wrote to the Editor of *Lancet* questioning the rate of detrioration in the placebo group. You will see that I'm not alone in this. Others are equally astonished by the placebo tricks in the medical literature. Listen to this:

The conclusion that cladribine favourably influences the course of chronic progressive multiple sclerosis therefore needs careful scrutiny.

Lancet 344; 537; 1994.

Magic of medical statistics! Never fails!" Choua chirped.

"Unbelievable!" I couldn't hold back. "Hard to believe that serious drug researchers make such mistakes! But, wait, what did the authors say in response to the letter. I'm sure *Lancet* asked the authors to comment on that glaring inconsistency."

"Nothing surprising there. The authors said something about their patients being very sick. Now I wonder why their patients were so sick," Choua said naughtily.

"Okay, you made your point," I shook my head with confusion. "Now, give me an example where the researchers change the placebo effect in the opposite direction. How do they enhance the value of the placebo so a holistic therapy looks bad by comparison?"

"That's simple too!" Choua chugged along. "Do you remember the New Zealand study published in the journal of the American Heart association? It claimed that EDTA chelation therapy does not work for patients who suffer from leg cramps and pain on walking short distances due to advanced plaque formation in their leg arteries."

"I don't remember the details. Tell me about it."

"That was equally astounding—or, as you put

it—preposterous!" Choua grinned broadly. "They worked the magic of medical statistics in the opposite direction. Listen to this:

> ***The proportion of patients showing an improvement in walking distance was not significantly different between the chelation group (60%) and the control group (59%)...Chelation therapy has no significant beneficial effects over placebo in patients with intermittent claudication.***

> *Circulation* 90:1194; 1994.

Wow! Fifty-nine percent placebo effect!" Choua threw the journal down with mock anger. "Have you ever seen a placebo response of fifty-nine percent? I don't know too many drugs that can give you that high a beneficial response. A remarkable study, isn't it?"

"Most remarkable, indeed!" I agreed. "I don't recall ever seeing such a high figure for beneficial effects obtained with a placebo."

"Magic, my friend, magic! This is pure magic of N^2D^2 statistics! They reported that sixty percent of the patient in the placebo group benefitted. Thus, the efficacy of EDTA chelation therapy was no better that that of the placebo. Pretty stuff! Isn't it?"

"There must be a mistake there some place. That can't be. How can the placebo benefit sixty percent of patients with advanced vascular disease?"

"Pretty stuff!" Choua chirped again. "Those who wanted

to tout a toxic drug that kills immune cells made their placebo patients deteriorate at six times the rate reported by others. So their drugs looked so much better when compared with the placebo. And those who wanted to put down EDTA chelation jacked up their number for beneficial effects of the placebo to fifty-nine percent. Amazing! It doesn't get any better, does it?" Choua bellowed loudly.

"It's not amazing. It's disgusting!" I nearly screamed.

"*Long live medical statistics! Long live drugs! Long live N^2D^2 docs!* Science has not failed medicine, medicine has..." Choua stopped in midsentence and briskly walked out.

Who ever saw a doctor use the prescription of his colleagues without cutting out or adding something?

Michel de Montaigne

Chapter 3

A Changing Medicine

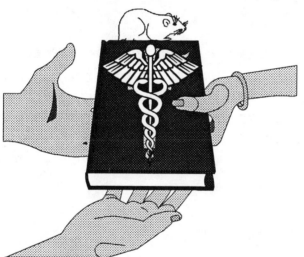

For A Changing Time

This is a time of profound change in medicine. The discovery that we can no longer use drugs to achieve optimal long-term clinical outcomes for sufferers of the dominant chronic health disorders is a fundamental breakthrough.

A great promise lies in what I call *energetic-molecular (EM) medicine*. EM medicine is based on a true understanding of the energetic-molecular events that separate a state of health from a state of disease.

EM medicine is founded on events that occur in molecules (and cells and tissues) before they are injured and changed, and not on the study of how dead and decaying cells and tissues look under the microscope after they have been damaged by a disease.

EM medicine has four faces: nutritional medicine, environmental medicine, medicine of self-regulation and medicine of fitness.

Rudolph Virchow, the father of modern pathology who published *Cellular Pathology* in 1858, liberated us from the restrictive tenets of gross pathology that hark back to medieval and ancient times. Cellular pathology, of course, gives us windows to injured tissues and cells *after* the fact. Now, knowledge of E-M dynamics of health and disease allows us to move beyond where Virchow could take us with his microscope.

While acute illness is likely to remain the preserve of safe surgery and potent drugs, chronic illness for enlightened individuals will become the province of EM medicine. For such people, drug medicine will succumb to nutritional and environmental medicines. And "limbic" fitness will prevail over current technology-oriented regimens. In fact, self-regulation is likely to move from the field of mysticism to the domain of science.

Indeed, we are moving toward the moment when the physician becomes a tutor and the patient a pupil.

All diseases are caused by accelerated oxidant stress. This may strike many as improbable—perhaps even as a nonsensical simplification of complex issues—but I have sound reasons for proposing this unifying theory of disease causation. I present extensive evidence for my viewpoint in the chapter Second Insight: Spontaneity of oxidation in Nature is the root cause of aging in humans and the root of all diseases. Increased oxidant stress on human biology is caused by factors in our internal and external environments. Chronic disease results from impairment of antioxidant defenses—related to poor nutrition—or excessive oxidant stress brought about by allergy, chemical sensitivity, environmental toxins, lifestyle stress and poor physical fitness. Susceptibility to recurring viral, bacterial and fungal infections, and parasitic infestation of the bowel develop when an individual's antioxidant—and, at later stages, immune—defenses are damaged by one or more of the above elements. Drugs are not an acceptable answer to these problems. Antibiotics, while essential for life-threatening infections, seriously damage bowel ecosystems and impair human defenses in many different ways.

WHAT IS HEALTH?

How is health defined in drug medicine? It isn't. The subject of what health is and what it may not be is scrupulously avoided in our medical schools, hospitals and physician offices. We glibly dismiss any reference to it by mumbling something unintelligible about physical, mental and emotional aspects.

But what are the physical attributes of health? How do we define mental health? What is emotional wholesomeness? I have attended tens of thousands of medical lectures since I entered King Edward Medical College in 1958. I do not recall ever hearing anyone answer these questions with any sincerity. Why?

I myself never reflected on this question in the more than 25 years when I worked as a disease doctor of drug medicine. I faced this problem only when my interest shifted from disease to health. I rendered my definition of what health is and what it isn't in the companion volume, *The Butterfly and Life Span Nutrition.* Here, I briefly define health again.

Health is being spiritual without any need to analyze what spirituality might be.

Health is waking up in the morning with a deep sense of gratitude—gratitude not for any accomplishment of the day before or for accumulations of yesteryears, *but for simply being.* An ENT surgeon from Greece recently attended my lecture at the meeting of the American Academy of Otolaryngic Allergy and expressed a common frustration, "But this is utterly new to my Greek thought." Well, if the concept of gratitude for simply being is foreign to us, we need to learn about it.

Health is waking up with a sense of energy, going through a day's work with that same sense of energy and returning to bed at night with it.

Health is as much energy before meals as it is after them.

Health is the ability to treasure personal time in silence—with family, friends or alone.

Health is two or three effortless, odorless bowel movements a day—without mucus and cramps.

Health comprises living, dynamic and vigorous bowel, blood and cellular ecosystems.

Health is an intact and functioning gateway of life—cell membranes that mark the boundaries between life within the cell and that which exists outside it in the blood. The cell membrane separates internal order of a cell from external disorder. It is a living, breathing, spongy and porous sheet that regulates the two-way E-M traffic between cells and the soup of life that bathes them.

The last two elements of my definition of health may seem tedious to some readers. I return to this core subject and present essential information at length in the chapter Second Insight: Spontaneity of Oxidation Is the Root Cause of All Diseases. Here, I wish to make a crucial point:

The essence of EM medicine is to seek a genuine understanding of the energetic-molecular dynamics of cells and tissues, and to reverse chronic diseases with nondrug therapies based on them. EM medicine promotes health with natural therapies that revive injured bowel, blood and cellular ecosystems.

It is not uncommon for me to see drug doctors criticize holistic physicians for their "unscientific" methods. The truth is that it is far more scientific to base restorative therapies for chronic disease on a genuine understanding of bowel, blood and cellular ecosystems than on mere symptom suppression with drugs that block normal physiological processes. Drug therapies for chronic disease—as necessary as they might be for symptom suppression—do not constitute restorative approaches.

WHAT HEALTH IS NOT

And now, I define what health is not. Health is not the mere absence of disease. Health has nothing to do with the frivolous notions of RDA and balanced diets of our nutrition experts. Health is not the euphoria of eating nor is it the denial of dieting. Health is not preoccupation with recycling past miseries, nor is it pre-cycling feared, future misery. Health is not living with regrets nor is it obsession with control in life.

I return to the question that I raised before submitting my definition of health: Why do mainstream physicians shun the subject of health? The answer is really quite simple: *None of the essential aspects of health I define in this chapter can be addressed with drugs.* There are no drugs that make us spiritual nor can they bring us gratitude and freedom from anger. There are no drugs for teaching us the limbic language of silence nor for putting out the oxidative fires of stress. Drugs cannot revive injured energy enzymes, nor can they repair damaged detoxification enzymes. There are no synthetic chemicals that can they upregulate energy and fat-burning enzymes. Drugs cannot restore a damaged bowel ecosystem nor can they strengthen a weakened blood ecosystem. Drugs cannot normalize disrupted energetic-molecular dynamics at the cell membranes. Indeed, the tools of modern medicine are singularly ineffective for coping with impaired physiologic processes that preserve health.

One Mission

A physician has but one mission: to alleviate suffering by reversing disease and promoting health.

It is a sad commentary on contemporary medicine in the U.S. that it is neither committed to reversing disease nor to promoting health. Disease can be reversed only by addressing the initial E-M events that separate a state of health from a state of absence of health—that is, the in between state of absence of health. Drugs can neither reverse disease nor promote health—notwithstanding their essential roles in saving lives in acute, life-threatening conditions, and in suppressing symptoms in chronic disease.

The twin goals of reversing disease and promoting health require nutritional, environmental, self-regulatory and fitness therapies.

Who is a better judge of whether a therapy works or not—a physician or a patient? Since antiquity, physicians have vigorously excluded the patient from assessing a therapy's effectiveness. Even to date, the dogma of disease doctors of drug medicine flatly denies that the patient's subjective sense about the clinical efficacy—or lack of it—has any true role in the research of drug therapies. In higher orbits of power, where drug medicine sets policies and procedures, patients' subjective evaluations are dismissed as *soft* data. The few physicians who do bring this subject up are regarded condescendingly, if not ridiculed outright.

In acute illness, indeed, the experienced physician is in a better position to be judge. The patient's judgment is often clouded by intense suffering, impaired intellectual function and fear of death. But does that hold for chronic illness? The best physician can only bring to his patient his knowledge and experience. One thing he can never do is *become* the patient. No amount of empathy, training or encounters with others' suffering can allow the physician to *feel* the pain of his patient. No sensory perceptions—no matter how sharply honed—can allow a physician to *know* the suffering of his patient.

We still have not invented any "sufferometer" that can quantify human suffering. We have yet to develop any "painometer" that can precisely measure the degree of pain. How does an orthopedic surgeon quantify a patient's pain? He can graph the muscle spasm with electromyography equipment. But can he measure the magnitude of suffering inflicted by a persistent spasm of the neck muscles? How can a physician truly judge the level of fatigue of his patient as he leaves his bed? Or his sense of dismay as therapies fail and promises do not hold up?

On a more mundane level, how can a physician judge better than the patient what dose of an herb gives him better sleep? Or what frequency of allergy injections give him the best relief? Or how often he needs extra support of oral or injectable nutrients to prevent the relapse of chronic fatigue?

In chronic illness, the patient is in a far better position to assess the outcome of a given therapy than the physician. Smart doctors—sharp with their statistics—may have trouble with this viewpoint; wise physicians will not.

As the physician and the patient become more enlightened, Choua often says, the clinical outcome evaluated by the patient will displace the frivolous double-blind, cross-over model of drug research that infatuate disease doctors at present.

Two Core Problems of Medicine

There are two core problems of medicine today:

First,

we try to solve 21st-century environmental and nutritional problems with 19th-century ideas of disease and drugs.

Second,

we have raised generations of physicians who know much about disease but little, if anything, about health. Indeed, contemporary medical journals are singularly silent on the matter of health and how it can be fostered. The prevailing dogma of drug medicine is utterly committed to keeping the sick incarcerated in the sickness mold.

The issue is not whether or not nondrug therapies work for chronic ecologic, immune and degenerative disorders. *They work*. Thousands of physicians have known that for decades. The challenge today is not to disprove their efficacy; rather, it is to improve the success rate of such natural therapies with continued innovation, and to document their efficacy with careful empirical observations.

Instead, the prevailing dogma of drug medicine is committed to eliminating all nondrug therapies in the United States. The postgraduate continuing education of American physicians is solidly controlled by drug companies. During the last 28 years of my work at Holy Name Hospital, I have attended more than a thousand formal lectures, mostly by speakers who were paid for by drug companies. Except for times when I was asked to substitute for a speaker who could not speak, and I spoke about matters of health, nutrition and environment, I do not recall a single speaker who discussed nondrug therapies. After all, wWhy would any drug company spend its money teaching physicians how not to use drugs?

Three Sciences

Science is the search for truth. Science is the observation of physical phenomenon. Science is self-correcting.

At an elementary level, one can look at science in three ways:

Science of observation
Science of empiricism
Science of controlled and reproducible experiments

SCIENCE OF SIMPLE OBSERVATION

The first science of simple observation is the purest of all sciences. It is the science of simple observation. It has no ulterior motive or hidden agenda except to state what has been observed. Each month my copies of *Nature* and *Science* contain articles written by physiologists, botanists, zoologists, biologists and paleontologists who describe their observations about the oxidative stress on various life forms, alive or long deceased. Sometimes their observations extend the current knowledge and at other times, they challenge long-established precepts. When such observations do not fit into the accepted body of scientific knowledge, they are not rejected simply because any high priests of the establishment declare them invalid. The crucial point is this: *An observation stands on its own merit.*

SCIENCE OF EMPIRICAL OBSERVATION

The second science of empiricism requires that we accept that which *works*. Apples fell down from trees long before Newton ever conceived his ideas of gravitational pull. People empirically knew that apples fell down and didn't fly up or sideways when they became ripe. Newton reflected on what he observed and that simple leap led him to propound his laws of gravity.

Folks in Pakistan have known for centuries that curries do not spoil so readily if they are prepared with turmeric. They accepted this as a valid empirical observation. Recent studies show that curcumin, the major yellow pigment in turmeric, is a powerful antioxidant and anti-inflammatory agent. So now we know how turmeric keeps curry dishes fresh for many hours.

The East India Company sent four ships to India in its first expedition in 1600. General James Lancaster provided lemon juice on his ship and it remained free of scurvy whereas the other three ships were badly affected by this disorder. This empirical observation was made long before vitamin C was discovered.

The ancients knew some remedies worked. Practical men demonstrated astute powers of empirical observations long before the modern concepts of science were articulated. They recorded the effects of many remedies after careful, repeated empirical observations. The Chinese and Indian Ayurvedic herbal medicines evolved over centuries. To this day, many of their herbal therapies are used worldwide by billions of people. I use many of them every working day in my office and validate their efficacy with science of empiricism.

SCIENCE OF CONTROLLED AND REPRODUCIBLE EXPERIMENTS

The explosive growth in the physical sciences that we have witnessed over the last 150 years has occurred largely as a result of controlled and reproducible experiments. An understanding of the laws of physics led to an understanding of energy and of properties of matter. Advances in analytical methods led to determination of chemical composition of natural substances and that paved the way for synthetic chemistry. Knowledge of biology and chemistry expanded into enzymes and genes. The field of molecular biology—in its infancy only a couple of decades ago—has mushroomed into an all-encompassing discipline. The impact of science on medicine, however, has been vastly misunderstood.

TRAGEDY OF SCIENCE IN MEDICINE

The artful practice of medicine takes lessons from biology.

I write in *Intravenous Nutrient Protocols in Molecular*

Medicine that human biology is an ever changing kaleidoscope of molecules. Health—at a molecular level—can be defined as a state in which oxidative stress on human tissues is effectively countered by their antioxidant defenses. Disease, by contrast, is a state in which oxidative stresses overwhelm the body's antioxidant defenses. The outcome of such dynamics is determined by the impact upon an individual's genetic make-up of molecules in his internal and external environments. The third essential element in this context is choice. I illustrate this schematically below:

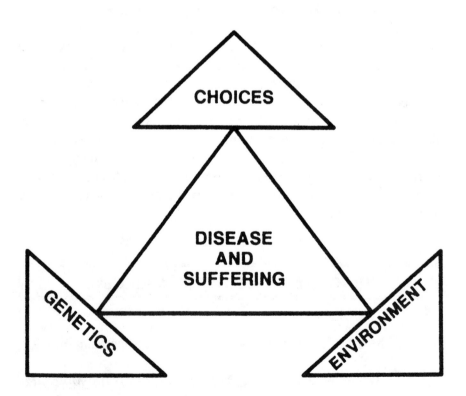

In biology, I write in *The Butterfly and Life Span Nutrition*, if we change something in one way, we change everything in some way. Different biologic burdens affect different people differently. Diseases change the function and structure of different tissues differently. Therapies affect different people differently. This must be accepted as the *core* philosophy of medicine.

The tragedy of drug medicine in the U.S. is this: Only that knowledge of biology that serves the drug industry finds its way into our physician offices, clinics and hospitals. There is little, if any, support for the knowledge of biology that can help us preserve health without drugs. In medical schools, there is considerable emphasis on basic sciences but, as we all know, young doctors abandon all interest in basic sciences as soon as they have access to prescriptions pads.

Medical science vehemently rejects the original two sciences: the science of observation and the science of empiricism. We physicians mindlessly prescribe drugs that we know are toxic and that in many cases, simply do not work. We vigorously call quackery all use of natural therapies that we know nothing about—and stubbornly refuse to allow their use even though they have been proven to be safe and effective by centuries of observation and empirical validation.

Tragically, science in medicine appears restricted to the application of double-blind cross-over models of drug research, while casting aside the biologic knowledge that by its nature leads to nondrug therapy. This practice persists in spite of the fact that the countless drugs deemed safe and effective by the *blessed* double-blind cross-over have in fact wrought havoc on human beings.

Four Predictions

I am an optimist. I believe the prevailing dogma of drug medicine will be challenged by a growing number of people. I believe that problems caused by our current infatuation with drugs will end as we become increasingly enlightened about matters of health and disease. However, I do not believe that everyone in medicine will readily see or agree with my precepts of EM medicine I describe in this volume. Some people may forever refuse to accept any responsibility for their health and insist on drugs for sheer symptom suppression. The disease doctors of drug medicine will continue to willingly provide them with the necessary prescriptions.

Four predictions—it seems to me—can be safely made about the future of medicine.

First,

ecologic, immune, degenerative and stress-related disorders will be the dominant chronic disorders of the 21st century.

Second,

these disorders will force the disease doctors of drug medicine to learn and use nondrug therapies for chronic immune and degenerative disorders. Patients, as well as physicians, will clearly see that problems caused by chemicals cannot be solved with more chemical drugs.

Third,

the emerging EM medicine will be a "participatory" medicine—a medicine in which the patient will actively guide the physician in energetic-molecular restorative work rather than simply accepting symptom-suppressing drugs.

Fourth,

self-regulation—and the hope and spirituality that always spring from it—will become an essential part of the mainstream management philosophy of all chronic disorders.

These four predictions do not arise from some far-fetched notion of utopia. Rather, these conclusions seem inescapable to me, as I reflect on the growing pandemic of hyperactivity and attention deficit disorders in children; chronic, disabling fatigue among previously active young adults; hormonal dysfunctions among young women; mood, memory and mentation disorders caused by multiple drug therapies among the elderly; and an ever-widening spectrum of eco-disorders among people of all ages. No miracles of synthetic chemistry can reverse these problems. As people become well informed about alternatives to drugs, they will demand the evolving EM medicine, and a new cadre of physicians will emerge to administer nondrug therapies.

Five Medicines

Medicine began as a sideline of ancient shamans—the men of spirits of the primitive era. It slowly evolved into medicine of gross organs—a profession in which therapies were used to approach problems of health as seen with examination of decaying and dead tissues. In the 18th century, the invention of the microscope ushered in the third medicine—histopathology. The microscope was now used to define diseases. The microscope was also employed to evaluate the efficacy of therapies used to treat those diseases.

Advances in synthetic chemistry brought on the fourth type—a medicine of enzymes, receptors, mediators, cell membrane channels and genes. The medicine of chemistry saves many lives. It is clearly at its best when it cares for those near death—*tail-end* medicine as I call it. It also endlessly prolongs the process of dying for many. This fourth medicine falters when it comes to preserving health and preventing disease—*front-end* medicine in my order of things.

We now look at the emerging possibility of the fifth type—energetic-molecular (EM) medicine which is based on the physics of health rather than on the chemistry of disease. This EM medicine is the true preventive medicine, focusing on the initial EM events that separate a state of health from a state of absence of health. This book discusses the fifth type of medicine.

Six Assumptions

The concept of RDA is not a valid concept. It is based on spurious data and erroneous conclusions. Indeed, I have often wondered how this frivolous idea could have lasted for so long. This concept is based on six insupportable assumptions:

First,

> *is the assumption that Nature created micronutrients only to prevent a handful of nutritional deficiency diseases.*

This amazing assumption is largely based on statistics obtained with animal experiments. How can the prevention of deficiency states in rats be equated with optimal metabolic requirements for humans?

Second,

> *is the assumption that micronutrients have no metabolic roles in preserving health and reversing chronic disease.*

This equally astounding assumption flies in the face of a huge body of clinical and experimental data concerning the metabolic roles of nutrients in health and disease. How can rat experiments, conducted to study deficiency diseases, provide guidelines for reversing disease and promoting health for humans?

Third,

is the assumption that studies conducted for weeks or months examining the effects of nutrients can yield valid guidelines for the entire human life span.

No one has ever investigated the metabolic effects of any nutrient in a population for its entire life span. Yet, I regularly hear nutritionists being criticized for prescribing doses of nutrients in excess of RDA values. How can rats given this or that nutrient for weeks or months be acceptable model for humans for seven, eight or more decades?

Fourth,

is the assumption that studies employing highly processed and unnatural foods can yield useful information for people eating natural, unprocessed and unoxidized foods.

The natural order of things requires us to eat what grows *where* we live—and what the land provides at *that* time. Our metabolism evolved slowly over eons to process natural food substances and cannot adapt rapidly to sweeping changes in our foods. Human digestive-absorptive enzyme pathways were not designed to process the plastic foods that we ingest. How can rats fed highly unnatural and purified foods in the laboratory be deemed appropriate metabolic models for humans who try to eat naturally?

Fifth,

is the assumption that human tissue ecosystems are immune to oxidative stresses that are destroying the ecosystems of planet Earth that surround us.

Every month medical journals publish papers linking degenerative diseases with functional micronutrient deficiencies, and every month they report protective effects of such nutrients. How do human ecosystems protect themselves against oxidative storms? Evidently with antioxidant nutrients. Yet, the practitioners of drug medicine ignore all that evidence and stubbornly cling to their irrelevant RDA notions. How can rats whose ecosystems are destroyed in laboratories—and who are sacrificed after the experimenters are through with them—be considered suitable biologic ecosystems for humans?

Sixth,

is the assumption—and this assumption follows as the expected consequence of the preceding five assumptions—that diseases can be treated only with drugs.

In the preface, I write that diseases heal with nutrients, not with drugs. This is elementary and so obvious that it is hard to see how anyone can fail to see this. It is ironic that when diseases are produced experimentally in rats, the idea of reversing those diseases with nutrients totally escapes drug researchers.

Medicine is artfully practiced only when it embraces the full knowledge of biology. We have a limited understanding of the healing response in man. There are simply too many variables in the healing phenomena. The statistics generated with rat experiments have little, if any, relevance to an individual patient.

Drug medicine compounds the error when it insists on interpreting these assumptions as a call for long-term use of drugs for chronic disease. Here, drug use statistics play havoc with reality. Ironically, drug medicine goes to great lengths to mask—or outright deny—statistics about drug toxicity, as it exaggerates the statistics about its long-term efficacy.

Seven Insights

Over the last several years of my research and clinical work, one or more events gave me some essential insights into health—dis-ease—disease dynamics. Seven such insights have dominated my thinking and my clinical management of patients. Each of these insights challenges a prevailing viewpoint regarding the pathologic basis of disease and the best ways of managing the clinical disorders they cause. These insights have also influenced my thinking in areas that at first glance appear unrelated to the disease in question. I now base all my EM medicine therapies on these seven issues, especially with regard to immune, metabolic and degenerative disorders. A discussion of each of the seven insights listed below follows.

1.   Absence of disease is not always presence of health.
2.   Spontaneity of oxidation in Nature is the true cause of aging in humans and the root of *all* diseases.
3.   Healing is a natural state of energy in tissue. Mind-over-body does not work; energy-over-mind does.
4.   Genes legislate life; the environment interprets the laws set forth by genes.
5.   The bowel and the blood are open ecosystems.
6.   Science has not failed medicine; medicine has failed science.
7.   Given an informed choice, a majority of people will prefer nondrug therapies based on *physics of health* over drug therapies based on *chemistry of disease*.

The seven insights were gifts to me from people who asked me to care for them in times of illness. Some evolved slowly after spending long hours listening to my patients describe their suffering, and others while peering endlessly at injured tissues through my microscope in search of some answers. Still others hit me like lightning. I vigorously tested each insight in various clinical settings. All my ways of caring for the sick are based on them. These insights have given rise to EM medicine that I describe in this and companion volumes.

Most of the precepts of EM medicine described in this volume have been tested and validated by many of my colleagues at the Institute of Preventive Medicine, Denville, New Jersey, and in the American Academy of Preventive Medicine. I hope the clinical therapies that arise from these insights, and the scientific principles on which they rest, will be considered by others—and validated, modified or refuted—in the best tradition of medicine.

Everywhere the old order changes
and happy they who can change.

Sir William Osler

I do not forget that medicine and veterinary practice are foreign to me. I desire judgment and criticism upon all my contributions. Little tolerant of frivolous or prejudice contradiction, contemptuous of that ignorant criticism which doubt on principle, I welcome with open arms the militant attack which has a method in doubting and whose rule of conduct has the motto "More Light."

Louis Pasteur

Chapter 4

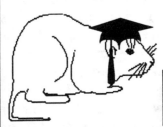

FIRST INSIGHT

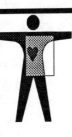

Absence
of
Disease
is not
always
Presence
of
Health

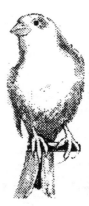

In 1982, on two consecutive July weekends, I lectured at two postgraduate immunology and allergy courses held in Jackson Hole, Wyoming. Rather than return home for the intervening days, I escaped to Yellowstone National Park. One day I went for a hike on a trail leading to the peak of Mount Washburn.

It was a warm clear day when I started. The trail meandered through lush meadows brimming with black-eyed susans and many other types of wildflowers. The flower fields blended with the blue-green hills at some distance, and the hills merged into the mountains on the horizon. Some bison herds were easy to spot in the distance. Sometimes I saw deer and large elk close by. These beings seemed at ease with hikers on the trail. Sometimes they seemed to acknowledge my presence among them with knowing looks, and sometimes with indifferent eyes. Chipmunks were everywhere, but their busy schedules didn't seem to permit any freedom to acknowledge or ignore anyone else. Every now and then I stopped to look at the butterflies. I found myself completely consumed by their dazzling displays of color and flight patterns.

I paused often to look up close at the low shrubs and tall pine trees, and to admire the mosaic of mountains in the distance, with the peaks partly lost in the mist. The frequency of my stops increased as I moved on. Soon I realized that I climbed quite a distance. The high altitude now made me aware of my breathing and increased the need for more frequent stops. I also noticed that there were some clouds above me, and the chill of the high mountain had replaced the warm glow of the sun below in the valley. There were neither bison, elk nor deer around now. At some turns, clusters of mountain goats looked at me, bulging haughtily from steep ledges.

I saw only a few other hikers after taking sharp bends in the trail. I asked one returning hiker how much farther I had to climb to reach the peak. "A couple of miles," he grinned, "but it's worth it. There's a watchtower at the peak, and you can warm up in the cabin for a while." A couple of miles! My legs suddenly felt limp. I thanked the hiker and moved on. Mountains always pull at me.

The last several hundred yards of the trail were dauntingly steep. Fierce, cold winds and the sheer, raw, unbearable beauty of the place stung my watery eyes. The cabin on the mountaintop gave me the warm shelter I had hoped for. I leaned against the glass wall and simply stared out.

My next memory of those moments on the mountaintop is one I will never forget. The words came from nowhere: *Diseases do not descend from mountains.*

Where did the words come from? Did I actually hear them? Or did I just imagine them? I do not know, but they shook me hard. I do not recall thinking for one moment about any part of my work in medicine on that trail. There were no thoughts of nutrition, allergy, chemical sensitivity, immunology or pathology. Biopsies of diseased tissues and causes of disease were furthest from my mind. There were no thoughts of genes, environment, no interest in searching for the truth or spirituality, and no notions of mind-over-body healing. Where did the words come from? And why on Mount Washburn of all places? *I do not know, but I do believe there is a time and a place for everything.* If that is unscientific, I plead guilty.

On the way down the mountain, my thoughts kept drifting back to the words I heard on the mountaintop. *Diseases do not descend from mountains.* Then, where *do* they come from?

I had examined more than 50,000 biopsies and surgical pathology specimens in the hospital by that time. Nearly every time I examined a microscopic slide and rendered a pathologic diagnosis I wondered where the disease came from. Where did it begin? More often than not I was left wondering, relying on medical texts that claimed the origins were unknown. Although there was a section in pathology or medicine texts devoted to discussion of the cause of a particular lesion, a description of the *initial* energetic-molecular event that triggered a given disease process was nearly always missing. With my microscope, I examined the tail end of the diseases, the ravages of a process that had clearly started much earlier.

WHAT CAUSES A HEART ATTACK?

What causes heart attacks? Of course, plaque formation in coronary arteries! What causes plaque formation? Of course, arteriosclerosis! What causes arteriosclerosis? Of course, cholesterol deposits in the blood vessel walls! Why do cholesterol deposits form there? There are risk factors: obesity, smoking, stress, hypertension and diabetes. How do these risk factors cause cholesterol deposits in the blood vessel walls? Well, they just do! The story of heart disease was related to me at medical school in this fashion.

The way back on a trail always appears to be shorter. It is interesting how perceptions of distance change between the way out and the way back in. Before I realized how much distance I had covered, I began spotting the deer and elk again. The chill of the high mountain air had lifted, leaving the warm glow of the sun. Diseases can only come from within us or from without. The thought amused me. Where else can they come from? I heard myself speak out loud.

Billions of words have been written to explain the cause of heart disease, the number one killer in the United States. Pathology and cardiology texts still say we really do not know what energetic-molecular events initiate the process that culminates in heart attacks. The books and journals literally contain millions of pages devoted to the many theories that have been proposed. There are chapters on multiple risk factors. But still there is no clear agreement among researchers and cardiologists about the cause.

SHAPES OF COLITIS

We excel in the classification of various types of chronic bowel disorders. We have spastic colitis, irritable bowel syndrome, inflammatory bowel disease, ulcerative colitis, Crohn's colitis, ischemic colitis, pseudomembranous colitis, collagenous colitis and microscopic colitis. (I remembered wondering about what a "non microscopic" colitis might be when I first heard the term *microscopic colitis.*) What energetic-molecular events trigger ulcerative colitis? Our gastroenterology texts are silent on this issue. What energetic-molecular events cause Crohn's colitis? We do not know. What about collagenous colitis and microscopic colitis? The answers are the same.

Diseases must arise from within! But what is the internal environment of man? What goes into his body and how do his genes regulate their disposition? While the answer seems simple—genes, foods and metabolism—the mind also has to do something with all that. Bad thoughts that populate the mind must in some way affect the gene-food-metabolism interactions —adrenaline surges, neurotransmitter outbursts, anger and hostility must also be factored in. So the internal environment is an integrated energetic-molecular kaleidoscope of gene-food-metabolism-stress interrelationships. My thoughts returned to my microscope.

TYPES OF ARTHRITIS

When I was a young pathologist, I knew of 23 different types of arthritis. Now I know of only three: 1) the arthritis of oxidative injury caused by wear and tear, 2) arthritis of oxidative injury caused by food and environmental triggers, and 3) arthritis of oxidative injury caused by microbes.

The rheumatology texts include descriptions of many types of arthritis of the young. We have rheumatoid arthritis, juvenile arthritis, migratory arthritis, arthritis of lupus, arthritis of Sjogrens' disease, arthritis of immune complex disease and Reiter's arthritis. What do I see with my microscope when I examine slides of joint tissues injured by arthritis? I see inflammatory cells and repair cells, and damaged synovium and cartilage that line the joint spaces. But what are the energetic-molecular events that cause rheumatoid arthritis? The answer is we do not know. What are such events in juvenile arthritis? The answer is we do not know. The answer is the same regarding the initial events in all other types of arthritis.

AUTOIMMUNITY IS IMMUNE BETRAYAL

What are autoimmune disorders? These are disorders in which the immune system of the injured person turns on his own tissues—a bit like an injured dog biting his master's child in confusion.

How many different types of autoimmune diseases do we see? Many. Is there a body tissue that is exempt from immunologic injury? Hardly. We see immune disorders of the thyroid, adrenal and pancreas glands; of lungs, liver, heart, kidneys and bladder; of skin; and of muscle and nerve tissues. In the thyroid gland we call them hypothyroidism (Hashimoto's disease and lymphocytic thyroiditis) and hyperthyroidism (Grave's disease). There are, of course, many other variants with different names. What energetic-molecular events set the stage for these disorders? The answers are the same: We do not know. In the adrenal gland, we have hypoadrenalism (Addison's disease) and hyperadrenalism. What causes these disorders? We do not know.

Down in the valley, black-eyed susans reclaimed the immediate environment of the trail. External environment! What makes up man's external environment? Air, water, organic and inorganic matter. So, how do air and water cause diseases? Bugs and pollutants, that is the usual party line. What about organic and inorganic matter? Acid rain leaches mercury and aluminum from the soil and dumps them into our drinking water. Almost one-third of the adult patients I see with chronic immune disorders have an increased body burden of toxic metals that directly poison their energy and detoxification enzymes.

Chipmunks are voracious eaters, and those I saw on the trail were busy foraging. Chipmunks hibernate in winter, using the extra body fat they accumulated during their busy months of summer eating. Nature has its own designs for weight regulation and for nutritional balance. We humans also eat voraciously, but we do not hibernate and lose our unnecessary fat overload as chipmunks do. We add to the body burden of fat by ingesting oxidized, denatured fats that clog our molecular pathways. Hibernating periods for people? Not a bad idea! Losing weight while we slumber peacefully would also be an escape from the unrelenting clutter of the cortical monkey. But humans do not hibernate. Perhaps we can use periodic fasting to achieve the same results.

ANTIBIOTICS ARE DESIGNER KILLER MOLECULES

Why do we make antibiotics? To kill microbes! What are microbes? Living beings! Can antibiotics kill one form of life without affecting another? Not for long!

To keep insects from eating our food, we kill them with insecticides—our designer killer molecules. What happens to the insecticides after the insects have been killed? Insects do not metabolize insecticides. The killer molecules must stay in our external environment. How does our industry pollute our external environment? Well, *they* don't think they do! Not many doctors believe there is any *scientific* evidence that pollutants cause diseases anyway. This is the principal reason why the mainstream doctors consider clinical ecologists quacks. How dare clinical ecologists look for the causes of disease in the environment and in nutrition? How dare they speak against drugs—the tools of our trade? Most insecticides are fat-soluble. Human brain tissue loves them, and loathes to give them up once it gets a grip on them. Detoxification of the body is easier said than done. Why do people not die from antibiotic and pesticide poisonings? They *do*—slowly, insidiously, from autoimmune and degenerative disorders, and without recognizing what has damaged their life-sustaining enzymes.

INJURED HORMONES: MESSED-UP MESSENGERS

What are hormones? Chemical messengers that help cells talk to each other.

Hormonal problems are forever increasing. Many people have cold hands and feet. Many suffer from sugar roller coasters—rapid hyperglycemic-hypoglycemic shifts that trigger adrenaline roller coasters. Many women suffer from PMS, irregular menstrual bleeding and endometriosis. So many have osteoporosis. What initial energetic-molecular events trigger the processes that cause these hormonal dysfunctions? We do not know. We use estrogens to treat osteoporosis—fully recognizing that bone loss is a far more complex process, and that estrogen carries several well recognized hazards. We use synthetic hormones to treat endometriosis. Yet we do not know the cause of it. Endometriosis is unheard of among tribal people living simple lives. When people from tribal cultures emigrate to Western countries, the incidence of endometriosis increases sharply. That observation may give some clues to the cause of endometriosis. But since those clues do not lead to any drug therapies, why bother?

NAME THE CANCER, PLEASE!

How many different types of malignant tumors do we have? Here we *really* excel. We are so clever at inventing new names for old cancers. In medical school I learned about 22 different types of malignant tumors of the breast. What are the initial energetic-molecular events that cause these tumors? Of course, our medical texts are silent on this critical question. Some cancers grow slowly while others spread quickly. Do we understand the biology of those tumors any better today than we did 30 years ago? No. Do we know why some cancers simply sit in their places for years, while others pulsate and strike at distant places with impunity? No. Do we wonder why lymphocytes (a type of immune cell) vigilantly guard against cancer spread in some instances and not in others? No. Do we know why some people who should die quickly fail to comply with the dogma of medical texts? Do we understand why others who should live for a long time with less aggressive malignant tumors die quickly? No. Does all this keep us from forever renaming old cancers in new ways? Of course not.

Now we have tumor markers—the joy of our cancer specialists. These are molecules produced by tumors that allow tumor specialists to name and re-name cancers in altogether new ways. Now our cancer specialists talk shop among themselves in ways that leave the general practitioners dumbfounded. Do these markers help us understand the tumor-host dynamics any better? I do not know many experienced pathologists who take such claims seriously. Cancer specialists are thrilled with this promise and talk animatedly as they stake out their new territories. These specialists have little tolerance for those who think there are viable alternatives to chemotherapy drugs. Tumor markers provide them with new tools with which to intimidate all those who may challenge them.

Some large elk bones by the trail ended my reverie. Where did the flesh go? Torn clean of the bones by predators—the food cycle! What will happen to the bones? Eventually, they will disintegrate into calcium, phosphorus, magnesium, boron and other minerals that will be recycled into other living beings. And so the food cycle will go on and on. Of all people, the Chinese have the clearest ideas of food cycles in nature. They bring up their children right, feeding them every part of the food, the meat, blood, skin, connective tissue of the joints and cartilage. It matters little whether the animal comes from the mountain or the sea. Everything is cycled *completely.* They eat their foods fresh, cooked quickly and served steaming hot. But the Chinese face new threats that I'm not sure they can cope with. (During a recent trip to China, we saw American fast-food outlets in all major Chinese cities. It saddened us to see Chinese toddlers digging their little white teeth into American-style deep-fried chicken, cheeseburgers and French fries. What was in that food? Oxidized fats, denatured proteins, starch soaked in a whirlpool of toxic fats, and large quantities of salt. If that does not ruin the taste buds of little Chinese children, I don't know what will. Are the Chinese strong enough to withstand the American marketing genius? I wondered.)

COOKED COLLAGEN: THE CHINESE PRESCRIPTION FOR HEALTHY SKIN INJECTED COLLAGEN: THE AMERICAN PRESCRIPTION FOR WRINKLES

The Chinese are gracious hosts. Robert Bradford, an eminent cancer researcher from San Diego, his wife Carole Bradford, my wife Talat and I got a glimpse of their hospitality during one of our trips to Liu Hua Qiao General Hospital, Guanzhou. Generals Xie Xiang Ao, M.D., Bing Wu He, M.D., and Mei Gong, M.D.—all senior members of the hospital staff—introduced us to many aspects of traditional Chinese concepts of nutrition and of cooking methods. The Chinese also believe in the wisdom of the Talmud: "Only after the Holy One, Blessed is He, created a remedy for the affliction did He send the affliction." General He told us that the animal feet and joints (with their rich content of collagen) are good for preserving the fair condition of the skin and for ailments of the joints.

I thought about my father, who increased the frequency of a collagen-rich dish made with well-cooked feet of sheep and goat whenever he felt out of sorts. Then I thought about the damaged tissues and scars I have seen in pathology specimens where plastic surgeons injected collagen for cosmetic enhancement. Some enhancement!

TO WHOM DO OUR CELLS BELONG?

When a child has strep throat and we kill the bugs with penicillin, where do the tiny carcasses of the bugs go? Who eats them up? What happens to the bits of their DNA and their enzymes? Injured bacteria are like rabid dogs. They ferociously attack human enzyme defense systems, such as the cytochrome P-450 system. Such bacteria—sometimes referred to as cell wall-deficient forms—are resistant to our antibiotics. They continue to damage a child's immune system long after his pediatrician thinks the problem is over. And what happens to viruses after they camouflage themselves within human DNA molecules where enzymes cannot reach them? Do our cells belong to us or to the viruses? How many types of infectious diseases are there? Thousands? Maybe more. How do bugs cause diseases? What are the initial energetic-molecular events involved in that process? We talk about specific infectious diseases caused by specific microbes, but do we know why the same microbe kills some people, makes others very sick, barely touches others, and leaves others totally unaffected? What do microbes know that we do not?

In the prevailing model of drug medicine, biopsies are performed to diagnose a disease, then treatment with the drug of choice follows—Choua's N^2D^2 medicine.

Where do diseases come from anyway? Do they actually come from Mount Olympus as in Choua's story? Or from mythical Atlantis, sunk deep in the Atlantic ocean? How do diseases arrive? Do they arrive neatly packaged and clearly labeled—the same way that our disease doctors of drug medicine treasure them. Do healthy cells ever go to sleep one evening and wake up sick the next morning? Is that how diseases begin? Do healthy cells ever suddenly pronounce themselves dead?

There must be something in between—something that separates a state of disease from a state of absence of health—a state in which there is absence of disease *and* absence of health. A person in this state knows he is not well, but the physician is not convinced that his patient suffers from any disease—the old all-in-the-head standby.

If a state of absence of health separates a state of health from a state of disease, then that must be our focus in preventive medicine. Could it be that the key to understanding the beginning of disease is in understanding the state of absence of health? Could it be the reason we do not understand the beginning of any disease in mainstream medicine is because we reject that such a state can exist?

ABSENCE OF HEALTH

This state of absence of health must hold the key to understanding where diseases might begin. Why is it that no one in medicine is interested in this state? Why doesn't anyone conduct research to define this state? Why isn't there any research funding for it?

People talk about doing preventive medicine with Pap smears, mammograms, colonoscopies and such things. But that is detecting diseases at early stages. Early detection is not the same disease prevention. True disease prevention must be based on a genuine understanding of the state of absence of disease before disease is present.

Near the parking lot where the trail began, I felt uneasy. I realized I had a slight headache. Aha! That's why we doctors don't like to think about where our diseases might come from—it gives us a headache. I spoke out loud. Drugs for diseases; that's so much simpler.

Back in my hotel room, I looked out. The water of Yellowstone Lake glistened and glowed under the rays of a low setting sun. I watched the water in silence for some time. On the way to the dining room, I realized the calm lake water had finally eased out of my mind the troublesome thoughts about diseases and the state of absence of health. My head was uncluttered, the headache gone.

****

On my return, I tried to relate my mountain experience to Talat. We were in the kitchen, she at the stove and I at the table. She listened to me patiently, turned and spoke softly,

"So? You got the word at the mountain that diseases do not descend from mountains! Where did you think diseases came from anyway?" She went back to her stove.

"You don't understand," I protested.

"Understand what? That diseases do not descend from mountains!" she said indifferently, without looking away from the stove.

"No! No! It's not that," I said with urgency in my voice.

"It's not that? So what is it then?" she turned and held my eyes.

"It's not that simple!" I said defensively.

"What's not that simple?" She looked a little puzzled.

"If we accept that diseases do not descend from mountains, then we have to search for their causes in our internal and external environments."

"What's wrong with that?"

"You don't understand."

"Understand what?" she asked with irritation.

"Don't you see! Searching for the causes of disease in internal and external environments is looking for answers in nutritional medicine and environmental medicine. And you know what drug medicine thinks of that."

"Quackery?"

"Yes. It isn't the sort of thing that..." I stopped in midsentence.

"Sort of thing that?" she pressed on.

"Sort of thing that one hears about in hospital conferences."

"What sort of things? Dizzy ideas on mountaintops? The type of ideas one might have when suffering from anoxia of high altitudes?" she laughed a little.

"Maybe," I mused. "But this simple idea challenges the fundamentals of drug medicine. It calls for a radically new approach to health and disease. We will need to break many intellectual barriers. We cannot hide behind disease names as we do now. Can you imagine what doctors would think if I said something like that at a hospital conference?"

"What?"

"That I have gone nuts."

"Have you?" she smiled impishly.

The concept that the absence of disease does not always indicate the presence of health should be the simplest to understand. Yet from extensive work with my colleagues in mainstream medicine, I know that in fact this is the hardest of all conceptual changes for them to make.

The truth of the matter is that the above simple notion strikes at the heart of drug medicine's dogma.

There are two principal reasons why we physicians are not interested in the absence of health. First, no drugs have yet been invented to cure the absence of health. Similarly, no surgical procedures have been developed for this purpose. Because we can only treat diseases with drugs and scalpels, and because no drugs and surgical procedures are yet available for treating the absence of health, we physicians have a problem. If we accept that the absence of disease is not always presence of health, and that we do not even understand what this state is, then it follows that someone else—such as nutritionist-quacks—have to care for such people with methods that do not employ drugs and scalpels. Oy vey!

LOSING FACE, LOSING REVENUE

How can we physicians accept that we do not understand

something as elementary as the absence of health? What a loss of face! We are supposed to be the healers—the preservers of health. For centuries, our predecessors claimed to be more interested in disease prevention than in curing diseases. Yet for decades, I have heard visiting professors unfailingly begin their lectures with a few words about disease prevention only to spend the following hour extolling the virtues of their favorite drugs—always the ones manufactured by the drug companies that paid for the lecture. And now this! We have to admit that there is something out there—absence of health—that cannot be managed with the miracles of our synthetic chemistry. And that we have to face the humility of watching some non-physicians take care of this problem. What a problem! What a loss of face!

The second problem created by this mischief of absence of disease is equally daunting for the disease doctors of drug medicine. If we were to acknowledge that the state of absence of health is a valid issue, and that non-physicians can effectively address it—and get paid for it—that would be a major loss of revenue for us, wouldn't it? It could carve out areas of rich profitability from our work. No! That mustn't be allowed. Why not simply dismiss the very idea that absence of disease is not always presence of health. Nip the evil in the bud!

We physicians are trained to stamp out diseases. Diseases are what we thrive upon. Diseases are what we make our livelihoods from. And diseases, we have been firmly taught, can only be treated with drugs or surgical scalpels. Any method of treatment that does not include the *scientific* use of drugs or scalpels, we have been warned over and over again, is quackery. A physician's reputation is his most treasured asset, (so went the cliche in medical school), and we must zealously guard it at all times. Quacks must be shunned! No. They must be banished, their licenses revoked. And if that doesn't work, there are prisons for such miscreants.

And so it is that we continue to pour billions of dollars into research that gives us two things: 1) new names for old afflictions (so we can claim to be *up* on current research); and 2) new and increasingly potent (and toxic) drugs so that we can be judged progressive. We are very uncomfortable with the idea that something may indeed lie between our diseases and the presence of health that is outside our realm of expertise—an area of absence of health, a pre-disease state of dis-ease. We contemptuously dismiss all concepts in medicine that do not inevitably lead to the use of one or more drugs. We relentlessly persecute—and prosecute—all those who espouse ideas of health outside the domain of drugs.

> ## ESTABLISHED DISEASES, WITH SOME EXCEPTIONS, ARE NOT SUDDEN DEPARTURES FROM HEALTH

The diseases of our times are burdens on biology—and heavy drains on our antioxidant defenses—caused by stress, poor nutrition, sensitivity to environmental pollutants, allergy, lack of fitness, and susceptibility to viruses, bacteria and other microbes.

Stress is an integral part of our biology. It is an ever-changing mosaic of interrelated energetic-molecular events. Stress and anaphylaxis, it seems, belong more to Chaos physics (the new physics of turbulence) rather than to the established Newtonian model. Nature designed the stress response for a survival advantage. Nature also gave us built-in mechanisms to switch off this reaction when it has served its purpose. But today's lifestyles are subject to unrelenting stress. Before we can turn off the stress reaction to one stressor, we are confronted with another.

Drugs cannot remove stress. Drugs are not acceptable long-term substitutes for Nature's own molecular balancing acts. Drugs only suppress symptoms and postpone the inevitable tissue injury inflicted by unrelenting stress.

Our nutrition is in double jeopardy. Our food is often depleted of nutrients. Each meal challenges our biology with pesticides, insecticides and antibiotics. Tissue damage caused by these elements, while slow to appear, is cumulative.

Drugs dull our sensitivity to subtle but progressive impairment caused by nutrition problems.

Moreover, in synthetic chemicals, we are wreaking havoc with the environment. The statistics for global environmental pollution are staggering. The incidence of environmental illness is rising at an alarming rate as is the occurrence of the classical hay fever type of allergy.

Drugs compound the problems caused by environmental illness and allergy.

Life in our time is robbing us of spontaneity in our physical activities. The recent emphasis on fitness is promising. Still, I see many athletically oriented young women and men who suffer from chronic fatigue. I do not think that athletics alone can spare us from the hazards of modern living. Drugs are not acceptable remedies for the lack of energy and vitality.

I close this chapter on a promising note. As physicians and people gain a genuine understanding of the energy dynamics of health and disease, there will be a growing emphasis on the critical distinction between absence of disease and presence of health. Such understanding will foster those practices that promote health. There will also be a promising growth of technologies that focus on early energetic-molecular events separating a state of health from a state of absence of health. I return to this subject in chapters Sixth Insight and Seventh Insight.

Chapter 5

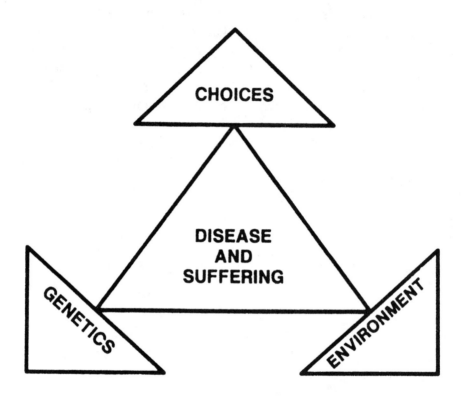

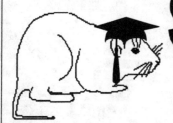

SECOND INSIGHT

Spontaneity of Oxidation
in Nature is the
True Cause of Aging
in humans and the
Root Cause of all Disease

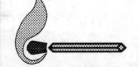

Prayer

is the best antioxidant

The scientific basis for this is simple:

Adrenaline is one of the most potent, if not *the* most potent, oxidant molecule in the human body.

Prayer and meditation is the best way to *down-regulate* adrenaline production.

Oxidation is Nature's grand design to make certain that no life form lives forever.

Oxidation—the loss of electrons, in scientific jargon—is a spontaneous phenomenon; it requires no outside prompts nor does it involve expenditure of energy. By contrast, reduction, the process that provides counterbalance to spontaneous oxidation, requires expenditure of energy. *The spontaneity of oxidation is—without any doubt in my mind—the basic cause of aging. Furthermore, accelerated oxidative molecular damage is the root cause of all illnesses.*

In medicine, it is prudent to shy away from theories that attempt to explain a large number of biologic phenomena by a single concept. The probability of being right would drop precipitously if anyone was to propose that *all* diseases are caused by the same fundamental event. And, yet, that is exactly what I propose in this chapter. I have many sound reasons for doing so. In this chapter, I marshall extensive evidence developed by a large number of researchers of oxidative injury as the cause of disease. I also present many of my research and clinical observations of accelerated oxidative molecular injury that eventually causes clinical disease. Finally, I describe direct evidence of oxidative injury to blood cell membranes and blood plasma proteins that—in my view—provide incontrovertible evidence to support my theory that all diseases are caused by accelerated oxidative molecular and cellular injury.

OXYGEN:
THE MOLECULAR DR. JEKYLL AND MR. HYDE

Oxygen launches, sustains, damages and terminates life. The essential molecular duality of oxygen holds the key to understanding human biology—how we stay well when we are healthy and how we get sick when we are ill. In clinical medicine, we usually have a clear understanding of the essential need for oxygen, but we rarely concern ourselves with the destructive potential of oxygen.

Living things that are capable of utilizing oxygen are composed of two families of molecules: 1) one family that makes certain that no life form lives forever. [I call these molecules aging oxidative molecules (AOMs)]; and 2) another family that makes sure that living beings have a chance to live out their normal life spans. [I call these molecules life span molecules (LSMs)]. The balance between AOMs and LSMs, in essence, is the basic equation of life.

Dr. Jekyll oxygen is molecular oxygen—atmospheric oxygen that sustains life. Mr. Hyde oxygen is nascent oxygen—atomic, toxic oxygen that kills life. The essential tragedy of our time is this: Our technology is rapidly turning life-sustaining, molecular oxygen into life-destroying, nascent oxygen. To solve the health problems caused by unbridled nascent oxygen, we use drugs that further increase its oxidant effects.

Below, I reproduce some text from *The Canary and*

Chronic Fatigue that will serve as a framework for a brief discussion of this essential issue:

A conversation I had with my research colleague, Madhava Ramanarayanan, Ph.D. (Dr. Ram) stands out vividly in my memory. In the late 1970s and early 1980s, Dr. Ram and I developed the IgE micro-elisa assay, for the diagnosis of inhalant allergy and the IgG micro-elisa assay, for monitoring the efficacy of immunotherapy for such disorders. We often had long discussions about where and how such allergies might begin. One day, Dr. Ram and I were going out for lunch, when he abruptly stopped and asked me to wait for him while he quickly changed the buffer for one of our research projects.

"Ram, what would happen if you didn't change the buffer?" I asked, without really looking for an answer.

"It wouldn't work that well," Ram answered without hesitation, as he walked to his refrigerator.

"Why, Ram? Why wouldn't the old buffer work well?" I asked.

"Because old buffers become stale," Ram replied.

"So? What's the problem with stale buffers?" I asked absent-mindedly.

"Stale buffers don't work well."

"Why don't stale buffers work as well?" I pressed.

I still don't know why on that day of all days I demanded answers to such mundane questions. Every child who has ever conducted a science experiment in school knows the answer. Everyone knows stale buffers don't work well, just like everyone knows fresh fruit tastes better than those that are overripe and spoiled. I didn't expect Ram to answer my question, and he didn't. Sometime during lunch, Ram suddenly asked me if I'd been serious about my questions concerning buffers.

"Yes, I am. Tell me why stale buffers don't work as well."
"Because they get oxidized," Ram answered.
"Why do buffers get oxidized?" I asked, still not knowing where my questions were going to take me.
"They just do!" Ram shrugged his shoulders.

We forgot about our seemingly trivial conversation on the capacity of buffers and the decreased capacity of stale buffers. But some days later, Dr. Ram casually asked me if I wanted to know why buffers get oxidized.

"Oh yes! Tell me, why do buffers get oxidized?" I asked.
"Because oxidation is a spontaneous process," Ram answered calmly.
"What? What did you say, Ram?" I felt a jolt.
"Oxidation is a spontaneous process," Dr. Ram repeated in his usual tone.

FRESH FRUIT SPOILS WITH TIME, BUT WHY DON'T SPOILED FRUITS GET UNSPOILED WITH TIME?

Buffers become spontaneously oxidized with time. Why don't oxidized buffers become spontaneously unoxidized with time? Fresh fruit spoils spontaneously with time, everyone knows that. Why doesn't spoiled fruit spontaneously get "unspoiled" with time? Why are the chemical changes involved in the oxidation of buffers and the spoiling of fruits unidirectional? Fish hooked out of water rots within hours at room temperature. Why doesn't the rotting fish spontaneously become "unrotten"? Cut, wet grass decomposes spontaneously in some days. Why doesn't the decomposed grass spontaneously "undecompose" in the days that follow? Butter turns rancid spontaneously. Why doesn't rancid butter later become "unrancid" spontaneously? And, for that matter, how is it that the word "undecompose" doesn't exist in the English language? At least, I don't remember anyone ever using it in spoken language or in writing.

These thoughts hit me with the force of a lightning bolt. These simple questions never arose in my mind during all those years of biology classes in high school and college. Nor did they take form during years of my search for the cause of disease, as I spent long hours studying microscopic slides. Now, for the first time, I suddenly saw the possibility of an answer to that most fundamental of all questions. *Oxidation is a spontaneous process—that means it requires no outside cues or external programming.* Fresh fruits get spoiled because they are oxidized spontaneously. Spoiled fruit doesn't get unspoiled because it doesn't have the energy reserve to do so. Butter when left at room temperature spontaneously turns rancid. Rancid butter cannot turn unrancid for the same reason.

THE GREAT KILLER MOLECULE

Oxygen is a killer molecule. Oxidant molecules are like little matches, ready to put things on fire when lit. A match can burn out the whole forest. How? It is ignited by oxygen, and the oxyradical formation triggered by this process perpetuates the process of burning. Nature designed life span molecules to provide a counterbalance to the oxidant molecules. These molecules prevent ignition by oxygen and hold in check other types of oxidant molecules. Living things generate these molecules so they can save themselves from immediate destruction by oxidant molecules.

REDUCTION REQUIRES EXPENDITURE OF ENERGY

The opposite of oxidation is reduction—a process by which atoms and molecules gain electrons. The "loss" by oxidation is balanced with the "gain" of reduction during life.

Living things live because they can expend energy. It is the energy of reduction that provides a counterbalance to oxidant stress, the essence of the aging process. How long the reduction arm of the redox reaction can hold in abeyance the oxidative arm determines how long a rose will bloom and how long an elephant will live. How effectively the reductive arm restrains the oxidative arm determines how fast we recover from a viral infection or from an incision made by a surgeon. The success of our antioxidant energy dynamics determines how well we cope with the progressive oxidant stress of environmental pollutants, allergic triggers, toxic metal overload, metabolic roller coasters, musculoskeletal stresses that arise from physical inactivity, and the potent oxyradicals released by the "fight or flight" stress response. This is the beginning of the state of dis-ease that when not corrected results in diseases.

OXIDATION IS NATURE'S GRAND DESIGN TO MAKE SURE NOTHING LIVES FOREVER

I wrote the above line in *The Butterfly and Life Span Nutrition* because this simple insight provided me with the scientific basis for my model of aging-oxidant and life span molecules. Aging-oxidant molecules exist to make sure no life form lives forever, and—when not counterbalanced—they cause premature aging and disease. Life span molecules promote health and prevent accelerated aging by holding in abeyance the aging-oxidant molecules. I included this statement in *The Ghoraa and Limbic Exercise* for the same reason—it allowed me to consider my own experience with different types of physical exercises in relation to the larger perspective of energy dynamics in human physiology. I include it here for the third time because this statement more than any other provides the sound scientific framework for my clinical work with chronic fatiguers.

OXIDATIVE THEORY OF AGING

Two main theories have been proposed to explain the basic chemical nature of the aging process in humans. In the 1950s, Bjorksten, a well-known chemist, proposed that tissues age when their proteins are denatured by a process called cross-linking. Proteins are thread-like molecules that are being constantly clipped into pieces and then assembled again. When the assembly of broken pieces is defective, the protein molecules may be pieced together in abnormal fashion, creating defective or cross-linked molecules. There is strong experimental support for this view. The question for me has been this: How do proteins get damaged in the first place? My unequivocal answer: by oxidative damage.

The second theory, which was put forth by Harmon, a well-known free radical researcher, held that free radical damage was the root cause of the aging process. Again, the question for me was this: How are free radicals generated? My unequivocal answer: by oxidative damage. Thus, I conclude that the true nature of the aging process is spontaneity of oxidation in nature. Several observations—some made clinically in my medical work and some others made in common occurrences of life—gave me a clear understanding of the larger role of oxidation in nature. I discuss the evolution of my thinking about the relationship of spontaneity of oxidation in nature to the root cause of degenerative and immune disorders at length in *The Canary and Chronic Fatigue*.

What is optimal nutrition for the entire life span? A low-fat, high-carbohydrate diet, as preached by some gurus of the dieting industry? A high-fat, no-carbohydrate plan that some others profess? A high-complex carbohydrate diet? A 60-20-20 diet? (60% starches, 20% fats, 20% proteins). A low-calorie diet? A low, low-calorie diet? A low, low, low-calorie diet? A rice diet? An ice-cream diet? There is really no limit to such absurdities.

Foods like people have life spans. Foods, like people, get injured. Foods, like people, get spontaneously oxidized. Indeed, the health disorders caused by denatured and processed foods are oxidative in nature. In my view, optimal food plans for the entire life span cannot be understood without holding spontaneity of oxidation in food substances as the centerpiece of all considerations. I devote the companion volume *The Butterfly and Life Span Nutrition* to this issue.

These questions and answers swirled in my mind's eye in flashes of images. Then other images followed. Images of damaged cells, decaying tissues, decomposed organs. The images of rancid butter merged with those of lipid peroxidation of fats in the cell membrane, and the images of decomposed cut grass mingled with those of decaying cells and dead tissues with pockets of pus. It was a high-speed kaleidoscopic view of injured things.

With time, I became convinced of the theoretical validity of my opinion that oxidation causes aging. I also recognized that the experimental and clinical data from diverse fields of inquiry in medicine and biology were entirely consistent with my viewpoint. It was now just a matter of time before I would recognize the oxidative nature of injury to the energy enzyme systems of human energy pathways. *It couldn't be anything other than oxidant molecular injury*. It was *that* simple.

Here, then, was the possibility for me to reduce the many complex issues of aging, nutritional and ecologic disorders and degenerative diseases to two simple manageable questions:

1. What is the energetic-molecular basis of the aging process in humans?

2. Could it be that the cause of all disease is related in some way to the basic nature of the aging process—and that different diseases are but different expressions of the same oxidative phenomenon? Genes may favor one or the other body organ to bear the brunt of accelerated oxidative

injury, but the essential nature of oxidative injury is the same.

In this chapter, I will relate how these two fundamental questions led me to regard all chronic immune, ecologic, nutritional and degenerative disorders in an altogether different light.

Oxidative Theory of Coronary Heart Disease

Drug medicine in the U.S. holds that the basic cause of coronary heart disease is not known, and assumes that it is an irreversible disease. Both are tragic errors.

I propose the theory that coronary artery disease *is* caused by accelerated oxidative injury, and it *is* reversible.

Cholesterol cats—the money men of cholesterol industry—have blamed coronary heart disease on cholesterol for decades. This theory has served them well. The business of cholesterol testing and cholesterol-lowering drugs has been enormously profitable for them. And there are more profits to be made in selling drugs for treating heart disease. When these measures fail—and they always fail predictably—the patient is passed on to coronary "angioplasterers" and coronary bypassers for their share.

Cholesterol-lowering drugs and other cardiac drugs used to manage coronary artery disease do not reverse coronary artery disease.

Coronary angioplasty—as necessary as it may be for a small number of patients with impending cardiac crises—does not reverse coronary artery disease.

Coronary bypass surgery—if it is ever truly necessary—does not reverse coronary artery disease.

These are crucially important messages for the sufferers of coronary artery disease.

Natural, unoxidized cholesterol is an innocent and an essential molecule. Why would Nature assign cholesterol so many essential roles in preserving the functional and structural integrity of cell membranes and in hormone synthesis if it were such an evil molecule? The cells that line the blood vessels do not have any receptors for natural, unoxidized cholesterol; they do have such hooks for oxidized and denatured cholesterol molecules. Natural, unoxidized cholesterol molecules are not found in the plaques that block arteries. Only oxidatively damaged molecules exist there. The blood of patients who have advanced coronary artery disease does not contain any antibodies against natural, unoxidized cholesterol; it does contain antibodies against oxidized cholesterol. There are yet other strong lines of evidence against the mistaken belief that cholesterol causes heart attacks. A small number of people with hereditary disorders who run blood cholesterol levels of several hundred mg/dl, of course, are exceptions to this. Their coronary arteries are damaged by the enormous overload of abnormal lipids in the blood. Again, none of the cholesterol-lowering drugs has ever been shown to prevent disease in such individuals.

Coronary artery disease is reversible. The effective strategies for this purpose include: 1) optimal choices in the kitchen; 2) slow, sustained exercise; 3) meditation and self-regulatory methods for slowing the heart; 4) avoidance of

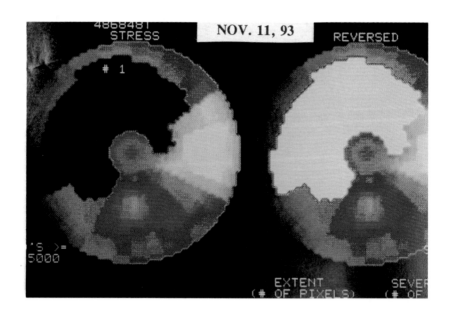

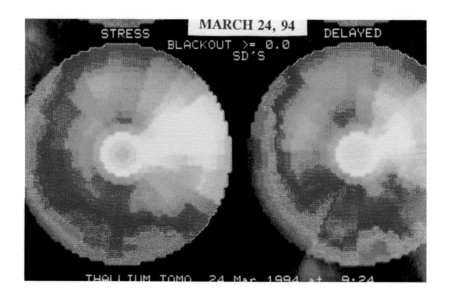

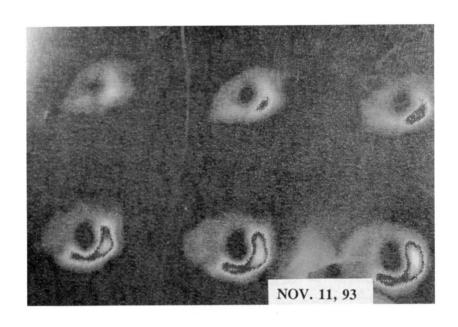

NOV. 11, 93

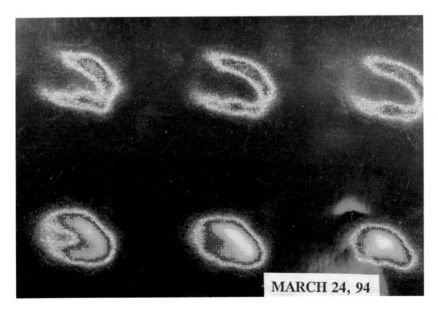

MARCH 24, 94

Below I reproduce the first (to my knowledge) photomicrographs of immunostained *Candida* yeast organisms in circulating blood of a patient with chronic fatigue. The yeast bodies appear dark with stain (identified with arrows) in the upper picture, while the organisms disappear in the lower dark-field picture (sugar in the yeast wall does not reflect light). The two bright bodies in both pictures are red blood cells which do not take up the immunostain. The lipid layer of these cells reflects light well and so they appear bright. For detailed description of immunostaining method, see page 454.

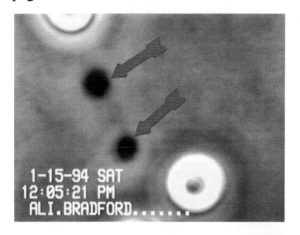

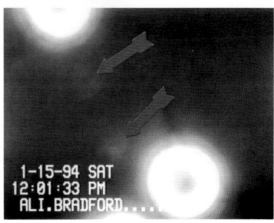

The three biologic profiles given below illustrate electromagnetic dynamics of health and disease: 1) a spiking, stressful, disease-causing, cortical profile (upper); 2) an even, health-promoting, limbic profile during autoregulation (lower right); and a composite profile showing conversion of limbic mode (right side) into cortical mode (left side) when autoregulation ends (lower left). For detailed descriptions, see pages 325-7.

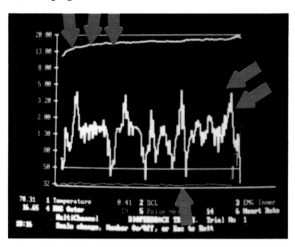

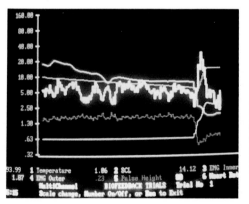

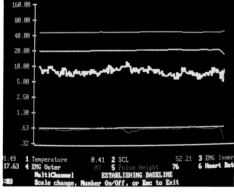

environmental triggers that cause adrenaline and neurotransmitter roller coasters; and 5) integrated programs to normalize the cell membranes of cardiac muscle and coronary arteries with intravenous infusions of EDTA (ethylene diamine tetraacetic acid) and related chelating agents as well as certain key minerals and amino acids.

I discuss this subject at length in the companion volume *The Chirri, Cholesterol Cats and Chelation for the Heart*. Here, I briefly illustrate the potential of chelation therapy with EDTA (ethylene diamine tetraacetic acid) for reversal of coronary artery disease with an actual case history.

A man in his early fifties underwent coronary angiography for angina attacks and was told he had nearly blocked off one of the main coronary arteries. The thallium scan showed defects in blood circulation to all walls of the left chamber of his heart. He was advised to undergo coronary angioplasty, which he declined. Instead, he chose to follow our heart disease reversal program.

The following table and pictures of his heart scans before and five months after beginning our program clearly demonstrate the reversal of his coronary artery disease.

REVERSAL OF CORONARY DISEASE: DEFECTS IN BLOOD SUPPLY BEFORE AND FOUR MONTHS AFTER BEGINNING A HEART DISEASE REVERSAL PROGRAM		
Area of Heart	**Before**	**After**
Anterior Wall	Present	Absent
Posterior Wall	Absent	Absent
Septal	Present	*
Inferior Wall	Present	Absent
Lateral Wall	Present	Absent
Apex	Present	Absent

* Small minimally reversing (radiologist's wording in the scan report)

At the time of this writing, the patient has been free of any angina attacks or other heart-related symptoms for more than 13 months after the above studies were performed.

A reliable method for evaluating the adequacy of blood circulation in the heart muscle is a thallium heart perfusion scan. In this scan, radioactive thallium is injected in the vein and scan pictures of the different parts of the heart are obtained at short intervals when thallium begins to enter the vessels in the heart muscle. Thus, the presence of thallium in the heart muscle scan indicates good blood supply. When plaque formation in the coronary arteries obstructs blood flow to any part of the heart muscle, the scan shows absence of thallium.

With modern scan technology, the presence or absence of thallium in the heart muscle can be graphically demonstrated with color pictures of the heart—red and orange colors indicating the presence of blood and black and blue colors showing absence of blood.

HEART SCANS BEFORE AND FOUR MONTHS AFTER HEART DISEASE REVERSAL PROGRAM

For the patient described in the present case history, thallium heart scans were obtained before and five months after beginning our total heart disease reversal program. Those scans are reproduced with explanatory comments on the next four pages.

In the thallium scan pictures shown on the opposite page, note the dramatic differences between the blood supply to the heart muscle before and after EDTA chelation therapy shown. The large black area in the pretreatment scan picture (November, 1993) represents a large area of the heart muscle that is totally devoid of blood. Such areas without any blood supply are in imminent danger of undergoing tissue death due to lack of blood supply—myocardial infarction in medical jargon—that causes acute heart attacks. In the postchelation scan picture (March, 1994), the red and yellow colors in the previously black area brilliantly indicate restoration of blood circulation to the endangered heart muscle. See color plates on page 210.

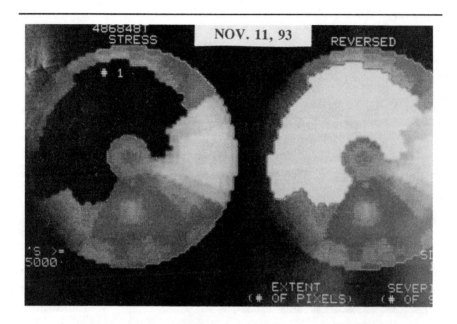

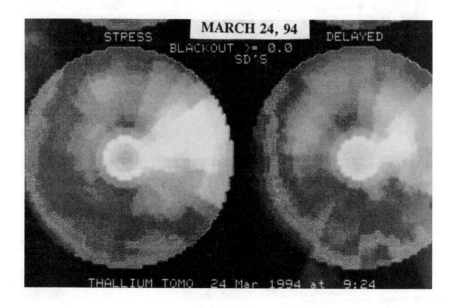

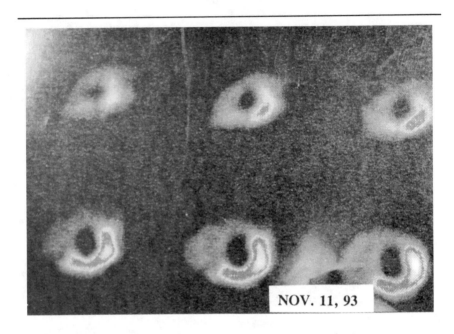

NOV. 11, 93

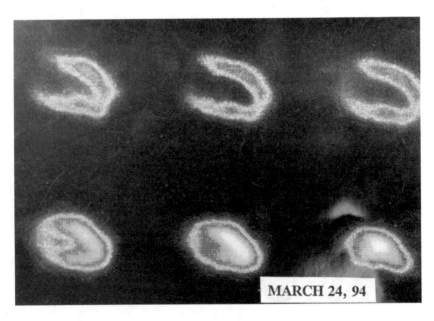

MARCH 24, 94

The two thallium heart scans shown on the opposite page represent pretreatment and postchelation color pictures of the various levels of the left heart chamber showing the status of blood supply. As in the first set of color scan pictures on the preceding pages, note the dramatic differences in the blood supply to heart muscle. The black and blue colors in the pretreatment (November, 1993) indicate absence or near-absence of blood circulation in most segments of the heart muscle. By contrast, the postchelation pictures show impressive restoration of blood supply to the once blood-starved heart muscle.

Not every patient should expect such a dramatic reversal of coronary artery disease in that short a period of time. Notwithstanding, it is a powerful, graphic demonstration of the potential benefit of a comprehensive, holistic heart disease reversal program that is based on a clear understanding of the true oxidative nature of the problem of coronary artery disease, and that includes effective chelation therapy.

I do not think that such a dramatic response can be attributed to a complete clearing of the plaques that clogged the main coronary artery. Rather, the observed changes are due to addressing all the issues of accelerated oxidative damage to the heart vessels. First and foremost, I repeat for emphasis, a good heart disease reversal program must focus on *normalization* of the energy dynamics at the cell membrane of the muscle, nerve and endothelial cells in the heart. Those are the sites at which oxidative damage jeopardizes life, and those are sites that our therapies must focus on.

I have had rather extensive experience with caring for patients with advanced coronary artery disease. To date, all those who closely followed the total program and were able to take 30 or more infusions have shown very satisfactory clinical responses. Specifically,

1. Absence of angina attacks or far fewer and less severe episodes.
2. Absence of heart palpitations or far fewer and less severe episodes.
3. Discontinuance of most cardiac drugs or a markedly reduced dosage.
4. Avoidance of coronary angioplasty or bypass surgery.

5. Increased depth of sleep.
6. A general sense of well-being.
7. Reduced fear of an impending catastrophe.
8. Decreased bowel transit time.

The last item may raise some eyebrows, but the integrity of the bowel ecosystem profoundly affects the cardiovascular status. For this reason, our heart disease reversal program puts special emphasis on restoring a damaged bowel ecosystem. I discuss this at length in the companion volume *Battered Bowel Ecology—Waving Away a Wandering Wolf.*

For general information, I include here brief comments about three patients.

An 82-year-old man with advanced coronary artery disease, history of multiple heart attacks and intractable congestive heart failure died nine days after receiving a single EDTA chelation infusion. I had some reservation for starting EDTA therapy under such circumstances. (His daughter asked me if I would have done so if he were my own father. When I said I would, she pleaded with me to do the same for her father.)

A woman in her mid-sixties consulted me for advanced coronary artery disease. She had undergone coronary artery bypass surgery a few years earlier. She lived under highly stressful circumstances, and continued to have angina attacks even after 11 infusions. She was persuaded by her cardiologist to undergo angioplasty. (Can angioplasty guarantee freedom from more attacks under these conditions? I seriously doubt that.)

A man in his early sixties suffered from extensive

obstructive lesions of his coronary arteries. He was advised to have an angioplasty. He learned about the chelation option and came to see me. He seemed very troubled by the fact that if chelation therapy was really of any value, why didn't the cardiologist do it. It is understandable how this question disturbs patients who do not know of any good program for reversal of coronary artery disease that employs EDTA chelation therapy, and who suddenly are forced to make a quick decision by their angioplasterers. I described in detail our total program and the role of EDTA chelation therapy, and asked him to return after he had discussed this option with his family and his cardiologist. I didn't oppose the idea of angioplasty for him. (Predictably, his cardiologist forcefully told him to avoid charlatans in medicine.) He was extremely distraught during the second visit, and expressed much frustration at being forced to make a critical decision on such short notice. He received one EDTA infusion and didn't return. Several months later, I learned that he suffered a heart attack several days after I saw him.

Patients with serious heart disease can ill-afford such conflicts. Discovery of serious heart disease is a highly stressful event. Conflict about the right choice can exaggerate the stress to dangerous degrees. Cardiologists, of all specialists, should be more sensitive to this conflict. Yet, a rare cardiologist has the courage to admit that he knows nothing about chelation therapy for heart disease, and advises his patients to seek proper advice from those well-versed in such procedures.

I know many readers—those who suffer from heart disease as well as those who care for patients with heart disease—will find the above comments disconcerting. It is indeed sad that this inexpensive and effective therapy is withheld while expensive procedures such as angioplasty and coronary bypass that do nothing to reverse the underlying cause of coronary artery disease are performed with high frequency and without impunity. The reader may ask the obvious question: If EDTA chelation therapy is really effective, why isn't it available to every patient with coronary artery disease. The answer is that their cardiologists are sadly misinformed about the clinical value of EDTA chelation therapy.

My patients often relate to me, in good humor, a question that their cardiologist frequently ask them: If chelation was really effective, why wouldn't I use it? Here are seven questions that I suggest patients ask their cardiologist who advise them against EDTA chelation therapy:

1. *Do you understand how coronary artery disease is caused at the energetic-molecular level?*
2. *Do you understand the physiologic basis of EDTA chelation therapy?*
3. *Have you ever attended a conference in which the results of EDTA chelation therapy were presented?*
4. *Have you ever treated any patients with EDTA chelation therapy?*
5. *Have you ever carefully assessed the clinical outcome of patients who received chelation therapy from other physicians?*
6. *Do you know everything that may be known about human biology?*
7. *Do you think it is moral or ethical for a physician to deny his patient a therapy just because he knows nothing about it?*

There are two chelation literatures: 1) A literature of

physicians like myself who observe good clinical results with EDTA chelation therapy in nearly all cases; and 2) A literature of drug doctors who never try this therapy themselves and are ever so ready to denounce it. A good exception was a recent mainstream report that reported clinical benefit in leg cramps while walking (claudication) with EDTA chelation (*Circulation* 90:1194; 1994). I relate Choua's comments concerning the placebo effects in this study in the chapter Prince Chaullah and Science in Medicine.

My clinical experience with this therapy has been most encouraging. I believe others will observe similar results—when chelation therapy is administered as part of a broad, holistic program for normalization of heart cell membranes that addresses all relevant issues of nutrition, environment and stress.

It is possible that with a much larger number of patients, my associates and I may not be able to maintain such an extraordinary record. But for now, our clinical charts are open for review by other physicians interested in our program (with necessary precautions to maintain patient confidentiality). As for the general public, any members of our rather large nursing staff may be consulted for verification.

I close this section with an interesting quote from the journal of the American Heart Association:

...there is an excess of cardiologists in this country. In the United States we have 6.5 cardiologists per 100,000 population; in Canada there are 2.5, in Germany 2.9; and in Great Britain 0.4 cardiologists per 100,000...despite more cardiac catheterizations, angioplasties, and coronary artery bypass procedures performed in the United States, the in-hospital death rate from acute myocardial infarction in the United States is similar to that of Canada.

Circulation 90:1102; 1994.

It is an eye-opening statement. But, of course, *Circulation* looks at the problem differently. On the following page, the journal recommends:

Reduction in cardiology training programs must be accomplished...An all-payer system should be established that will fully fund all accredited postgraduate medical education positions.

The journal is clearly not interested in the issues of appropriateness of therapy. After admitting that many unnecessary procedures are performed in this country, it focuses on issues of the number of cardiologists and the best payment system.

Oxidative Theory of cancer

The dogma of drug medicine holds that cancer results from gene mutation, and *assumes* that once such mutation occurs, it is irreversible. This viewpoint is tragically erroneous.

In this section, I briefly describe my theory that cancer is caused by oxidative molecular damage. Such damage may involve some genes as well as nongenetic cellular molecules such as enzymes that seam together DNA and RNA molecules from their components. Other nongenetic molecules such as proteins with regulatory roles may also be involved. This theory is consistent with my opinion that all diseases, except those triggered by trauma, are caused by oxidative damage. I will discuss this subject at length in a future volume of this series. Here, I briefly outline my theory and marshall evidence for it from diverse lines of theoretical, clinical and experimental observations.

Several cancers are associated with nutritional factors. Environmental factors have been incriminated in the cause of others. In experimental animal models, many types of cancers can be produced with viruses and carcinogenic chemicals. This is an age of gene manipulation, and enormous sums of money are committed to gene research each year. Some genes—oncogenes, as they are commonly called—are thought to trigger cancer formation. Certain genes—P 53 and related suppressor genes—have been ascribed protective roles against cancer. At present, the concept that genetic changes are irreversible and that genes govern cancer formation and growth is firmly entrenched in the drug medicine dogma. All efforts at cancer control are directed at developing new chemotherapy drugs and antibodies to destroy cancer cells.

Notwithstanding billions of dollars spent on cancer research, and a yet larger number of words written to publish the findings of such research, this approach has not worked nor does it have any chance of working. (Hodgkin's disease and some uncommon tumors are a few exceptions to this general rule.)

The fundamental question remains unanswered. What causes cancer? Cancer specialists invariably shrug and dismiss this question as both impertinent and an unwanted distraction in their pursuit of killing cancer with chemotherapy drugs.

GENES PRESERVE HEALTH, GENES MAKE EVOLUTION POSSIBLE

DNA in human cells provides the blueprint for approximately 60,000 proteins. These molecules are essential for human life in all its stages: at birth, during spurts of growth in infancy and childhood, immune defense against infections, wound healing, digestive-absorptive functions, energy and detoxification pathways, and eventually for decomposition and disintegration of tissues after death.

If DNA was copied flawlessly every time, there would have been no evolution—to evolve is to change and no change can be maintained for a long time except through a change in DNA configuration. Without DNA alterations, today we would have the same DNA as our genetic ancestors over three billion years ago—and the same physical characteristics as single-celled microbes that existed then.

If DNA is copied with a mistake, each copying error carries the risk of fatal structural or functional derangements. A common example of such an event is miscarriage—the spontaneously aborted fetus show evidence of DNA damage in most, if not all, instances.

Every second that passes, the DNA in each cell of your body is being damaged. Chemical bonds are breaking, DNA strands are snapping, and nucleotide bases are flying off. Each cell loses more than 10,000 bases per day just from spontaneous breakdown of DNA at body temperature. Meanwhile, many cells are dividing and therefore copying DNA, and each copy introduces the possibility of error.

Science 266:1926; 1994

Translation: Each DNA molecule in the body has 10,000 chances in a single day of becoming cancerous. Of the estimated 100 trillion cells in the body, we can conservatively assume that at least one in hundred cells in the body of a child—one trillion in all—divides every day. Since each break, loss or alteration in a DNA base can potentially cause cancer, it follows that a child may have as many as 10,000 trillion chances of a developing a cancer cell on a given day. Why, then, doesn't every child die of a cancer during childhood?

DNA copying occurs with an astounding accuracy—on the average, only three base pair mistakes are thought to occur when copying 3 billion base pairs of human genome (*Science* 266: 1925; 1994). This mind-numbing copying accuracy is assured by the most extraordinary DNA repair system composed of several enzymes. Thus, the reason all of us do not have cancer at all times is the enormous capacity of our DNA repair enzyme systems.

*This explains the primary difference between the philosophy of oncologists and holistic physicians. An o*ncologist strives to kill the last living cancer cell with chemotherapy drugs even when he knows that his therapy seriously damages patient's DNA repair enzyme system. Indeed, this explains how chemotherapy substantially increases the risk of second cancer. The holistic physicians, by contrast, seeks to facilitate body's own healing ability—or, in our present context, the DNA repair system of enzymes.

A CANCER CELL IS AN OXYPHOBE

In the early part of this century, Otto Warburg won the Nobel Prize for his studies that revealed that a cancer cell dislikes oxygen—is an "oxyphobe". It predominantly uses anaerobic metabolism in which little, if any, oxygen is utilized. His findings provide the molecular basis of biooxidative therapies such as ozone hemotherapy and hyperbaric oxygen therapy. It also explains the efficacy of a rather ingenious approach of directing oxygen-hating microbes such as clostridium to cancer where they relish cancer cells. Warburg further proclaimed that once a cell turns to an anaerobic mode—and hence becomes cancerous—it can never revert back to the normal aerobic mode. In other words, the cancerous transformation is a one-way street, and hence is irreversible. This, of course, fits into the prevailing notion that cancer at the cellular level is irreversible.

Warburg was right on one account (predominantly anaerobic, glycolytic mode of metabolism in cancer cells) but quite wrong on the other (the notion of irreversibility). Many studies, including those of surface charge normalization cited above, invalidate Warburg's view of irreversibility.

A CANCER CELL IS HIGHLY CHARGED

A cancer cell accumulates electrons on its cell surface. Excess electrons give its cell membrane a very strong negative surface charges—often two or more hundred times stronger than the -2-4 microvolts of healthy cells. Like charges repel. In a fight for space and privileges, however, the weak negative surface charge of an immune cell is no match for the highly negatively charged surface of a cancer cell. It is easy to see how the weak defending immune cell would be literally expected to be blown away by the ferocious cancer cell. This indeed happens. A cancer cell uses the strong surface charge as an effective electromagnetic shield against the attacking immune cells—unless of course, a cancer is vastly outnumbered by immune lymphocytes that band together to effectively sequester and cordon off the cancer cell. In some slow-growing cancers, I often see a band of immune cells forming a stout wall against cancer cells.

In 1949, highly negative charges were reported in cancer of the cervix (*Am J Obs Gyn* 57:274; 1949). Ten years later, control of the tumor by normalization of the surface charge on cancer cells was documented in mice (*Science* 130:388; 1959). This was an exciting possibility of turning a cancer cell back into its noncancer form by changing the surface charge. Many physicians in foreign countries jumped at this chance and developed charge neutralization technologies.

Why has the enormous potential of this simple method of reverting cancer cells back to health been totally ignored in the U.S.? I can only speculate.

First, in the United States we are incarcerated in the destructive mode of thinking—we like to poison cells with chemotherapy or burn them with radiotherapy. Surface charge neutralization is restorative, not quite fit for our consumption.

Second, we seem to have an aversion to using simple, low-cost physical methods of treatment of cancer.

Third, we are not inclined to look favorably at therapies developed in foreign countries—the old and arrogant not-invented-here (NIH) syndrome.

It is ironic that it costs some hundreds of dollars to build surface charge neutralization machines, but it would require hundreds of millions of dollars to get FDA approval to use such a machine. How well does charge neutralization technology work? Many foreign physicians have told me of good clinical responses in many instances. I return to this subject in the chapter, seventh

Insight.

A CANCER CELL BREATHES OXIDATIVE FIRES

Cancer cells—like the mythic Chinese dragons—breathe oxidative fires. They produce prodigious amounts of hydrogen peroxide—one to two hundred times as much as is produced in non-cancer cells. Indeed, even immune cells at the height of activity during their attack on microbes do not come close to cancer cells as regards the amounts of hydrogen peroxide produced.

Cancer cells—like the Greek crabs after which they are named—send out tiny projections that are in reality tentacles of oxidative coals, ready to light up the plasma proteins in oxidative flames. These projections are made up of tiny bits of the cell membrane as well as the cell soup of cancer cells. Frequently, these tentacles get pinched off, form complexes with clotting proteins such as Factor VII, and ignite the oxidative flames that engulf other clotting proteins such Factors IX and X. (Factors VII, IX and X are among the substances that are essential for normal blood clotting.) The end result of these reactions is that the cancer cells get surrounded by fibrin nets that protect them from natural killer and other immune cells that normally search and destroy errant cells including cancer cells. These reactions also break contact of cancer cells with other malignant cells that surround them. Thus, cancer cells are freed and begin to travel to other parts of the body, looking for new sites to seed and flourish.

Each cancer cell floating free in the blood, lymph and

tissue carries simmering oxidative coals, ready to burst into oxidative flames at the slightest provocation, thereby triggering further oxidative reactions.

> ### SIMPLE MOLECULES SELF-ASSEMBLE INTO AMINO ACIDS; AMINO ACIDS SELF-ASSEMBLE INTO FUNCTIONING PROTEINS

I have considerable difficulty accepting drug medicine's prevailing gene theory of cancer and the attendant notions of the irreversibility of cancer. There are several fundamental observations in chemistry that challenge assumptions made in the gene theory.

Do genes really control everything? If so, where do genes come from? In their famous 1953 experiment, Stanley Miller and Harold Urey of the University of Chicago subjected simple molecules such as ammonia, methane, hydrogen and water in a flask to repeated cycles of heating, electrification and cooling—conditions that are thought to have existed when life began on planet Earth. The experiment produced a crimson-colored primordial soup, rich in amino acids. Amino acids, of course, are the building blocks of proteins, including enzymes.

In subsequent years, origin-of-life research has been focused on the fundamental chemical mechanisms of prebiological molecules. Notable among these studies are those of Sidney Fox who clearly demonstrated that under primordial conditions, amino acids could self-assemble into proteins—without the intervention of genes. The next important step was to demonstrate whether or not proteins so formed could assemble themselves into tiny protein microspheres—the precursors of cells as we know them today. Experiments clearly showed that this assemblage does occur.

If the reactions within a sphere help make macromolecules, then we're talking about a cage in which thermal proteins could help build nucleic acids like RNA or DNA. Perhaps thermal proteins can also help synthesize true proteins...through this type of mechanism, cellular evolution could have arisen from microspheres.

Biologist Aristotle Pappelis
Quoted in *Science News* 146:59; 1994

I include these brief comments about the origin-of-life research to support my view that molecules have their own minds—their own sense of natural order of things. Simple molecules, such as ammonia and water, larger molecules, such as amino acids, and complex molecules such as proteins (including) enzymes, can assemble and disassemble themselves without any organizing influence of genes. Such observations challenge the notions of irreversibility of cancer cells of drug medicine.

Where does cancer begin? What are the initial energetic-molecular events that turn a healthy cell into a cancer cell? How does a cancer cell go into nonoxygen-utilizing mode—become an oxyphobe? How does it begin to produce prodigious amounts of hydrogen peroxide? How does it accumulate electrons on its surface and become strongly negatively charged?

AN OXYPHILE TURN INTO AN OXYPHOBE

Each cell has the biochemical machinery for behaving as a cancer cell. Each cancer cell has the capacity for "normalizing" its behavior. What is the evidence for my viewpoint?

A cancer cell is an aerobic healthy cell before it becomes a predominantly anaerobic cell—as a result of oxidative injury to its DNA, DNA repair enzymes and possibly some regulatory proteins according to the oxidative theory I propose in this volume. How does that happen?

In *The Canary and Chronic Fatigue,* I describe the evolution of aerobic (oxygen-utilizing) microbes from earlier anaerobic (nonoxygen-utilizing) life forms. The later aerobic microbes retain the DNA necessary for anaerobic existence of their predecessors. Thus, all an oxygen-utilizing cell requires to switch into a nonoxygen-utilizing mode is a reversion to its primitive mode. Does this ever happen? Of course, it does! A common example of this phenomenon is when a colon cancer cell reverts back to its earlier form, recalls a forgotten memory and begins to make CEA—carcinoembyonic antigen material used to diagnose colon and other cancers. Another common example of this phenomenon is when well-differentiated cancers lose their differentiation and become de-differentiated. Ontogeny follow phylogeny is the common scientific expression for such regression.

What turns a healthy "oxyphile" cell into a oxyphobe? Oxidative injury. I consider this a logical and inescapable conclusion drawn from a vast body of experimental and clinical data and my strong intuitive sense about it. I know this may be dismissed as sheer speculation by many, but I'm certain this viewpoint will be proven right in time.

EACH CELL IS A CANCER CELL, NO CELL IS A CANCER CELL

This is not a frivolous play on words. If a cancer cell was incapable of reverting back to its healthful form, the human race would have gone extinct a very long time ago. No child would have survived his childhood. What is the evidence for this?

Earlier in this section, I quote from *Science* a rate of 10,000 base hits inflicted on DNA in each cell in a day. Then I calculate the rate at which the cells in the body of a growing child will sustain DNA injury that can lead to clinical cancer. There are estimated 5,000 trillion chances that a DNA base hit that is not promptly repaired will develop into clinical cancer. Thus, within the energetic-molecular (E-M) perspective of DNA base injury, it can be defensibly argued that each cell is a cancer cell and that no cell is a cancer cell.

In my view, nothing in cancer theory and practice should be held more important than this. As I write earlier—and it bears repeating—this simple statement brings into sharp contrast the two opposing views of cancer therapies: the supportive and normalizing approach of the holistic community, and the destructive and "denormalizing" approach of chemotherapy.

A CANCER CELL
AND ITS MICROENVIRONMENT

The term tumor doubling time indicates the rate at which tumors double their size. A medical student left her book on my table. The opened pages showed some data about tumor doubling times for various types of cancer and included the following table:

Tumor Doubling Time of Breast Cancer	
Tumor in breast	14 weeks
Tumor in lung	11 weeks
Tumor in soft tissues	3 weeks

Until that time I never reflected on this subject. I learned about different rates of growth of cancer in primary and metastatic sites many years ago. Like the medical student who left her book on my table, I rote-learned the data for examination and never wondered about the cause of this phenomenon. In mainstream gene-dominated thinking, this subject is as readily dismissed as are all other subjects that support the nondrug philosophy of empirical medicine. But, on this occasion I wondered: Why should the tumor grow so slowly in the breast, less slowly when it metastasizes to lungs and so rapidly when it spreads to the soft tissues? If cancer is truly a genetic rebellion as we are told over and over again by oncologists, why do the rebellious genes behave so differently in different tissues?

My explanation is that cancer cells actively read their cellular microenvironment at all times—and respond to them appropriately. In the breast tissue, a breast cancer cell reads energetic-molecular (EM) events in its environment and adjusts to it, as its environment reads the cancer cells and responds to EM events taking place within that cell. This ongoing EM interaction influences the rate of growth of a cancer cell and determines the tumor doubling time. The cell microenvironment may curb tumor growth or allow it to expand luxuriantly.

The microenvironment of a breast cancer cell has had considerable time to respond and gear up to quell the mischief of the cancer cell, and so curtails its supply of nutrients to the deviant cell. The microenvironment of the cell also resists being polluted by the emanations of the cancer cell—it would rather let the cancer cell wallow in its own filth. The same does not hold for the microenvironment of the cancer cell in soft tissues to which it metastasizes and in which it finds its new home. The healthy cells in soft tissues are ill-prepared for an assault by the deviant cancer cell. Unrestrained by its new neighborhood, the cancer cells goes haywire, steals nutrients from its unsuspecting neighbors and multiplies rapidly. Thus, the tumor doubling time of breast cancer in soft tissues is more than four times faster than when it is still confined to its native mammary microenvironment.

The next question that arose in my mind was why shouldn't a breast cancer cell grow equally rapidly in the lung. The answer to that question was as forthcoming as in the case of the soft tissue. A cancer cell, as I describe earlier in this section, is oxyphobic and does not fare well in the presence of abundant oxygen. Its metabolic mode is predominantly glycolytic or sugar burning, with little or no utilization of oxygen. Thus, even though the lung microenvironment is not primed up to restrain the growth of an invading breast cancer cell, high oxygen tension in the lung does not allow as rapid growth of the cell as in soft tissue.

I include the above comments for one specific reason: to emphasize the dynamic interaction between the cancer cell and its microenvironment and to make a counterpoint to the prevailing theory that cancer behavior—and our concepts of therapy—should be seen only in light of the notion of irreversibility implied in the gene theory of cancer.

CANCER IS REVERSIBLE

Why do cancer cells develop a strong surface negative charge? This simple question arose in my mind sometime ago. Evidently it can happen in two ways: 1) Cancer cell membranes accumulate negatively charged electrons in response to changes in their environment; and 2) They do so in response to metabolic changes taking place within them, such as speeded-up anaerobic metabolism that increases acidotic stress and excessive production of hydrogen peroxide. Since free-floating cancer cells metastasize freely—multiply and flourish—in otherwise healthy tissues, it seems probable that the strong negative charge develops on the surface of the cancer cell in order to provide a counterbalance to a strong positive charge within it.

Next came the expected question: If reversal of a strong

negative surface charge results in tumor regression, is that not clear evidence that the cell innards might also respond to changes in the surface charge? In other words, cancer is a *reversible* phenomenon. This provides additional challenge to the prevailing dogma that cancer is caused by mutated genes, and that genes, once mutated, cannot become "unmutated." Slowly the concept evolved in my mind that cancer represents abnormal growth and replication behavior of the cell in response to changes in its electromagnetic and biochemical micro-environment—*and that such abnormal growth behavior is reversible if the micro-environmental factors that caused it to become errant are removed.*

WHY DOESN'T THE STOMACH PRODUCE INSULIN? WHY DOESN'T THE PANCREAS PRODUCE ACID?

Consider the following simple statement: The stomach cells that secrete acid have the full complement of genes as do the pancreas cells that produce insulin. What keeps the stomach cells from producing insulin? What prevents acid production by the pancreas cells?

When a woman finishes her menstrual cycle, bleeding and tissue shedding leave behind gaping holes in the inner lining of the uterus. The leftover endometrial cells then multiply to repair the holes. How do they know when to multiply? By orders of the genes that control cell growth is the likely answer from physicians. If such cellular growth were to proceed unrestrained, that would be the beginning of cancer. (Indeed, too much cell growth caused by estrogens leads to hyperplasia, and eventually cancer.) How do the cells know when to stop? By order of the same genes, is the probable answer. The simple question in my mind is this: How can genes do all that unless they are able to *read* their microenvironment? The genes must be capable of adapting to the unique circumstances of the cell in which they are contained.

What I address above is the central aspect of biology: that molecules, genes, cells and body tissues continually sense their microenvironment and respond to them in ways most suitable for their survival—as well as for the survival of the whole organism. This means there are two sides to the cancer story: 1) How the energetic-molecular and cellular microenvironment changes; and 2) How genes respond to their altered environment.

MOLECULAR MECHANISMS SUPPORTING THE OXIDATIVE THEORY OF CANCER

In the context of the cause of cancer, two types of genes are important: 1) proto-oncogenes (precursor genes) that, in general, act as driver genes, and stimulate cell growth and differentiation for specific structural or functional purposes, and 2) tumor-suppressor genes which, in general, act as brakes, and prevent excessive cell growth. It is known that proto-oncogenes in normal cells can be disfigured by injury causing deletions (missing parts), point mutations, translocation and rearrangements (parts of genes taken out and put back in wrong locations). Any or all of such changes can turn a proto-oncogene into an activated gene. How are genes damaged? This question continues to be vigorously —and needlessly, in my opinion—debated among the academic community. I say needlessly in my opinion because genes can only be damaged oxidatively in the larger, natural order of things I describe in this volume. I knew that ever since my core idea of spontaneity of oxidation being the root cause of all diseases took form in my mind. Below, I include brief comments about molecular research that fully validates the prediction I made many years ago.

*We found that hydroxyl radicals generated
by stimulated leukocytes (white blood cells)
and iron caused eight different types of
modified DNA base damage...We found
that stimulated leukocytes, cigarette smoke,
and purine and xanthine oxidases were
each capable of activating the K-ras
proto-oncogenes into transforming
oncogenes. Our data support the following
model of oxidant-induced carcinogenesis:
Leukocytes or cigarette smoke releases
superoxide anions and hydrogen peroxide.
Hydrogen peroxide can subsequently
diffuse into the nuclei of cells, react with
iron that is either bound to or in close
proximity to DNA, and generates hydroxyl
radicals. Once generated, hydroxyl radicals
can cause DNA base damage and DNA
strand breaks, which can cause oncogene
activation and/or tumor-suppressor gene
inactivation.*

> *Oxidative Processes and Antioxidants: Their
> Relation to Nutrition and Health Outcomes.*
> Ross Products Div., Abbott Laboratories
> Columbus, Ohio 1994

Translation: In the presence of iron, oxidant molecules

produced in the body and those in cigarette smoke cause cancer.
I have no doubt that future research in this area will corroborate
the findings of the above research studies, and will further validate
my oxidative theory of cancer.

****

(Iron, like oxygen, fascinates me. During the early 1980s,
my colleagues and I published a series of papers about the toxic
effects of iron overload on the heart, liver, adrenal gland and other
body tissues [Ali.M. et al, *JAMA* 244:343; 1980; *Lancet* i:652;
1982; and *Arch Pathol Lab Med* 106:200; 1982]. We learned then
that iron-overloaded patients had a higher incidence of cancer.

During a recent visit to the American Museum of Natural
History in New York, I found myself facing *Ahnighito,* a 34-ton
fragment of a meteor brought to the city by Robert Peary in 1895.
The exhibit legend told how Eskimos used to travel long distances
to take pieces of the meteor rock for use in their axes. The meteor
rock, they knew, comprised almost pure iron. That shook me hard:
Iron, like oxygen, was abundant in the primordial soup from which
life arose and which I was reminded of by *Ahnighito*. How utterly
fascinating that Nature assigned both molecules dual, Dr. Jekyll-
Mr. Hyde roles in human biology. We cannot live without oxygen
and our tissues cannot obtain oxygen without iron in red blood
corpuscles. Yet, oxygen and iron-induced oxyradicals also
powerful life terminators, and cause premature aging, diseases and
cancer. What marvels of biology! I discuss the role of iron in
increasing the incidence of heart disease among postmenopausal
women in the chapter Fourth Insight dealing with environment and
genes.)

HORMONAL THEORY OF CANCER

Some hormones cause cancer, others prevent it. The best example of this phenomenon is estrogen and progesterone. Estrogens drive the endometrium—the inner lining of the uterus and cause it to proliferate excessively, a condition called endometrial hyperplasia. If high doses of estrogens are given over a long period of time, the endometrial cells pushed beyond their endurance turn rabid—the beginning of cancer of the uterus. Indeed, many women were given cancer of the uterus by their doctors by relentlessly pushing estrogen therapy before the relationship between estrogens and cancer of the uterus was recognized. The effect of estrogens on the cells of the breast glands is similar.

Progesterones counterbalance the estrogenic overdrive and so protect the endometrial lining from the carcinogenic effects of estrogens. This is the reason why today both estrogen and progesterone are prescribed together.

How does the capacity of some hormones to cause cancer fit in with my oxidative theory of cancer? It is totally consistent with my theory. Hormones cause cancer by overdriving the tissues that respond to their messages. Overdriven cells—cells that are actively multiplying to meet the demands put upon them—are very vulnerable to oxidative stress. In this context, the biologic response of rapidly replicating cells is similar to the probability of limb injury in toddlers driven by their curiosity to explore new places.

VIRAL, CHEMICAL AND MYCOTOXIN THEORIES OF CANCER

The known causes of cancer include radiation, hormonal agents, environmental chemicals, microbial toxins such as mycotoxins and viruses. Does the oxidative theory of cancer proposed here conflict with any of such data or theories? I do not believe so—though I recognize clear proof of this is lacking in some areas at this time.

In the following section dealing with how viruses cause cellular injury and clinical infection, I cite studies unequivocally demonstrating that such viral injury is oxidative in nature, and can be clearly prevented by appropriate antioxidant measures.

In the past, viral injury has been thought to be much more important in the cause of cancer than other agents. Indeed, 20 to 25 percent of all human cancers have been attributed to viruses. I think future studies will show the causative role of mycotoxins produced by about 500,000 different species of molds that share planet Earth to be much more important. For example, in one study hepatitis B antigen was detected in eight of 38 primary cancers of the liver, whereas aflatoxin—a highly toxic substance present in peanuts among other foods—was found in 27 cases (*J Med* 18(1):23; 1987).

CHEMICAL CARCINOGENS
AND OXIDATIVE THEORY

The carcinogenic effects of a large number of chemicals are well established. Since the 18th-century observations that chimney sweepers develop cancer of the testes because of exposure to carcinogenic soot, many chemicals have been suspected of causing cancer in different organs of the body. Lung cancer in smokers, bone sarcoma among technicians in the radium industry and bladder cancer in rubber industry workers are well-known examples.

Why are some body organs specifically vulnerable to certain chemicals? Because of genetic predisposition. How do chemicals cause cancer? By oxidant injury. As in the case of carcinogenic hormones, chemicals that cause cancer also hit actively growing cells the hardest. Indeed, this is the basis of using chemotherapy drugs. Cancer cells, of course, are rapidly growing cells, and so are especially vulnerable to the oxidizing effects of chemotherapy drugs. This phenomenon also explains why chemotherapy damages the bone marrow—in all cases, albeit to varying degrees. The cells lining the mouth and the bowel also have a high turn-over in health, and so are more vulnerable to the toxic effects of chemotherapy.

OXIDATIVE THEORY OF CANCER EXPLAINS MANY UNEXPLAINED ELEMENTS

On the day I finished the first draft of this chapter, David Landers, M.D., a good friend and a past Director of Gynecology and Obstetrics at our hospital, came to review the pathology slides of a case. The patient was a 44-year old woman, when he removed and I diagnosed a highly aggressive ovarian cancer in 1974. The cancer had already broken through the surface of the ovary—an extremely poor prognostic sign (in mainstream thinking), since it indicates the spread of the tumor to the various crevices of peritoneum that line the inside of the abdomen like a continuous sheath. It is generally accepted as an indication that the cancer is beyond surgical cure. The patient was given radiotherapy after her surgical wound healed. Three years later, Dave explored her abdomen as a "second-look" operation and found no evidence of residual neoplasm.

Now, in 1994—twenty years after the initial surgery—I diagnosed cancer on a needle aspiration biopsy of a small area of tissue thickening around the rectum observed with a CAT scan. What puzzled Dave most was that he had been aware of this area of thickening for a few years. It hadn't changed in its measurements and caused no discomfort for the patient. A few days later, he removed the thickened tissues along with the segment of rectum that the tumor had invaded. I asked my staff to pull out the 1974 tumor slides and compared them with the tumor excised in 1994. Except for some color fading in the slides of the initial tumor, the two tumors looked *exactly* the same.

I asked Dave how might we understand such a case. Were there any clinical clues to the behavior of the tumor? It was a highly malignant tumor that broke through the surface of the ovary twenty years earlier, seeding the abdominal cavity. In 1977, the operative search for any residual tumor was negative. Where did the present tumor come from? If it was there all those years, why did it remain dormant—deep in the pelvis—for so long? Dave knew that the tissue thickening—a now proven and highly malignant cancer— was there for a few years. What was holding it back? Immune surveillance? That's the usual answer. But what caused the immune surveillance to break down in some people and not in others? Dave offered advancing age as a possible explanation.

I recalled a 94-year-woman who had an advanced infiltrating carcinoma of the rectum. Four years earlier at the age of 90, she developed an aggressive cancer of the endometrium that spread to surrounding tissues. She was not expected to live, but she did. At the time of rectal surgery, there was no evidence of recurrent cancer of the uterus. So much for age!

I believe cancer, at an energetic-molecular level, must be regarded as a disturbed interface between the cell and its microenvironment—the cell behaves as cancer in response to an assault on its senses. The chemotherapy model of cancer treatment requires that every last cancer cell must be destroyed—a goal that is neither theoretically valid nor clinically feasible. *This is the fundamental flaw with the prevailing thought among oncologists.* Not every cancer cell needs to be killed—some may be coaxed into behaving like noncancer cells.

SPONTANEOUS REMISSION OF CANCER

In medical terminology, spontaneous remission of cancer refers to exceptional and unexplained partial or complete disappearance of cancer without medical intervention. This phenomenon fascinates me for five reasons:

First,

Nature admits to no exceptions. What we consider exceptions in biology are part of the natural order of things. Healing, I write earlier is as integral to life as is injury. There is nothing exceptional about a cancer cell reverting back to a "normal" noncancerous behavior. None of us would have been alive if it didn't occur.

Second,

spontaneous remission of cancer is Nature's expression of her willingness to yield its secrets of cancer healing—of how a cancer cell can change its EM dynamics back to a state of health. The notion of spontaneous remission as an happening without cause is frivolous—the cause is not hard to know if we turn from a disease model of thinking to a serious study of the EM basis of health—dis-ease—disease dynamics.

Third,

spontaneous remission of cancer offers a solid base of hope—both for the patient who suffers from cancer and for his physician. It is not an uncommon occurrence. Even if it happened only once, it still firmly establishes the possibility.

Fourth,

spontaneous remission of cancer opens the door to all nondrug, restorative therapies that are known to facilitate the healing response in the human body.

Fifth,

on the negative side, few things make mainstream physicians in the cancer community so uncomfortable as the subject of spontaneous remissions of cancers. They consider it an annoying distraction from their daily business of pouring drugs into patients who suffer from cancer.

In this context, it is interesting to note that the National Cancer Institute held a conference on the subject of spontaneous remission at Johns Hopkins Medical School in 1974. The NCI didn't think the subject was serious enough to require any follow-up conferences—probably because it found no drugs that could facilitate spontaneous healing. In 1976, the Institute published a monograph covering the proceedings of that conference. That monograph is out of print—why throw good money after the bad!

How rare are spontaneous remissions when defined as

tumor regression without chemotherapy? The answer depends on who you ask. Physicians who specialize in nondrug, natural cancer therapies will cite a very large number of cases to support their view that cancer remission without chemotherapy or radiotherapy is not uncommon. Most oncologists will dismiss such claims as blatant lies.

Spontaneous Remission: An Annotated Bibliography published by the Institute of Noetic Sciences, Sausalito, CA (1993), lists 1,051 case reports published in peer-reviewed medical literature. What percentage of the actual cases does this number represent? It's anybody's guess. Spontaneous remission is not at all an uncommon evebt in the experience of pathologists, and I know that it is a rare pathologist who prepares a formal report for publication of such cases. That volume includes a graph showing a steep rise in the frequency of medical reports of spontaneous remissions during the last four decades. Notwithstanding, this number represents a very small percentage of the true number.

Patients whose advanced cancers spontaneously regress challenge the deepest beliefs of most oncologists and radiotherapists, though they will probably vehemently contest this statement. Usually they dismiss this subject as insignificant and irrelevant to their work, and mutter something about the immune system. On occasions, some of them find this idea useful. Many patients refuse chemotherapy recommended by oncologists, and later the patients return months or years to tell them of their success with nondrug therapies. When confronted with that awkward situation, the idea of spontaneous remission comes handy—it explains away case histories that do not fit into their chemotherapy model.

What is spontaneous remission of cancer? It is a war

against cancer that the body's own EM dynamics, antioxidant defenses and DNA repair enzyme systems win—it's that simple! The subject of spontaneous remission is of great interest to me and my colleagues in empirical medicine, because it gives us clues to what therapies we might choose to facilitate the physiologic healing processes that normally control cancer—disallow deviant behavior of cancer cells and coax the errant cells back to a healthful mode. *This is the core philosophic principle of empirical medicine when it offers its nondrug therapies for the management of cancer.*

Everyone knows or has heard of people who were expected to die of cancer in several months or a few years but who defied the medical prognosis and underwent spontaneous remissions. I know of hundreds of patients who had limited cancers that could be surgically removed, and so had little reason to die of the tumor. Yet, they succumbed quickly. I also know of many patients who lived for decades with cancers that had been originally pronounced terminal. What can one make of such cases?

THE CHINESE APPROACH TO CANCER

During one of our trips to China, we met Professor Wang Wanlin, Director of Strait International Salvation Hospital and of Shaxi Province Association of Traditional and Western Medicine. He is a hematologist who runs a cancer hospital outside Guanzhou (Canton). We were dumbfounded to learn that his success rate with acute childhood leukemias is over 85%. Such statistics are not to be believed anywhere. I stared blankly at his face as he related case history after case history with a gentle smile on his face. He uses a mixture of twelve Chinese herbs and photofluorescence (light therapy performed by drawing a blood sample, exposing it to certain wavelengths of ultraviolet light, then transfusing the blood back). He further told us that on some occasions he does use very small doses of chemotherapy drugs. The first two therapies allow him to drastically reduce the amount of chemotherapy drugs and so cut down on the drug toxicity. I kept thinking about the children who died of leukemias and on whom I had performed autopsies. I didn't know whether to call Professor Wang a pathological liar or to feel sorry for the children who died of drug toxicity.

At the Japanese-Chinese Friendship Hospital in Beijing, Professors Chen Shao-wu and Zhou Shu graciously gave several hours of their time and presented many case histories of cancer control with bioelectric therapies and Chinese herbs, used in conjunction with certain copper and iron salts. *Are the Chinese consummate liars?* I wondered. *Or are they really onto something important about cancer control?* Why are we Americans denied these therapies? How far will our silly notions of science in drug medicine take us before we come to our senses?

Why is such clear evidence of the reversibility of cancer ignored in drug medicine? The answer, it appears, is largely because the notion of reversibility underscores the role of the environment in the genesis and propagation of cancer. And, there are no drugs for restoring the cellular environment; there are no drugs for normalizing the abnormal surface charge of cancer cells. There are no drugs for relieving excessive oxidative stress on cells. Such therapies clearly are the domains of holistic medicine. And those holistic quacks must be rigorously kept away from patients with cancer. Business as usual!

THE PROMISE OF GENE THEORY OF CANCER WILL ALWAYS BE HOLLOW

The gene story of cancer causation will always be incomplete, its promise to patients with cancer will always be unfulfilled. I have three important reasons for making this dire prediction.

First,

the rate at which genes are oxidatively damaged by progressive global oxidant stress will always far exceed our ability to detect, let alone repair, injured genes.

Second,

genes legislate life; the environment interprets the laws set forth by the genes. The gene theory completely misses the increasing role of growing global pollution, functional nutritional deficiencies and unrelenting stress on health.

Third,

the gene theory of cancer completely denies the essential restorative nature of natural, nondrug therapies for cancer.

I discuss this subject at length in the chapter Fourth Insight: Genes legislate life; the environment interprets the laws set forth by them. Here, I include an interesting quote:

> *The last two decades have been a wild and exciting scientific ride in the cancer research community...But one sobering note, almost all in the field say, is that despite the remarkable progress made in understanding the genesis of cancer, the work so far has had little impact in the clinic.*
>
> *Science* 266:1944; 1994

I have only one reservation about the above quote: It describes the impact of gene research in the clinic as *little*. I assert that it has *no* impact in the care of patients who develop cancer. How can it? Genes form but only one side of this equation. The cancer research community totally ignores the other side. Hundreds of billions of dollars of public money have been spent on cancer research and treatment without any gains in the clinic. I will make another prediction: After we spent thousands of billions more, the results will be the same. Consider the following quote:

> *We are losing the war on cancer...The main conclusion we draw is that some 35 years of intense effort focused largely on improving treatment must be judged a qualified failure.*
>
> *N Eng J Med* 314:1226; 1986

Qualified failure! Now, let's see if the government of the United States disagrees with the *Journal.*

> *However, the extent of improvement in survival for specific cancers is often not as great as that reported. One reason is that biases artificially inflate the amount of 'true' progress...improvements in patient survival have been most dramatic for the rarer forms of cancer and least dramatic for the more prevalent cancers. As a result, even though the absolute numbers of lives extended is considerable, this number remains small relative for all cancers.*

> *Cancer Patient Survival—What Progress Has Been Made?* General Accounting Office of the
> United States of America, March, 1987

Number remains small for all cancers! How could it not remain small? After all, the therapies in the prevailing model of treatment are destructive, not restorative!

I have been a student of medicine for thirty-seven years. How many times have I heard of great miracles of synthetic chemistry that promised a cure of cancer? Did anyone of them prove to be a safe cure? Not one! This is the sad record of the work of our cancer community that is ever so vigilant against alternative nondrug therapies—ever so committed to eradicating all competition.

Does that mean we should abolish research in genetics? Not at all! Every month, gene research opens new windows into the energetic-molecular dynamics of health—dis-ease—disease continuum. My essential point in this discussion is that: When gene research provides us with a sound scientific basis for employing nondrug therapies for normalizing cancerous behavior of cells, we must commit as much energy and funds to those nondrug, restorative therapies as we do for destructive chemotherapy.

DETECTION OF CANCER IN INCIPIENT MOLECULAR STAGES

The scientists say they can quickly develop a test for screening healthy people for the incipient stages of most kinds of cancer ...The test is based on several recent advances in molecular biology, including the new insight that cells slip into the uncontrolled growth known as cancer through defects in specific enzymes that monitor and control cell division.

The New York Times October 11, 1994

Screening healthy people for incipient stages of cancer!

That would be a great advance for physicians like myself who believe cancer is reversible and who vigorously address all elements that impair antioxidant and immune defenses. The essence of EM medicine is to put the primary focus on human defenses and approach the local disease only in a secondary way—tend the soil with greater energy and put less emphasis on the seed. (Just as a farmer diligently tends the soil and does not worry about the seed once it is selected.) Thus, we focus on environmental and nutritional factors, stress and problems of physical fitness.

How would that affect the drug doctors? What measures will they take when a new test gives information about cancer in its incipient stages? Will they radiate the incipient cancer? Will they radiate the whole patient? How will they find where the cancer is in its incipient molecular stages? Will they try a surgical approach? What body organ will they sacrifice for the molecular incipient stages of cancer? Or will they employ chemotherapy? I know that some oncologists might look at the test as a windfall—many more people who will require chemotherapy. But will it really work that way? Will people mindlessly let their antioxidant and immune defenses be shattered by chemotherapy for cancer in its incipient molecular stages, when there is no sign of cancer in a physical sense?

Or, would oncologists approach this problem the same way they do when patients show abnormal blood protein spikes that indicate an evolving bone cancer called myeloma? Some patients who consulted me for such protein spikes were told by their oncologists to wait until the bone cancer can be diagnosed with a biopsy and chemotherapy can be administered. Of course, they rejected such advice.

The thought that molecular biologists are ready to give us tests to detect cancer at pre-cellular, molecular incipient stages both frightens and excites me. I am frightened when I realize that millions of people will be given chemotherapy, or told to wait patiently until chemotherapy can be justified by a later stage of cancer. Evidently, they do not believe that cancer in incipient stages can be reversed with restorative approaches. I am excited when I recognize the enormous potential of reversing such incipient molecular stages of cancer with comprehensive nondrug therapies.

We have to be cautious about talking about a universal screening test being just around the corner...early diagnosis does not necessarily mean the test will prolong life.

The New York Times October 11, 1994

The above statement is a revealing comment from another cancer expert asked to comment on the test by the *Times*. He clearly understands why I am frightened by the aspect of a new screening test for incipient cancer in the hands of drug doctors.

I am an optimist. As the general public becomes better informed about the basic facts of incipient cancer and the nondrug therapies that enhance immune disorders, rather than chemotherapy that destroys our defenses, they will use such information to make the right choices.

The test reported by the *New York Times* detects the

incipient stages of cancer by detecting "junk DNA" in body fluids—called junk because its function is not known at this time. I'm sure that junk DNA is especially vulnerable to miscopying—due to oxidative injury during cell division and DNA replication, though scientific proof of that is not yet forthcoming. The test employs a technique known as polymerase chain reaction (PCR) that permits rapid identification of tiny bits of DNA.

The principal strengths of my oxidative theory of cancer —which holds that a cell behaves as a cancer cell when its innards are oxidatively damaged, and that cancer is essentially a reversible phenomenon—are the following:

First,

It proposes a unifying concept of the genesis of cancer that provides a sound scientific basis for the mechanisms of action of various agents that are known to cause cancer.

Second,

It puts forth a basic model for integrating various therapeutic approaches that have shown efficacy in controlling cancer growth and spread.

Third,

It offers a viable alternative to the prevailing strategy of launching attacks on cancer cells that are more destructive to the patient than they are to cancer cells.

I have no doubt that future research in the cause of cancer, and the management of patients who harbor cells that behave in a cancerous way, will be along the way I describe in this chapter. The tragedy in this area of medicine is this: The oncology community has turned its back on all therapies except those that dangerously poison the whole person, and has strived to outlaw all therapies except those it espouses. Some enlightened oncologists do recognize the problems I address here.

Clinical oncologists cure an occasional patient with a hematological malignant condition or a germ-cell tumor but spend most of their time practicing palliations.

Lancet 343:495; 1994

The idea that the root cause of cancer is accelerated oxidative stress—and that the behavior of cancer cells *can* be modified for better clinical outcome—is not a delusional plausibility of an idealogue. All this is not wishful thinking on my part. I have seen far too many cases of successful management of cancers without chemotherapy to think otherwise. I am certain that enlightened patients who suffer from cancer will demand from their physicians a more enlightened view of what cancer is and how best to manage it without therapies that are more destructive to them than to the cancer they harbor. I see a tidal wave of change.

Oxidative Theory of Viral Diseases

Drug medicine assumes that where there is a disease, there must be a bug, and where there is a bug, there must be a drug.

Disease doctors of drug medicine have had a field day with viruses. There has been infatuation with the Epstein-Barr virus (EBV), the unremitting joy of chronic fatigue syndrome specialists. God knows how many millions of people have been administered toxic antiviral drugs in the hope of eradicating the virus. The EBV, of course, is a cunning rascal, burying itself into the host DNA to protect itself from toxic drugs, and then striking out at opportune times—when the host defenses are down due to poor nutrition, stress, antibiotic abuse, and drug therapies to suppress symptoms caused by environmental factors, and unrelated bacterial and viral infections.

Then there is cytomegalic virus (CMV). Some drug doctors are as fond of this virus as they are of EBV. They have their own arsenal of antiviral drugs. Of course, the herpes virus is everyone's favorite.

How do viruses injure tissues? By oxidative injury. Firm evidence for this was reported by Oda and colleagues of Kumamoto University, Japan, in 1989. They studied the ability of mice to survive severe infections caused by the influenza virus. For this purpose, they compared unprotected mice with two subgroups of mice protected by weak and potent antioxidants—with short-lived superoxidase (a weak antioxidant) and superoxide dismutase made long-acting by pyran conjugation. All unprotected mice succumbed to influenza infection, while 90% of them survived when protected with strong antioxidants. The weak antioxidants protected about 20% of the mice. (*Science* 244:974; 1989.)

It is clear that in the case of viral infections, the lines between drug doctors and holistic doctors are equally and sharply drawn. I see the best clinical results when such infections are managed with full supportive measures. The liberal use of antioxidants, including judicious use of vitamin C infusions, is not only rational from a theoretical standpoint but also effective from a clinical standpoint. It is rare for my associates and I to resort to antibiotic therapy for common viral infections. Nothing in medicine works in all cases. But after trying both approaches, I find the drug approach dismally lacking.

Oxidative Theory of Chronic Fatigue

My current interest in the basic cause of chronic fatigue, is in reality, a continuation of my search for the initial energetic-molecular events that turn a state of health into a state of absence of health, then into a state of disease. During this period, I diligently searched the medical and biology journals for any information that would disprove my evolving concept that the spontaneity of oxidation in nature is the true cause of the aging process—and is the root cause of chronic fatigue. I published my theory that chronic fatigue is caused by accelerated oxidative molecular injury in the *Journal of Advancement in Medicine* (6:83-96; 1993). In that article—reproduced in the companion volume, *The Canary and Chronic Fatigue*—I marshalled extensive experimental and clinical evidence for my theory, including a large number of scientific citations.

Electrons are those tiniest packets of energy that are in perpetual motion within atoms and molecules—restless and bursting with a desire to break loose. Whenever I see young people rebelling, I wonder how can it be any different? It is the nature of living things to want to break loose — in this, electrons are no different from teenagers. In this fundamental equation of life, an amoeba is no different from a dinosaur, nor a lowly shrub from the loftiest of giant sequoia trees. At atomic and molecular levels, life reduces itself to this simple pattern. Living things age, die and decay because they cannot forever control the loss of electrons and energy contained within them. What would be expected if the rate of the energy loss were accelerated? Fatigue! This, indeed, is what happens when a world-class sprinter literally collapses at the finish line, then recovers, usually within minutes, because of his conditioning. What would be expected if this rate of energy loss were accelerated *chronically*? Chronic fatigue! What would be expected if the normal oxidative pathways were relentlessly overdriven by allergic triggers, chemical sensitivities, designer killer molecules in our antibiotics and pesticides, oxidants in pollutants, metabolic roller coasters of sugar and neurotransmitters and the powerful oxidant molecules of stress? Unrelenting fatigue—chronic fatigue!

I relate here one other image that I described in *The Canary and Chronic Fatigue,* which is still as sharp in my mind as the day I first saw it.

Sally M., a woman in her early forties, consulted me for disabling fatigue. She'd led an active, energetic life except for some allergy symptoms. However, following an attack of a "virus infection that did not clear up for weeks," she developed persistent fatigue. When she consulted me, she suffered from intractable abdominal bloating, muscle aches, joint stiffness, headaches, severe PMS symptoms, mood swings, and memory and mentation problems. On the second visit, when I reviewed her laboratory results and prepared to start my nutritional and allergy treatment protocols, she complained of "wormy" feelings in her breast, "electric shocks" in her left flank before eating and a "sinking feeling" in the pit of her stomach after meals. Sometimes she felt "blue" and sometimes "angry and hostile." Conscious of the fact that such symptoms are often dismissed by physicians with a fondness for the old "all-in-the-head" label, she hesitantly asked me if I thought she was losing her mind. Two of the three physicians she consulted before seeing me found nothing wrong with her and advised her to see a psychiatrist. Indeed, medical texts have no disease labels that fit these symptoms.

I saw Sally's anguish one day during one of my ghoraa runs (my morning limbic run). In a flashing image, I saw Sally curled up on the ground, consumed by a fire of "molecular rage." Her body heaved as she struggled to sit up, then it collapsed. I saw her body quiver with bursts of adrenaline, cholinergic fly balls, and neurotransmitters, turning and twisting upon themselves. I saw molecular fireworks. I saw oxyradicals in a feeding frenzy, poking gaping holes in her cell membranes. I saw a hemorrhage of magnesium and potassium molecules through the leaky cell walls. I saw calcium molecules flooding the cell innards and suffocating their life span enzymes. I saw violent whirlpools of energy waves. There were cortical electrical sparks all over her body, as if all her tissues were being shorted. Bursts of adrenaline. Pools of lactic acid. Spiking potentials of membrane phospholipids. A death dance of oxyradicals. Sally's body chemistry was in a pyrotechnic state. Her cell membranes were shot full of holes. Sally made another attempt to rise, convulsed and collapsed.

So that is it. That is what severe fatigue is. It is lacerated cell membranes. It is violated cell innards. It is the hemorrhage of magnesium and potassium. It is mitochondrial enzymes within the cells drowning in a calcium flood. It is the agony and death of cells. But first and foremost, it is a state of high oxidative turmoil—a Fourth of July chemistry. I consider evidence of oxidative damage to the structure and function of cell membranes as the strongest direct support for my theory. In one of my studies, I observed that up to 80% of red blood cells in patients with chronic fatigue showed deformed structure of the cell membrane (*Am J Clin Pathol* 94:515;1990). Remarkably, most of these cell membrane deformities were corrected after patients were given 15 grams of vitamin C intravenously. Many essential issues concerning chronic fatigue are discussed in the companion volume, *The Canary and Chronic Fatigue*.

Oxidative Theory
of Autoimmune Disorders

In a series of articles, published in the early 1980s by the American Academy of Environmental Medicine, I proposed my theory that all autoimmune disorders are essentially caused by accelerated oxidative molecular injury. At that time, even my colleagues in environmental medicine, who are used to looking at new theories without preconceived notions, received my theory with polite silence. (I learned years later the reason for their silence: They thought the idea was far too speculative.)

Since then, a growing number of experimental studies have conclusively demonstrated that the initial events in the injury to the immune system are oxidative in nature. Changes in the immune cell counts and the presence of antibodies directed against an individual's own cells and molecules are clearly secondary events triggered by initial oxidative injury.

Strokes are unusual in young people. A case of a stroke that caused paralysis of the right arm and right leg in a 35-year-old woman was once presented at our hospital. The primary care physician and his consultants aggressively searched for the cause of the stroke in the young patient. The woman suffered from two miscarriages in the past. An association between a history of miscarriages and stroke due to a clotting disorder—hypercoagulability of blood in pathologic jargon—had been described. A large number of scans and laboratory tests were ordered. Tests for lupus anticoagulant and antibodies against some fats called cardiolipin turned out to be positive, establishing the presence of an autoimmune injury.

During the discussion period, I asked, "What tests were done to define the nature of autoimmune injury in this case?"
"None!" came a resounding answer from the speaker.

In N^2D^2 medicine, discussions of the autoimmune injury go only as far as the use of steroids. The discussion moved on to the use of anticoagulants and other drugs in the case management.

Nowhere does the fundamental difference between the dogma of drug medicine and the philosophy of holistic medicine come into sharper contrast than in the management of autoimmune injury. Drug medicine relies solely on drugs that suppress the immune system. For example, to treat such disorders, steroids and other immunosuppressants that further damage the immune system are used. An acute autoimmune injury, such as that seen in the young patient with stroke and paralysis, calls for aggressive attempts to support the immune system. This entails sound nutritional and ecologic approaches and effective methods of self-regulation. Drugs are not the answer, except for short-term symptom relief. However, U.S. physicians, with rare exceptions, are neither trained nor equipped to undertake nutritional and environmental therapies.

Oxidative Theory of Rheumatoid Arthritis and Other Types of Autoimmune Arthritis

Free radical production within the inflamed joints in rheumatoid arthritis is markedly increased *(FASEB J, 2:2867; 1988)*. Such radicals are produced by the activation of immune cells, which release mediator molecules of inflammation in response to allergic foods, sensitizing molds and environmental pollutants. Free radicals then perpetuate the cycle of oxidant injury. Environmental triggers cause greater oxyradical production that increases the inflammatory response in tissues which, in turn, decreases host tissue resistance to the trigger.

Oxidant molecules damage hyaluronic acid in synovial joint fluid in rheumatoid arthritis (*Science* 185:529; 1974). Injection into the inflamed joints of superoxide dismutase—an effective first-line defense antioxidant enzyme in human tissues—reduces inflammation in rheumatoid arthritis *(Oxidative Stress* Sies, H,. Ed. Academic Press, New York, 1985, 403)*.

Of greater interest to physicians interested in nondrug therapies of rheumatoid arthritis—and other autoimmune types of arthritis such as psoriatic arthritis, lupus arthritis, juvenile arthritis—are natural substances that inhibit free radical production in joints. A good example is inhibition of NADPH oxidase enzyme by Picorhiza kurroa plant *(Free Rad Biol Med* 8:251; 1990)*.

Oxidative Theory of Pancreatitis

J.M. Braganza and colleagues of Manchester Royal Infirmary have published extensive experimental and clinical data that clearly establishes oxidative injury as the pivotal effector of pancreatic cell injury (multiple citations included in *The Pathogenesis of Pancreatitis*, Manchester University Press, 1991). They and others have shown that increased oxidative stress occurs in various body organs of experimental animals within 30 minutes when inflammation is induced by various agents. The injured pancreas begins to repair the damage by activating immune cells including white blood cells and scavenger cells called phagocytes. Oxidative bursts that occur within such immune cells—as a result of cell membrane activation—add to the direct oxidative stress of the inducing agents. In the case of the pancreas, such oxidative stress turns simple edema of the pancreas into pancreatitis and hemorrhagic necrosis.

Braganza and colleagues also studied how the increased oxidative stress associated with pancreatitis in their patients affected the status of vitamin C. They end the abstract of their paper with the following:

It is included that the stress of an acute intra-abdominal crisis is accompanied by a nonspecific decrease in the plasma level of vitamin C. In acute pancreatitis early and profound oxidative stress compounds this problem by denaturing the available vitamin. There may be a case for the judicious parenteral administration of ascorbic acid to patients with acute pancreatitis to boost plasma antioxidant defence.

British Journal of Surgery 80:750; 1993

Following an excellent discussion of how vitamin C counters the increased oxidative stress of pancreatitis—and eventually is depleted—the authors recommend that an intravenous injection of vitamin C should be considered for patients with this potentially fatal condition to reduce excessive oxidative stress.

There is a large body of data that show increased oxidative stress in patients with pneumonia, heart disease, bowel disorders and in a lesion of a host of other body organs (*Ann Int Med* 107:526; 1987). Notwithstanding such extensive findings, the researchers always stop short of the logical conclusion: That increased oxidative stress in all these conditions is but an expression of spontaneity of oxidation in nature—and that oxidation is the true cause of these diseases.

Thus, since oxidation is the true cause of these diseases, the rational approach to treatment must be holistic, integrated, nondrug therapies that are designed to reduce oxidative stress. (Evidently, surgical approaches and potent [and toxic] drugs are necessary in acute, life-threatening conditions.) So why is this not done? Because disease doctors of drug medicine are not trained in holistic, nondrug, nutritional and environmental therapies.

Oxidative Theory
of Hepatitis, Appendicitis, Nephritis, Pneumonia and Cholecystitis

Consistent with my theory that all diseases are caused by oxidative injury, I propose that hepatitis, appendicitis, nephritis, pancreatitis, cholecystitis (inflammation of the gall bladder), and inflammations of other body organs are caused by oxidative injury. At first blush, this proposal may seem to put my credibility in doubt. However, I have sound scientific reasons for including these diseases in my oxidative theory.

The evidence that the tissue injury in different types of viral hepatitis is caused by oxidative stress can be derived by scientific studies that I cite earlier in the paragraphs dealing with viral injury and oxidative stress.

Scientific evidence clearly linking appendicitis, nephritis and cholecystitis—to my knowledge—has not been reported. I have no doubt that such evidence will be forthcoming when this subject is investigated with good research studies. To support my viewpoint, I draw upon the observations made for pancreatitis. The basic pathologic mechanisms of injury in such inflammations in the various body organs are similar.

Oxidative Theory of Cataract

The eyes are designed to see using light. Light causes oxidation—photooxidation as it is commonly referred to. Predictably, they are exposed to the risk of photooxidation of the lens proteins—that make up 98% of the lens solid mass—at all times they are in use. Nature made lens proteins extremely long-lived compared with proteins in other body organs. Still, with passing years, photooxidation and the oxidant stress of oxygen takes its toll. Damaged and denatured proteins accumulate, form clumps, precipitate and cause lens opacities. Nature has its way of protecting vulnerable tissues. How does Nature do it?

Drug medicine assumes that cataracts can neither be prevented nor reversed. The usual advice to a person with early signs of a cataract is to wait until the cataract is fully developed and then have the lens removed with surgery. Some enlightened drug doctors now recommend a multivitamin tablet for such patients.

I believe vitamin C is the least toxic and most effective of all antioxidants in human systems. So I would expect that Nature would use this molecule to build a special antioxidant system for the lens proteins. Indeed, it is so. The lens level of this vitamin is as high as 60-fold the level found in human plasma (*Curr. Eye Res.* 10:751; 36).

Glutathione is another powerful antioxidant molecule. Lens glutathione levels are several times the levels found in blood

(*Arch. Ophthalmol* 109:196; 1991). Predictably, the amounts of vitamin C and glutathione are lower in cataractous lenses (*J. Klin. Oczna* 38:477; 1968). In some clinical studies, persons with the lowest intake of vitamin C had an 11-fold risk of developing cataracts as those with the highest intake (*Am. J. Clin Nutr.* 53:3520S; 1991). The risk of cataract has also been associated with lower levels of other antioxidants such as vitamin E and beta carotene (*Ann. N.Y. Acad. Sci.* 570:372; 1989).

The lens substance is also rich in antioxidant enzyme systems including glutathione peroxidase/reductase, catalase and superoxide dismutase. All such enzyme systems actively protect lens proteins from oxidative damage and formation of cataracts.

All these antioxidant systems of the lens, however, have a limit. Advanced stages of cataract do require cataract surgery.

Oxidative Theory of
Sugar-Insulin-Adrenaline Roller Coasters

In the natural biologic order of things, no molecule used by the organism is ever a killer molecule or a villain. In oxidatively damaged and disrupted biologic systems, however, some molecules clearly assume the role of killer molecules, and insulin and adrenaline in excess are good examples of such bad players.

The problems caused by sugar overload are pervasive in the United States today. Essentially they consist of sugar-insulin-adrenaline roller coasters that trigger a variety of reactions including mood swings, weakness, jitters, anxiety, sweating, lightheadedness, palpitations, nausea and occasional vomiting. These roller coasters can—and do—exaggerate other symptoms such as those caused by stress, PMS, thyroid and adrenal hormonal imbalances and chronic bowel disorders. I discuss this subject at length in *The Butterfly and Life Span Nutrition.*

Insulin—the principal hormone that regulates sugar metabolism—is a misunderstood molecule, both for its role in health and in diabetes.

People often think that insulin production in Type II diabetes (the common type seen in adults) is reduced. In reality, the exact opposite is true. Insulin supply in the majority of diabetics is actually increased. The real problem is that insulin production is ill-timed so that the diabetic does not have enough when he really needs it—within minutes of eating his meals—and has too much of it later when not needed. Diabetes, of course, is an energy disorder caused by oxidative injury to enzymes in tissues that use insulin such as muscle cells, and to receptors in pancreatic cells that make insulin and glucagon—the hormone that provides a counterbalance to insulin. I cite two examples to illustrate this:

The function of enzyme Na^+K^+ ATPase is impaired in Type II diabetes. This enzyme regulates the passage of sodium and potassium across the cell membrane and so plays the pivotal role in preserving the healthy electrical charges at the cell membrane.

In Type II diabetes, a genetic receptor abnormality at the membrane of muscle cells interferes with the transport in and out of sodium, calcium, potassium and magnesium so that sodium and calcium flood the cell innards and potassium and magnesium leak out. This—it seems to me—is the essence of the so-called problem of insulin resistance.

It should be evident from the above two facts that in the clinical care of patients with diabetes, we ought to focus on molecular and cellular oxidative stress in our attempt to regulate blood sugar. In the hundreds of lectures on diabetes that I have attended over the years, I have yet to hear a diabetes specialist mention this. So it is that an excess of sugar, the principal energy molecule in health, becomes a killer molecule when the cell membranes are oxidized and denatured. Insulin, the essential hormone of sugar metabolism, becomes a bad player when the membrane receptors that regulate its entry into the cell are oxidized and denatured. In drug medicine, we only talk about drugs to control high blood sugar levels.

Oxidative Theories
of Diabetes and Alzheimer's Disease

A report in the April 21, 1994 issue of *Nature* makes my case eloquently.

Abnormal, oxidatively damaged proteins called beta-amyloid proteins occur in the brains of people who suffer from Alzheimer's disease. The tangled fibers made up of such proteins literally choke the neurons and nerve fibers trapped in them. Such telltale signs of cell death are called neurofibrillary tangles or plaques. Four years ago, Yankner and co-investigators at Harvard Medical School published an important paper showing that beta-amyloid proteins indeed are toxic to nerve cells. Predictably, that report triggered a flurry of activity in the drug industry to develop drugs that inhibit plaque formation in the brain and prevent Alzheimer's disease. There were the expected pronouncements of an imminent drug breakthrough for this dreadful disorder.

No one bothered to ask the basic question: If Alzheimer plaques are caused by oxidatively damaged proteins, why would any drug for this disease fare any better than thousands of other drugs that have failed miserably for other oxidative degenerative disorders in the past?

Now comes another important research report—from the same research team—that extends their earlier observation about a similar protein in another disease, Type II diabetes. The report showed how the islet cells of the pancreas that produce insulin are choked by fibrils composed of amylin—a peptide very similar to beta-amyloid. It is also an important article because it documents what many of us have suspected for a long time: that Type II diabetes is a degenerative disorder caused by some oxidatively injured protein(s). The presence of amyloid protein deposits in the pancreas of diabetic patients were first reported as early as 1901.

Just as researchers are now scrambling to develop and test agents designed to prevent the formation of beta-amyloid plaques as a potential treatment for Alzheimer's disease, so may they now begin to develop agents for preventing the formation of amylin deposits in the pancreas. It is estimated that at least 12 million Americans suffer from Type II diabetes.

Focus News from Harvard Medical, Dental & Public Health Schools April 29, 1994

I, of course, have heard such proclamations over and over again during the last 35 years. There is not a single drug used by the disease doctors of drug medicine that has proven to reverse ecologic, immune and degenerative disorders over the long term. Now, should that stop anyone from the prophecy game of drug medicine?

There is a profound irony here! Type II diabetes is

essentially a disease of sugar overload that stresses the insulin-producing cells of the pancreas in genetically predisposed persons. (Type I diabetes—the type seen in children and young adults—is caused by fulminant immune damage to islet cells in the pancreas.) Most nutritionist-physicians succeed in the nondrug management of some cases of Type II diabetes. If drugs may not be discontinued altogether, at least the drug dose can be substantially reduced. How can we rationally address problems caused by massive sugar overload? By following the principles of nutritional medicine. Oops! Those nutritionist quacks again!

Alzheimer's disease is a dreaded disorder that causes memory loss and dementia. This disease has a very strong link with high aluminum content of the brain tissue. The overload of neurotoxic metals such as mercury, lead, nickel and others can be fully expected to add to the injury caused by aluminum. Most people with Alzheimer's disease also show evidence of poor circulation due to plaque formation in the brain blood vessels. In view of these considerations, what therapy can be expected to be most beneficial for patients with Alzheimer's disease? A therapy that takes toxic metals out of the brain tissue and a therapy that improves the blood circulation to the brain. What therapy eminently accomplishes both goals? EDTA chelation therapy. Oops! Those chelation quacks again!

Is beta amyloid protein found in plaques of Alzheimer's disease a product of oxidative damage to natural proteins present in the brain? Objective scientific evidence for this has not yet been published. So it remains speculative on my part at this time. However, I have absolutely no doubt that such evidence will be forthcoming with future research in this area.

When proteins are oxidatively damaged, they cannot be

"un-oxidized" by drugs to undo the tissue damage caused by them. The only real chance we have of reversing such lesions is to prevent further oxidative damage and to facilitate recovery using Nature's own way of replacing oxidatively damaged proteins with newly synthesized, unoxidized proteins. The problem for drug doctors is that such a philosophic approach is considered unscientific and so unworthy of the scientists at the National Institutes of Medicine (NIH). Why? Because quacks were there first. The NIH syndrome thrives in our universities.

Oxidative Theory of
Cell Membrane and Plasma Damage

I draw the strongest support for my theory that accelerated oxidative molecular injury is the root cause of all disease from direct microscopic evidence of oxidative damage to blood cell membranes and blood plasma proteins. In this section, I include some comments about two sets of personal observations about these phenomena:

The oxidative damage to blood cell membranes seen in states of accelerated oxidative injury; and

The oxidative damage to blood plasma proteins seen in states of high oxidative damage.

In one of my research studies, I examined the effects of intravenously administered vitamin C on the form and function of blood cells. For several reasons discussed in the earlier sections of this chapter I expected vitamin C to exert some beneficial antioxidant effects on such cells. This expectation notwithstanding, I made a startling observation during the first series of experiments. One of the first blood samples 1 examined in this study was taken from a patient in the middle of a severe food sensitivity reaction. When seen with a high-resolution phase-contrast microscope, nearly all his red blood cells showed varying degrees of cell membrane deformity. That was the first time the term *oxidative storms* arose in my mind—red cell membranes were being literally bent out of shape by such storms. Blood samples, taken soon after finishing an IV drip of 15 grams of vitamin C, showed restoration of the cell membrane shape in more than half the cells. I then examined the blood samples of several other patients suffering from a variety of immune disorders before and after vitamin C drips. As a group, these patients showed cell membrane deformities in up to 80% of red blood cells (*Am J Clin Pathol* 94:515; 1990). Vitamin C drips restored the normal shapes of such cells in more than 50% of instances.

With the two photomicrographs reprinted on the next page, I illustrate the functional and structural changes in red blood cells caused by oxidative stress, and the reversibility of such changes with intravenous vitamin C infusion. The red blood cells appearing in the upper photomicrograph show several patterns of irregularities and elongation. The membranes of some cells show sharp angulation, crinkling and spiking caused by accelerated oxidative stress. Some cells are clumped together due to adhesiveness caused by oxidative injury. The lower photomicrograph shows how deformed structure of red blood cells is restored by an intravenous vitamin C infusion. Note how all cells are well-sepearted from each other. (In health, cells are seperated from each other by a weak surface negative charge which is altered by oxidative stress.) Vitamin C, of course, is the principle water-phase antioxidant of human blood.

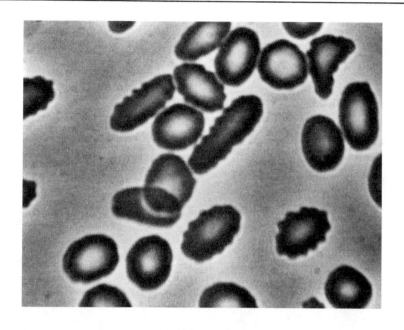

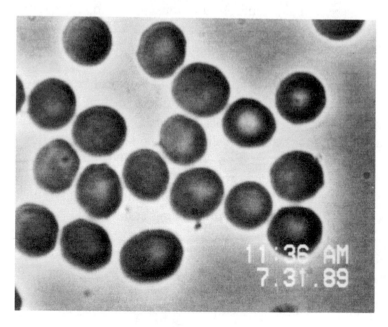

The results of these early experiments—limited as they were in their scale—convinced me that the phenomenon of cell membrane damage caused by oxidative stress was related to health or absence of it in a very fundamental way. The cell membrane separates internal order of the cell from external disorder. I discuss this at length in the companion volume *The Canary and Chronic Fatigue*. It seemed to me then that it was only a matter of time before I would see validation of my observations in many other studies performed by other researchers. This, indeed, did happen.

OXIDATIVELY MODIFIED PROTEINS CLOT THE BLOOD AND PLUG THE HOLES IN BLOOD VESSELS

The second set of observations relate to the patterns of oxidative damage to blood plasma proteins seen in blood samples of patients in states of accelerated oxidative damage.

When a little girl falls down and lacerates her elbow, why does her wound bleed for a few minutes and then stop bleeding? It happens because blood clots and seals the tears in the blood vessel walls. If the natural mechanism that shuts off bleeding were not there, any small laceration could prove fatal. Indeed, this is the case in hemophilia and related bleeding disorders in which extensive bleeding from trivial internal and external injuries to blood vessels can create life-threatening conditions.

How does blood clot? In a simplified—yet scientifically valid—way, blood clots when oxidative injury turns some soluble blood clotting factors into an insoluble meshwork of threadlike fibrils. Blood clotting factors, I indicate earlier, are proteins that largely function as enzymes. These proteins are especially sensitive to oxidant molecules generated when the endothelial cells (lining the inner surface of blood vessels) are injured and set off oxidative bursts.

Phlebitis—clot formation in veins—often occurs in patients with cancer. I remember this question when I took my examination for the diploma of Fellow of the Royal College of Surgeons in England in 1966. No one ever probed the biochemical link between cancer and phlebitis then. Nor did I ever reflect on this phenomenon. The question in the examination was asked primarily to emphasize the need for searching for occult cancers when patients developed unexplained phlebitis.

Chemically sensitive patients often bruise easily. Not uncommonly, young patients with such disorders develop unexplained phlebitis. It is commonly believed that environmental pollutants circulating in the blood are toxic to endothelial cells. I do not remember anyone ever exploring the biochemical reactions underlying such phenomena in any of the hundreds of conferences on environmental medicine that I attended. Nor did I either.

The idea that oxidative sparks might put the blood plasma on fire first came to my mind when I began my studies of the microscopic changes in the blood of patients with chronic ecologic and immune disorders. Earlier in this section, I described the changes in the shape of red blood cell membranes that were reversed with intravenous vitamin C drips. In those studies, I observed that blood plasma congeals in a variety of patterns, some of which can be clearly related to the degree of oxidative stress. Furthermore, these abnormal patterns of plasma congealing can be reversed with appropriate antioxidant therapies. Indeed, this is an excellent—and in my opinion the best—method for assessing the clinical efficacy of antioxidant therapies.

Ascorbic acid (vitamin C) prevents platelet aggregations by norepinephrine, collagen, ADP and ristocetin.

Am J Clin Pathol 95:281; 1991

In a follow-up to my red blood studies, I turned my attention to the effects of vitamin C on blood plasma and platelet function and structure. Platelets are tiny blood corpuscles that clump to form a meshwork with fibrin fibers as alluded to earlier. In the laboratory, we study blood coagulability by examining the way platelets clump when they are exposed to oxidizing agents such as adrenaline and collagen. I discovered that platelets clump much more quickly in patients with serious ecologic and immune disorders, and that such clumping is slowed down when these patients are given vitamin C drips. In the report cited above, I documented the ability of vitamin C to prevent platelet clumping induced by a variety of oxidizing agents. Next came a totally unexpected finding: Drops of weak vitamin C solution quickly broke up the platelet clumps—a finding of readily apparent and enormous significance to those who suffer from coronary artery disease. (Abnormal platelet clumping is one of the early events in coronary artery occlusion, with blood clotting that leads to heart attack.) For this reason, I think vitamin C is a far better preventive agent than aspirin for heart disease.

The following two graphs show the clumping effect of oxidative stress on blood platelets and the reversal of such effect by vitamin C. Four lines in the upper graph illustrate the patterns of platelets aggregation (clumping) when they are exposed to the oxidant stress caused by the addition of adrenaline, ADP, collagen and ristocetin. The lower graph shows how addition of vitamin C (shown by arrow) breaks up those platelet aggregates and platelets seperate from each other, as do red blood cells in photomicrographs shown on page 284. These observations led me to my conclusion that vitamin C is a far superior "clot-buster" than aspirin is for patients with coronary heart disease.

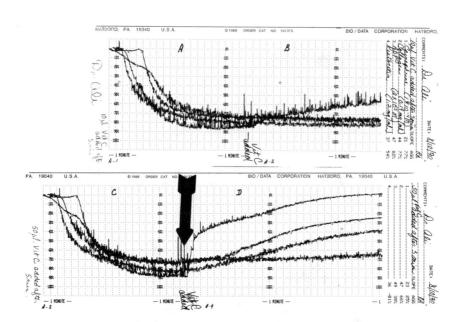

The following two photomicrographs show evidence of oxidative injury to plasma proteins. The upper picture shows clumping of red blood cells caused by accelerated oxidative injury to blood proteins in a patient with an acute viral infection. Arrows in the lower picture show irregularly shaped dark masses composed of oxidized proteins in a patient with persistent chronic fatigue.

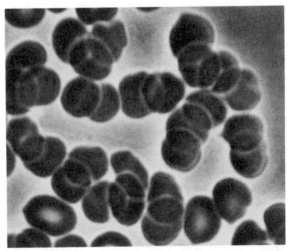

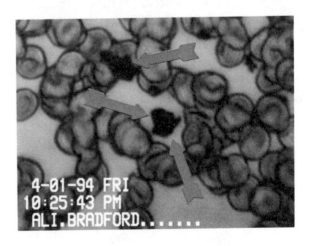

Robert W. Bradford, the eminent cancer researcher and a close friend, has described these patterns of plasma congealing in great detail. I refer the reader to an excellent monograph *The HLB Blood Test as an Indicator of Oxidative Injury and Disseminated Intravascular Clotting* published by Bradford and colleague, Henry W. Allen. (Bradford Research Institute, Chula Vista, California, 1994.)

OXIDATIVE SPARKS PUT BLOOD PLASMA ON FIRE

Disseminated intravascular coagulation (DIC) is a bleeding disorder that proves fatal unless it is aggressively managed with heparin, a commonly used blood-thinner that prevents clotting. For decades I heard and used this term in my hospital work without ever recognizing the role of oxidative injury.

(As I write this section, I look up the section on DIC in the 5th [1994] edition of *Robbins Pathologic Basis of Disease,* the best known pathology textbook in the world. I read a detailed discussion of DIC but find no reference to oxidative injury. It really doesn't surprise me, but it does give me the reason why my colleagues in drug medicine never think of oxidative injury when they treat acutely ill patients with this serious condition.)

What therapies can be expected to offer the greatest hope of survival for patients with acute, life-threatening DIC? Of course, well-designed antioxidant therapies, including IV drips containing vitamin C, magnesium, potassium, zinc and other nutrients. Oops! Those vitamin C quacks again!

How is DIC caused? How do oxidative sparks put the blood plasma on fire?

DIC is a disorder characterized by abnormal patterns of blood clotting in blood vessels and episodes of hemorrhage in various tissues. It can be acute and life-threatening or chronic with slowly developing episodes of bleeding or blood clotting. DIC may be associated with the following:

1. Cancer: Oxidative coals in cancer cell tentacles ignite the oxidative flames of coagulation. Mucus released from some types of cancer can initiate this process as well.

2. Infections with bacteria, fungi and parasites: Immune cells literally use oxidative bursts to destroy microbes and parasites.

3. Allergic and chemical sensitivity reactions: Histamine is released from the mast cells when the offending agent triggers an oxidative response in these cells. Recurrent allergic reactions and persistent chemical reactions literally create oxidative storms that damage cell membranes, as described in the preceding sections, as well as put plasma proteins on fire.

4. Trauma: Direct injury to cells lining blood vessels releases coagulation factors that trigger oxidative sparks to congeal blood proteins in order to stop bleeding. Such oxidative sparks, unless put out rapidly by antioxidants, cause self-flaming oxidative fires.

5. Toxic exposures: Oxidation is the primary method in which the body tries to detoxify injurious chemicals, as in the

case of trauma.

6.   Miscellaneous conditions such as heat strokes, drugs that cause intravascular breakdown of red blood cells, vasculitis and others.

CAMP FIRE COALS TURN INTO A WILD FIRE

What is the common denominator in all the conditions listed above?

To understand this, we need to return to the subject of spontaneity of oxidation in Nature. How do coals simmering in a camp fire turn into the leaping flames of wild fires? This is because the breeze fans the coals into sparks that fly and ignite dry twigs in the vicinity of the camp fire. Lighted twigs, in turn, put the dry wood on fire. Winds turn such small wood fires into roaring wild fires. Spontaneity of oxidation turns tiny oxidative bursts in living cells into oxidative fires that put the blood plasma on fire in precisely the same way.

Oxidation is the first defense Nature has bestowed upon living beings against foreign molecules and alien microbes. In health, oxidative defenses are triggered by an external challenge and are fed and perpetuated by the phenomenon of spontaneity of oxidation. Oxidation also brings into action antioxidant defenses so that oxidative flames are quenched as soon as their work in coping with external threats is completed. However, if antioxidant defenses have been exhausted by chronic, unrelenting demand, the oxidative storms rage unabated, leading to the development of

---

DIC. A similar situation develops when the antioxidant defenses are depleted due to enormous demands put on them by acute oxidative insults. The same basic equation of life holds true in all these circumstances: the redox reaction, the balance between oxidative needs of the body and the antioxidant defenses. Oxygen plays its dual role of molecular Dr. Jekyll and Mr. Hyde.

ANTIOXIDANT HEALTH AND DISEASE PREVENTION

How do we reverse the molecular disarray that is disease? How do we preserve—and restore, when damaged—the molecular mosaic that is health? By reducing the utilization of our antioxidant reserves—life span molecules in my lingo—and by upregulating the ability to replenish those reserves after periods of excessive utilization. The former goal can be achieved with self-regulation and meditation, and by reducing exposure to aging-oxidant molecules in our internal and external environments. The latter goal can be met with optimal choices in the kitchen and with protocols of nutritional medicine and fitness medicine. What binds these four disciplines together is the common thread of molecular dynamics. The clinical application of these molecular dynamics to the treatment of disease is the practice of molecular medicine.

WHAT IS THE BEST METHOD FOR ASSESSING OXIDATIVE INJURY?

Many methods have been used to assess oxidative phenomena. Chemists usually measure the oxidative reactions in the laboratory by measuring the activity of enzymes that facilitate or block oxidative-reductive reactions—the redox cycling as it commonly called in chemistry. Examples of such enzymes include superoxide dismutase and catalase enzymes.

In medical research, investigators have used measurement of ethane and pentane gases that are produced as a result of oxidation of fatty acids. The use of such chemical methods in medical research declined rapidly after some initial excitement, largely because these methods are cumbersome, and their applications are not suitable for hospitals or physician office laboratories.

From a purely theoretical standpoint, direct examination of the blood cell membranes and blood plasma should offer the best opportunity to assess oxidative damage for several valid reasons:

First,

the blood forms the first line of defense against oxidative stresses, and so would be expected to show evidence of accelerated oxidative damage before any other body organ.

Second,

the blood is an easily accessible body tissue for sampling.

Third,

the study of blood for assessing oxidant damage is far less expensive than any other method. Microscopes are available in all laboratories and no other equipment is necessary.

Fourth,

the examination of blood gives an immediate assessment of the oxidative index, and the efficacy of therapies used for a given patient can be accurately and readily evaluated.

It is profoundly ironic that mainstream medicine has turned its back on this simple diagnostic procedure. Indeed, the handful of holistic physicians who use this method are often persecuted for it by their state licensing boards. I write about the sad story of two such physicians in chapter eight.

THE MOST TEST:
MICROSCOPIC OXIDATIVE STRESS TEST

"Most" is my term for microscopic oxidative stress test. My researh colleague, Dr. Robert Bradford, a pioneer in this field, uses the term LBA (live blood analysis) for the same purpose.

In the first part of the Most test, a drop of patient's blood is taken by a quick finger stick and a thin smear of blood is prepared on a glass microscopic slide. A glass coverslip is then put over the smear to protect it from oxidant injury by the ambient oxygen as well as dehydration.

In the second part of the Most test, multiple circular imprints of another drop of blood from the same finger stick are prepared by gently touching the finger with the blood drop with three glass slides, one by one. These blood imprints are allowed to dry and then examined under a microscope.

The term ROS—reactive oxygen species—is part of the standard chemistry nomenclature. Earlier in this chapter I discuss at length how ROS inflict molecular and cellular injury and cause disease. In the Most test, the focus is on how ROS injure cell membranes and cause visible evidence of oxidative damage. Thus, the cells may agglutinate (clump), may lose their normal smooth, regular outline and become deformed, or show spiking and crinkling. The Most test also focuses on blood plasma proteins that are oxidatively injured and congealed or precipitates.

The photomicrograph shown below was taken during the Most test performed on the blood of patient with lung cancer with metastatic spread to the liver. It shows oxidatively damaged red blood cells clump together so that no cell is separated from other cells as is seen in health and is shown in photomicrograph on page 283. The irregularly shaped, pale-white, fluffy objects found between the clumped red cells represent "oxidative plaques"—plasma proteins congealed and clotted by oxidative injury. These changes can often be reversed—albeit for a short time—by intravenous vitamin C infusion.

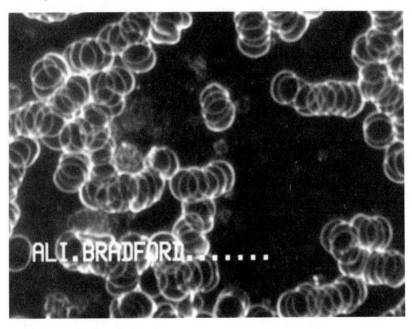

SPONTANEITY OF OXIDATION AND
THE HEALTH—DIS-EASE—DISEASE CONTINUUM

The spontaneity of oxidation in nature—and its essential role in the health—dis-ease—disease continuum—has been one of the most important insights I have gained in over 35 years of medical study. In this chapter, I use examples of major chronic degenerative and immune disorders to support my theory that accelerated oxidative molecular injury is the fundamental cause of *all* diseases. Target organs change in different people, but that does not distract from the validity of the core idea.

Exercise requires energy, and energy in the body is produced by the oxidation of food materials. It follows that exercise must also increase oxidative stress. How do we reconcile this to the enormous and proven benefits of exercise? I address this issue in the companion volume *The Ghoraa and Limbic Exercise.*

Health, in molecular terms, is the molecular mosaic that balances life span molecules against aging-oxidant molecules; disease, a state of energetic-molecular disarray in which AOMs overwhelm LSMs and that culminates in accelerated oxidative molecular injury. This is a simple yet profound view of the chemistry of life. It is also the strongest possible scientific defense of holistic medicine.

ALL ANTIOXIDANTS ARE ALSO OXIDANTS

Sometime ago, a woman consulted me for chronic disabling fatigue. She told me she had received 200 grams (200,000 milligrams) of vitamin C intravenously twice a week for the preceding three months under the care of another physician. I asked her if she knew what her physician had hoped to achieve by such massive doses of this vitamin. "He plans to root out the Epstein-Barr virus which is the cause of my problem," she replied. I explained to her the Epstein-Barr virus (EBV) becomes incorporated in our own DNA molecules and that it was simplistic to think that the virus can be eradicated by vitamin C drips regardless of the dose administered. Indeed, such massive doses are likely to worsen her condition. Her husband agreed with me but she didn't. Three months later, she completed a course of over 9,000 grams—over nine million milligrams of vitamin C. At the end of that period, her EBV antibody was not lower than where it had been at the outset of therapy and she showed no improvement.

A HOSE OF LIQUID ANTIOXIDANTS

All antioxidants are also oxidants. Otherwise, all we would have needed to treat all diseases would have been a large hose of liquid vitamin C, E, A or any other antioxidant. Nature does not subscribe to such frivolous notions.

A man begins to clean his oven with a pile of clean rags. The oven is black with soot and charred foods. One by one, he uses a clean rag to clean a part of the oven and then rather than throw away the dirty rag he puts it back into the dirty oven. When all clean rags have been dirtied, he begins to reuse the dirty rags, carefully putting them back into the oven. What will be the end of this story? All the soot and charred food would be still in the oven and the oven would be dirty. Something identical to this happens when we flood the human biologic systems with antioxidants.

Antioxidants and oxidants in the body play both sides of the field. When an antioxidant is used to neutralize an oxidant molecule, it becomes oxidized in the process. Thus, each molecule of ascorbic acid (vitamin C) turns into a molecule of hydroxyascorbic acid which is an oxidant—precisely the way a clean rag cleans a part of the dirty oven and in the process becomes dirty itself. It loses its capacity to clean the oven any further. Indeed, it becomes a dirtying agent.

It is easy for anyone to test the validity of this statement with direct study of the oxidative damage to blood proteins and blood cell membranes with a high-resolution microscope. Indeed, Dr. Robert Bradford, a good friend and an eminent cancer researcher of Chula Vista, California, and I have confirmed that large doses (25 grams or more) of vitamin C given intravenously twice a week actually increase the oxidative stress rather than reduce it.

This is the scientific basis of my frequent advice to my patients to meditate and pray for calming the oxidant storms that arise from adrenaline surges caused by stress of modern life. I discuss this subject further in *The Ghoraa and Limbic Exercise.*

> **WHAT'S WRONG WITH MY THEORY THAT**
> **SPONTANEITY OF OXIDATION IS**
> **THE CAUSE OF ALL DISEASES?**

This question preoccupied me for several years. This is a simple theory—easy to comprehend, easy to test with established scientific knowledge. Yet, it has such profound implications for a model of health for individuals as well as nations. So, what's wrong with it? The question repeated itself over and over. But, as I mention earlier, every month my copies of *Nature* and *Science* carried reports of oxidative stress on living beings that fully validated my viewpoint.

During the past fifteen years, I also read a large body of scientific reports that vehemently argued against the role of oxidative stress in the cause of human illness. I quote below from a comprehensive 1993 review of this subject:

However, because free radical-mediated changes are pervasive and often poorly understood, the question of whether such species are a major cause of tissue injury and human disease remains equivocal.

Critical Reviews in Toxicology
23(1):21-48; 1993

Pervasive, yes! Poorly understood? This quote is taken from the abstract of the review on the first page and illustrates the main mistake practitioners of drug medicine make. (The author of the review article is a pharmacologist.) They cannot see the difference between the low-rate *physiologic* oxyradical activity and the *pathologic* effects of accelerated oxidative molecular injury. They fail to see the globally increasing oxidant stress on human biology. The author continues:

...free radical-mediated changes are often not injurious but rather merely reflect homeostatic mechanisms...The extent of this involvement (free radical injury in rheumatoid arthritis) must not be overstated inasmuch as the underlying cause of this disease is certainly autoimmune in nature, and thus antioxidant therapy will be treating only a symptom.

Critical Reviews in Toxicology
23(1):35: 1993 (Parenthesis added)

An astounding statement from someone who should know better! What comes first, free radical injury or autoimmune injury? Evidently, the author has never reflected on where autoimmune disorders might come from. Mount Olympus? Choua would have asked.

All autoimmune injuries are first free radical injuries before they become immune injury. Electron transfer events that trigger free radical formation are the *initial energetic-molecular events* that separate a state of health from a state of absence of health. Molecular and immune cellular injury occurs when the generation of free radicals is accelerated and uncontrolled.

> *...there is no firm link between this oxidative event and atherosclerotic disease.*
>
> *Critical Review in Toxicology*
> 23(1):36; 1993

Yet another mind-boggling statement! I suppose our pharmacologist friend will change his opinion as soon as FDA approves a drug touted to reduce oxidative stress on LDL cholesterol and on the scavenger cells in vessel walls that accumulate such oxidized and denatured cholesterol.

Yearning for Immortality

I close this chapter with some brief comments about human vulnerability to spontaneity of oxidation in nature and the law of oxidative death.

> *I want to prove...that the boundaries set by the gods are not unbreakable.*

Gilgamesh 5,000 BC

There is considerable interest in physical immortality at this time. Some Gilgamesh cousins—the *New Age* gurus of physical immortality preach to their flocks that humans can attain physical immortality and live for ever—if only they would buy *their* videos, take *their* workshops, join *their* retreats and eat *their* exotic potions. (What a horrible thought! To continue to live long after our children and their children, and our friends and all their children are gone!)

I do not know much about physical immortality. It is quite evident to me that life for all living beings does end, for some earlier than for others. I will readily change my point of view if I see at least one life form live forever. For now, I continue to believe that no living being capable of utilizing oxygen is really exempt from the immutable law of oxidative death.

Simplification without much knowledge is simplemindedness; much knowledge without simplicity is not much different.

Chapter 6

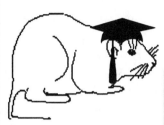

THIRD INSIGHT

Healing is
a natural state of energy.
The Mind-over-body
<u>does not work</u>;
An Energy-over-mind
approach does!

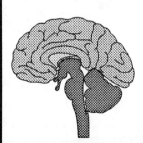

Life is energy—and all living beings are energy beings.

When life begins, it begins to end. Living beings begin their decline at birth. Thus, the process of living is at once the process of aging and dying as well as that of healing. The injury-healing cycle endures as long as life exists—and healing is a natural state of energy.

The subject of healing energy fascinates me—and should interest everyone who cares for the sick.

At an intellectual level, the energy of living beings is simple to comprehend. When we turned the great cities of Hiroshima and Nagasaki into rubble, we fully realized the power of atomic energy. And, of course, the human frame is nothing but billions of ever-changing atomic kaleidoscopes. It should naturally follow that all life is essentially an energy function—all living beings—a single-celled amoeba, a flower, a child, and a dinosaur—are energy beings. Moreover, the energy of each being is irrevocably linked to the energy of other beings. It is all one grand *network*. This is not merely a theoretical concept. It is a core concept for all who care for the sick.

Although it is unthinkable to dissociate "energy" from healing, the word invites derision in medical circles. I clearly recall how much hesitation I felt before I used this word in my medical writings for the first time.

Why? We physicians associate the word *energy* with faith healers, witches, charlatans and mystics. We are bitterly irritated when we hear such people make claims of success that are nothing more than blatant lies. Thus, the word *energy* in medicine is linked to ignorance, abuse and fraud. This linkage is unfortunate because in our ignorant animus against healing without drugs and scalpels, we turn our backs on a subject worthy of serious study. Thus, we relinquish our role in an area that is of overriding importance in clinical medicine.

DO MIND-OVER-BODY APPROACHES REALLY WORK?

Notwithstanding the rather limited and temporary benefits of positive thinking and affirmation, I have seen no evidence that mind-over-body approaches to healing work. In contrast, energy-over-mind approaches heal. I observe evidence of that every Wednesday evening during self-regulation training sessions. When the clutter of the thinking mind is put to rest, the energy that constitutes us is free to guide us.

Our infatuation with mind-over-body healing is a relatively recent development. Since man became aware of the healing response in injured tissues, he has been interested in the energy phenomenon. Since antiquity, people have explored the various dimensions of the healing phenomenon, and have entertained the question of how to facilitate a natural healing response in injured tissues. To date, I can find no records showing that the ancients ever succeeded in using their minds to order healing in tissues. I have never seen convincing evidence from any faith healers, mystics, shamans and the modern gurus of the mind-over-body industry indicating that they found a way *to use their thinking minds to prod the nonhealing tissues to heal*—at least in the physical ways that can be *observed* with a microscope or assessed by other chemical and physical means.

This is not to say that miracles do not happen. I *know* they happen. I have seen miracles take place among my patients thousands of times. But miracles are energy phenomena. I have yet to see proof that miracles can be brought about by clever thinking.

CAN THE MIND COAX INJURED TISSUES TO HEAL QUICKER, OR DO TISSUES HEAL FASTER WHEN THE MIND IS STILLED?

In many well-documented cases, the course of illness appears to have been radically altered certain measures taken by the sick. The question that intrigues me is whether the observed benefits resulted because the mind ordained the injured tissues to heal or because injured tissues were spared the disease-promoting activities of the thinking mind. Do diseased tissues regenerate more expediently when they are relentlessly driven by schemes concocted by the thinking mind? Or do they heal more quickly when the unrelenting mind is stilled?   Before the thinking mind can heal hurt tissues, it must first understand how healing occurs. For the mind to fix a healing problem, it must first know what that healing problem is. The issue is not that the phenomenon of healing can be facilitated. It clearly can be. The question is what, if any, role does the thinking mind play in the healing response. It amuses me that those who speak the loudest of their mind's ability to heal are the people who seem to have the least understanding of the healing response in distressed tissues.

"IT JUST HAPPENS, DR. ALI, HONEST, IT JUST HAPPENS."

A very large number of patients tell me they can control migraine attacks, asthma episodes, colitis and other disorders with mind-over-body healing. Some tell me that they can heal chronically painful backs with their minds. Such stories are of intense interest to me. I never doubt that these people are telling me the truth. What I pursue vigorously is *how* they use their minds to heal the body. How do they persuade their tightened arteries to let go so that they might get some relief from migraine pain? How do they plead with, coax or simply order their spastic bronchial tubes to open so they can breathe without using drugs? How do they convince their ulcerated colons to cease from episodes of cramping and bleeding? How do they use their minds to tell irritated, rebellious muscles in their backs to loosen up?

To date no one has ever answered such questions. When questioned, my patients become defensive, making statements such as:

"Dr. Ali, I can often control my asthma attacks," the patient proudly tells me.
"That's wonderful! How do you do it?" I ask.
"You know how, don't you?"
"No, I really don't."
"Well, with mind control." He smiles.
"Tell me how you do mind control."
"With mind-over-body healing."

"How do you do your mind-over-body healing?" I persist.

"You know! The mind-over-body approach." He becomes a little tentative.

"Tell me how you do your mind-over-body approach to asthma?" I press him. "I mean, how do you use your mind to send messages to the bronchial tubes to open so that air can get in?"

"Well..." The patient stops in midsentence.

"Yes..." I coax him.

"I... I... I don't know how..."

"Just think about it. Try to recall how you do your mind-over-body thing. I'm very interested in that."

"It just happens, Doc."

"Of course, it happens. But I need to understand how it happens. If you can teach me how you do it, then I can teach your method to my other patients who suffer from asthma."

"It just happens, Dr. Ali, honest, it does happens."

"Of course, it does!" I reassure him.

"You really don't believe me, do you?" he asks.

"Of course I do," I assert. "Every Wednesday I spend three hours with my patients teaching them self-regulation. So I do know it works. I just want to know how *you* do it."

"Maybe I can't explain it, but it *does* work."

"I know! I know! I don't doubt you for one moment."

"So you do believe mind-over-body works."

"I didn't say that, did I? It would have been different if we really could use our minds to do such things. But how do we know it is the working of the mind if the mind does not even know what it is? How can we say we use our mind to do something our mind doesn't even understand?"

"How else do you think it works?"

"I don't know. Perhaps because you have intuitively found a way to shut off your thinking mind—keep the cortical monkey out. Perhaps because tissue energy shuts out the mind so that the natural healing state of energy in injured tissues can do what Nature designed it to do—heal. Perhaps because the natural state of the bronchial tubes is to stay relaxed and open. That's what they do when they are left alone—when the ceaseless demands of their thinking minds are blocked by the healing energy of irritated bronchial tubes. Isn't that what asthma sufferers tell us? Stress makes their asthma worse."

"You mean it is not the mind that heals? It's something else? Something other than my thinking mind?" he asks, perplexed.

"Isn't that what you just told me?" I retort.

THE MIND OF AN OSTEOBLAST

Fractured bones heal without taking cues from the thinking mind. To my knowledge, osteoblasts—the bone cells that multiply and lay down new bone for the healing of fractured bones—do not have much respect for mind-over-body healing.

Consider wounds healing in healthy little children, vigorous adults and active elderly individuals. Suppose a two-year-old girl, a 42-year-old woman and a 92-year-old woman trip over a stone and fracture their wrist bones. Whose broken bones will heal the fastest and whose will take the longest? Predictably, the child's broken bones will heal in the shortest time and the elderly woman's will take the longest. Now let us factor in the conventional mind-over-body approach. The child does not even know that such notions as mind-over-body healing exist, makes no attempt to engage in it, and yet her bones heal the quickest. The 92-year-old woman should have the most knowledge, and should have all the necessary time to put the mind-over-body healing method to the test. Yet, she will have the most difficulty, and in most instances, can be expected to have incomplete bone healing even under the ideal circumstances. How do we reconcile these everyday observations with the mind-over-body theory?

The osteoblast cells in the two-year-old girl burst into activity and merrily go about their business of mending broken bones, following their own energy signals, totally oblivious of what her mind may or may not dictate. Cells revved up with healing energy cherish their autonomy. The healing cells in the 42-year-old woman will follow a different pace and heal the bone slowly. The osteoblast cells of the 92-year-old woman will lay out new bone in their own leisurely way, sensing no need to acknowledge any of the exhortations of the clever, thinking mind.

NONUNION IN PEOPLE, MALUNION IN ANIMALS

As a young surgeon in training, first in Pakistan and later in England, I saw many cases of nonunion of fractured bones. Nonunion refers to a condition in which fractured bones do not heal even when set and immobilized in a cast. For some reasons, the natural healing process is arrested in this condition. (Impaired blood circulation, poor nutritional status and prolonged immobilization are some of the causes of nonunion.) Malunion refers to cases in which the two broken ends of the bone unite but do so in a crooked way.

The subject of nonunion often summons references to the

healing phenomena in primitive cultures and in wild animals. Fractured bones heal among tribal cultures in which broken bones are set and splinted without using modern technology, though the broken bones often heal with malunion—in a malaligned fashions. Similarly, fractured bones always heal in the animal kingdom, though predictably producing crookedly healed bones. Nonunion is a rare phenomenon in nature. By contrast, nonunion is not very uncommon after the broken bones are immobilized in casts. Thus, there is a clear distinction between healing of fractured bone under natural circumstances with minimal or no interference and healing of broken bones under conditions of forced immobilization with orthopedic techniques. Nonunion is a price we pay for introducing the mind of man to the natural healing response in bone.

Obviously, I do not make a case here for not using modern orthopedic techniques on fractured bones. I do not advocate that we accept crookedly healed bones. I include here brief comments about the conditions of nonunion and malunion of fractured bones to illustrate my essential point: The thinking mind cannot force healing on osteoblast cells. These cells will do what Nature designed them to do. They lay down new bone and mold and remold such bone in response to healthy stresses of life so that the end result is a healed bone. Children's broken bones usually heal quickly. The mended bones model and remodel themselves continuously. X-rays of such bones, taken several months after the healing response began, show perfect bone structure so that someone unfamiliar with the case would not even suspect that a fracture had occurred. The thinking mind clearly plays no role in such bone healing.

My essential point in this brief discussion of bone healing is that while the mind can interfere with bone healing, it cannot initiate or speed the healing response in broken bones.

THE ADRENALINE PUMP
AND THE MIND OF A GAZELLE

Nature gave us the fight-or-flight response as a survival technique. When the mind perceives a threat, a large number of reflex reactions—outside the mind's control—gear the body for response. The heart races to pump more blood for maximal effort; the lungs hyperventilate to bring inhale more oxygen to sustain the effort; the pupils dilate to see more; and the muscles are held taut for maximum efficiency. The fight-or-flight response is elicited by bursts of adrenaline from the adrenal gland. I devote the companion volume *What Do Lions Know About Stress?* to this subject.

A leopard crouches behind the bush and slowly approaches a gazelle grazing in a meadow. When the leopard can no longer hide its approach, it lunges forward toward the gazelle. The prey sees a flashing image, freezes for a moment in shock, then breaks into a frenzied dash. The flashing image has been processed by the gazelle. Almost instantly an adrenaline surge sends a barrage of molecular messages that thrust the body into a dance of survival. Some minutes later, the exhausted leopard gives up the chase, and the gazelle escapes. Within moments, the chemistry of the gazelle begins its return to a normal state, as the adrenaline peak ebbs and the related flight molecules break down. Does the gazelle use its mind to control its body and return its Fourth-of-July chemistry to a health-restoring steady state energy?

EARLY MAN
AND THE BODY-MIND-SPIRIT TRIO

I am fascinated by the ancient records of spiritual healing. In all cultures and in all segments of mankind's history, there is clear evidence of spiritual healing. Methods change, but the essence of healing does not. It is also clear that such healing was always an energy phenomenon, though its essential nature escaped critical intellectual scrutiny—as it continues to do to date. If spiritual healing is hocus pocus—as my colleagues in drug medicine believe—how could it survive for millennia? Fads in medicine come and go. Why did the essential mystery of spiritual healing endure?

How did early man come up with his body-mind-spirit trio in the first place? It is easy to understand why he thought about the first two. He had bodily senses, and he could think, imagine, hope and dream. But why the third element? How did he know that the third element of the spirit existed? After all, whatever he could think about or imagine comes under the jurisdiction of the mind. No matter how wide the swing of his imagination or how vast the reach of his mind, it was all an intellectual function. How did he dream up the very notion that the spirit existed? Indeed, the very thought of the spirit is well within the confines of the thought process. By definition, the spirit must be accepted as beyond our physical senses and beyond all intellectual faculties.

The primitive healer closed his eyes and went into an altered energy state for the healing ritual. The shaman of today does the same. Closed eyes and the rhythm of the drums allowed the ancient to escape the confines of the thinking mind. It is the same with the shaman and others who take this healing approach.

MUSIC AND HEALING

Music sustains. Music alleviates suffering. Music heals. How does music do all that? How does music reverse a disease process?

Is musical transformation an intellectual function? Did Mozart and Beethoven engage in highly intellectual functions when they composed? I doubt if any singer in the history of mankind has been listened to more frequently than the Indian singer, Lata Mangeshkar. It has been estimated that more than a billion and a half people in India, Pakistan, Bangladesh, Far East, Middle East, South Africa and many other countries listen to her songs regularly. Certainly, Lata is heard more frequently in New York City taxis than any other singer. (More than 80 percent of the taxis in the city are driven by Pakistanis and Indians.) Lata has the singular quality of reaching the core of her listeners. I doubt if any singer has ever alleviated more human suffering with her/his words than Lata has. Does she use her mind to exert her healing influence? Or, does she harness the mental faculties of her listeners to order their injured tissues to shape up—and heal themselves? "Man, if you gotta ask you'll never know," Louis Armstrong replied when asked what jazz is. Thomas [Fats] Waller spoke of the same dimension when asked to explain rhythm: "Lady, if you got to ask you ain't got it." Healing, like music and rhythm, cannot be explained or understood—it can only be *known*. The gurus of the mind-over-body industry do not seem to know this.

THE MIND CREATES THE FOURTH-OF-JULY CHEMISTRY, HEALING ENERGY EXTINGUISHES THE OXIDATIVE SPARKS.

The mind can light up the oxidative sparks of anger, resentment and hostility, but the clever designs of the thinking mind cannot extinguish such sparks. I see evidence of this phenomenon every working day. An occupied mind—the cortical monkey in autoregulation lingo—loves to recycle misery. It thrives on packaging and repackaging past hurts. When that is not enough, it precycles feared, future misery. It turns a natural state of healing energy into turbulent Fourth-of-July chemistry. It mercilessly drives the energy enzyme pathways of the body, literally short-circuiting human energy systems. Unable to cope with the unending demands of the thinking mind, the energy-depleted and exhausted tissues succumb. The clever-thinking mind succeeds in its relentless pursuit.

WHY ARE WE PHYSICIANS MIFFED BY THE MIND-OVER-BODY APPROACH TO HEALING?

This is an interesting question. Physicians make their livings treating diseases, but their sincerity is widely questioned in the U.S. today. Notwithstanding such cynicism, a vast majority of physicians are hard-working, caring and compassionate professionals. Physicians *do* want their patients to get better. What could be safer, less expensive and convenient than mind-over-body healing for physicians? Unfortunately, most physicians are too wedded to drug medicine to reflect on this simple question.

Most advances of Star Wars medicine took place in the later part of this century. Before that, we physicians had none of the high-tech tools of our trade. It would have been the most natural thing for us to engage in the mind-over-body healing approach. So why didn't we?

It may be argued that physicians were not seduced by mind-over-body healing because it would have disempowered them—put the patient in charge of the healing process. It would have minimized the importance of the physician's role in the care of the sick, and it might have denigrated their herbs and lancets. Indeed, implicit was the clear risk that success in mind-over-body healing might put them out of commission. There is, however, a problem with this theory. Clearly, there were physicians in the past whose commitment to the well-being of their patients was unequivocally sufficient to consider this approach—if for no other reason than that mind-over-body healing has no serious adverse effects.

So why didn't physicians engage mind-over-body healing? I believe the real answer is that they found it simply doesn't work—notwithstanding rather limited benefits of positive thinking and affirmations of health. Even in modern times, we have known that what is being touted as mind-over-body techniques are petty intellectual games.

There is another interesting aspect to this subject. If mind-over-body healing really worked, we physicians would have known this better than any other group. We would have certainly adopted the method for personal use and for treating our family members. The reality is quite different: We physicians, as a group, probably use more drugs for our own infirmities than any other large group of professionals. If the mind-over-body approach really worked, certainly we, more than any other group, would have put it into personal use.

Injured molecules, cells and tissues heal spontaneously when they are spared the clever healing schemes of the thinking mind. I discuss this simple truth, that perceptive individuals in the healing profession have known for thousands of years, at length in the companion volume *The Cortical Monkey and Healing.*

PSYCHOSOMATIC AND SOMATOPSYCHIC MODELS OF DISEASE ARE ARTIFACTS OF OUR THINKING

Diseases are burdens on biology. Human intellect and human body organs are integral parts of the human condition. To separate them, as Socrates lamented, is to negate the completeness of the human condition.

Our technology has rendered irrelevant the debate on the psychosomatic and somatopsychic nature of diseases. Advances in behavioral biology and experimental psychology have put these two disciplines on a collision course; a complete merger between the two is simply a matter of time.

Hope is an energetic-molecular event. So is dejection.

Neuropeptide research is closing in on defining emotions and behavior as chemical sequences. The French philosopher, Teilhard de Chardin, dreamed of the day when man's technology would conquer oceans and winds and begin to explore the energy of love. We are seeing the dawn of that day.

Self-regulation with an energy-over-mind approach brings forth profound energetic-molecular changes in human biology. In *The Limbic Dog and Directed Pulses* and *The Pheasant, Suffering and Limbic Breathing*, I describe various biochemical and electromagnetic changes that I have observed with autoregulation methods in my patients. Clinically, many of my patients can control asthma and arthritis, lower blood pressure in hypertension, and normalize overactive and underactive thyroid glands with consistency and predictability.

It is unusual for me to see a patient who is unable to learn how to alter one or more electrophysiologic responses during his very first training session with me in our autoregulation laboratory.

Clinically, I see far superior results with energy-over-mind approaches than are possible with positive thinking and affirmations. I have not seen the mind-over-body gospel work. Many of my patients revers their chronic diseases when they learn how to quiet their minds, perceive their tissue energy, and *allow the tissue energy to guide them*. Tissues evidently know their business, and do respond. We need only to learn how to shut our thinking *cortical minds* and limbically perceive the healing energy of that larger *presence* that surrounds each of us at all times. This is not simply a clever play on words. Molecular and tissue repair are visceral and limbic-energetic functions. Injured tissues do heal with their innate energetic pathways, when we keep the disruptive influences of the thinking mind (cortical monkey) out of their healing ways.

AUTOREGULATION

The terms *autoreg, autoregulation, self-regulation, cortical* and *limbic* appear throughout the volumes in this series. This is is a short note about how these words took form.

In my early clinical work, I developed stress management techniques for patients with chronic indolent problems. Since the patients' conditions seemed to resist the standard prevailing medical methods, I found myself teaching them how to slow their hearts, open their arteries and dissolve their muscle tension. In medical terminology, these activities are referred to as autonomic functions, so it seemed logical to use the term *autonomic regulation*. My patients abbreviated the term to *autoreg*.

I soon realized my patients desperately wanted me to teach them effective methods for self-regulation and facilitating natural healing. I also recognized that self-regulation went far beyond any ideas of autonomic regulation, and started a search for a simple term that declared my purpose. Again my patients solved the problem. They stayed with the term autoreg, as I experimented with different words. In the end I decided to follow their lead.

Looking back, my work with autoregulation evolved in the following sequences: stress management, autonomic regulation, self-regulation, and aspects of hope and spirituality in the healing response.

AN ESSENTIAL LESSON

One of the essential lessons my patients taught me is this: Slowing the heart rate, keeping the arteries open, and slow, even breathing profoundly affect our mood and state of mind. These basic methods of autoregulation are very effective in dissipating anger and anxiety, even when that is not our intended purpose. But that is just the beginning. Autoregulation reveals the path of self-regulation and healing. A passage through the realms of self-regulation inevitably ushers a person to higher states of awareness and consciousness.

BEYOND POSITIVE THINKING

Positive thinking, as desirable as it may seem on the surface, is still thinking. My work with very ill patients has convinced me that positive thinking alone is not sufficient to transform one's biology from a cortical state of turmoil to a calm, steady, regenerative limbic state.

It is cruel to advise a patient to think positively when he is in the throes of intense suffering.

Early in my work with autoregulation, a simple and useful conceptual model for autoregulation evolved in my mind. In this model, human biology exists in two basic but overlapping states:

1) a state created and sustained by a superficial part of the brain—neocortex in scientific jargon—in which a person stays head-fixated, forever planning and scheming; 2) an energy state in which the body tissues escape unrelenting censors of the thinking process—the tyranny of the mind—and revert to a natural, regenerative state.

I learned from personal experience and by working long hours with my patients that it is extremely difficult, if at all possible, to be in the healing mode unless we can halt the thinking mind. In the thinking mode, it is unlikely that we can allow ourselves to be led by the gentle guiding energy that exists within us—and that surrounds each of us at all times.

Beyond these two states there is yet another state: the spiritual state. I write about this third state in *The Canary and Chronic Fatigue* and other companion volumes.

THE CORTICAL MODE

The cortical mode counts, computes and competes. It censors and cautions. It controls and constricts. It assesses and analyzes. It wavers and warns. It imposes chronic thinking on us. And with its unrelenting chatter, it causes stress, impaired immunity and leads to a state of absence of health—a dis-ease state. The dis-ease state, if not reversed, damages tissues and causes disease. I discuss these issues more fully in the companion volume *What Do Lions Know About Stress?*

THE LIMBIC MODE

I use the term *limbic mode* to refer to a native state of healing energy. The limbic mode cares and comforts. It soothes and pampers. It gives and accepts affection and love. It creates images of health. It heals. In the limbic mode, our biology is in a steady state, assuring the continuity of basic life functions. It keeps the rhythm of the heart, arterial pulses, muscle tone, breathing cycles, and other essential life functions in order.

In the limbic model of healing, we learn to perceive the healing energy of living tissues and simply allow the superior wisdom of this energy to guide us. There is no attempt to use the mind to order the injured tissues to heal. (Injured tissues do not seem to have much respect for our clever-thinking schemes anyway.)

In the biologic profiles shown on the following pages, I illustrate the patterns of electrophysiologic stress I observe in the cortical mode, and how these patterns change when an individual escapes the tyranny of the mind and by slipping into the limbic mode.

The biologic profile given below illustrates a disease-causing cortical mode of the functions of various body organs. The sensing electrodes attached to the patient indicate electromagnetic expressions of spasm of the arteries (single arrow), stress on the heart as shown by wide swings in the heart rate (two arrows) and a high skin conductance (three arrows). See color plates on page 210.

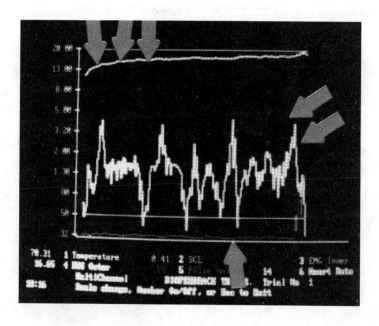

The biologic profile given below illustrates a limbic,
healing, physiologic mode. The sensor electrodes indicate body
organ functions as follows: yellow line, skin conductance energy;
red line, arterial pulse; bright white line, heart rhythm; green line,
forearm muscle sensor; and blue line, upper arm muscle sensor.
Note how all tissue energy sensors show smooth, even, resting
(and healing) patterns. See color plates corresponding to the black
and white picture given below on page 210.

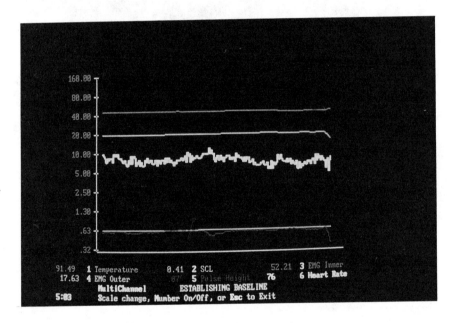

The biologic profile given below illustrates how a restful, healing limbic mode during autoregulation (left side of the graph) turns into a stressful, disease-causing cortical mode when autoregulation is interrupted (right side of graph). The colored electrode sensor lines show energy patterns in various body organs as follows: yellow line, skin conductance energy; red line, arterial pulse energy; bright white line, heart rhythm; green line, forearm muscle energy sensor; and blue line, upper arm muscle sensor. Note how the red artery sensor line dips suddenly as the subject switches from limbic to cortical mode. The heart, muscle and skin energy lines begin to show stressful patterns soon after. See color plates on page 210 for photograph corresponding to the black and white picture shown below.

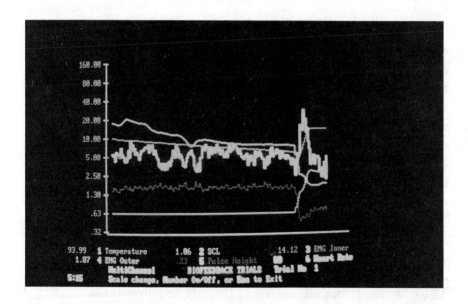

AUTOREGULATION IS SELF-REGULATION WITH HEALING ENERGY

Autoregulation, as defined in this volume, is an *energy-over-mind* approach to freeing the natural healing response from barriers imposed on it by the thinking mind. All living beings—cells, tissues and body organs—are energy beings. In autoregulation, we simply allow ourselves to be guided by the innate energy of living beings. Before we can do that, however, we need to learn how to perceive the patterns of energy in our tissues, whether healthy or sick.

In my clinical work, I use elaborate computerized electromagnetic technology to demonstrate to my patients how energy patterns in the body are determined by the way we look at the world around us—and how they change when we successfully banish the thinking mind and allow ourselves to be led by such energy. Machines do not heal—and biofeedback technology is no exception. There is, however, considerable value in demonstrating objective, measurable, and reproducible electromagnetic changes during autoregulation. The technology clearly documents that the energy patterns in the health—dis-ease—disease continuum are real. It appeases the cortical monkey by giving it a taste of its own medicine.

I chose the term *cortical* because the cortical brain is the seat of most, if not all, activities that are required for calculating, computing, cautioning, creating images of stress and overdriving injured tissues. Unless checked, this culminates in disease.

Needless to say, we need all those functions as well—but not for healing purposes.

> ## SELF-REGULATION TECHNOLOGIES CHANGE; SELF-REGULATION PRINCIPLES DO NOT

The science and technology of modern medicine have made it possible for any person to see his disease at microscopic, electrophysiologic and molecular levels. A person can *know* the true nature of his illness at microscopic and submicroscopic levels. He can understand the nature of tissue damage by seeing how damaged tissues look.

A person can become intimate with his disease at an electrophysiologic level by examining his biologic profile—a live, dynamic composite picture of graphs showing the function of his internal body organs on a computer screen. In my autoregulation laboratory, I show patients how they can alter their own biological profiles with simple exercises.

A person can familiarize himself with his disease at a cellular level by examining his cells' reactions to different molecules. I show this to patients using high resolution video technology.

Injured molecules, cells and tissues all heal with energy—in autoregulation, we simply allow this energy to harness itself for healing functions.

Different technologies offer different advantages. What

needs to be held constant is a clear view of our goals, an awareness of the energy in our tissues, a desire to attend to our tissues and *listening for healing* rather than *talking for control.*

AUTOREGULATION IS NOT HEALING WITH COUNSELING, ANALYSIS, REGRESSION, HYPNOSIS OR BIOFEEDBACK

Compassion comforts. All methods that a professional uses to console a suffering individual are acceptable as long as the goal of short-term relief does not thwart the long-term recovery process. In my view, the very essence of long-term recovery is in *knowing* the true nature of the suffering and in following a path that frees a person from dependence on another. As for those who provide care, the essence of that caring is showing the way to total recovery. Thus, for the professional, the goal of all disease-reversal and recovery programs is to teach the patient ways of self-reliance—in matters of nutrition, environment, fitness, language of silence and energy perceptions. I consider it a failure on my part if I do not succeed in helping a patient see this clearly. I am a realist who has learned that long-suffering patients need enormous support before reaching the physical relief and clarity of vision for the future that I describe here.

Regrettably, counseling, analysis, regression, hypnosis and biofeedback—as they are often practiced today—sink the patient deeper and deeper into dependence on the therapist. In many cases, these therapies offer little more than cortical traps. Most of my patients received such therapies for many years before they consulted me. It takes very little time and training for them to see the difference between talking for control and being guided by their energy for healing. Talking in most instances is a mere recycling of misery, the language of silence is liberating.

PLACEBO, HYPNOSIS AND SELF-REGULATION

There is one fundamental difference between the placebo effect or hypnosis on one hand and self-regulation on the other.

When a person is relieved of his suffering with the placebo effect or hypnosis, it happens without his knowing the true nature of his suffering. The effects of both approaches invariably cease after some time.

****

When autoregulation relieves a person's suffering, he comes to a biological-intuitive understanding of his condition. The longer he stays with self-regulation, the more profound and lasting the benefits.

I illustrate this essential difference by citing an example: A physician gives his patient a placebo (starch capsule) and tells him that the medicine in the capsule will cure his headache. The placebo works, and the headache indeed is relieved. Because the patient in this case was tricked into thinking that the starch capsule in the placebo was an effective remedy, he did not understand the true nature of things. On those occasions when patients discover the truth, they naturally feel as if they have been victimized.

A hypnotist treats a patient suffering from a migraine headache. The hypnotic suggestion works, and the headache is relieved. The patient associates the hypnotic trance with some sort of a spell, albeit a helpful and healthful spell. This patient is not much better than the one enjoying the placebo effect, insofar as his understanding of the true nature of things is obscured. In both cases, the patient learns to depend on the therapist. With each migraine, the dependence grows while the benefits of the therapy diminish. I have seen no exceptions.

Self-regulation is a path to independence. Hypnosis and placebos lead to dependence on someone else. Neither hypnosis nor placebos enlighten the patient as to the true nature of his suffering.

I am not opposed to hypnosis for temporary relief of symptoms, but I do not accept it as a legitimate long-term approach to chronic suffering. Self-regulation, and self-regulation alone, can take us to the gates of the spiritual world which we must enter on our own. It is that spiritual world that gives us enduring relief from the suffering caused by disease.

IT'S TOO SIMPLE

Ken Gerdes, M.D., of Denver, an internist and a close friend, was among the group of physicians who attended my first autoregulation workshop for physicians. He wrote to me on his way back to Denver. He thought my discussion on the molecular basis of aging, accelerated aging, potential for intervention and treatment of disease with autoregulation was rational, logical and scientifically sound. Further, he had no difficulty accepting the clinical results that I was seeing with my autoregulation methods. "I have been thinking about it all day," he wrote, "I am troubled about one thing. It's too simple."

During the first two years of my work with autoregulation, I was also troubled, sometimes deeply troubled, about the utter simplicity of the principles and practice of autoregulation. As I closely observed more and more of my patients resolve their various chronic diseases without drugs, I recognized I had to make a choice:

I could dismiss as apocryphal the accounts of my patients (consider them innocent, or worse, deceitful) and stop my work in self-regulation.

Or,

I could accept self-regulation as a valid medical discipline that gives us predictable clinical results, and continue my work to advance this field.

I chose the second option.

After I gave my very first autoregulation workshop for physicians, three of the 14 physicians from this group incorporated autoregulation in their clinical practice. After each subsequent workshop, I received calls from physicians affirming the benefits of one or more features of autoregulation.

This ongoing peer review is most valuable to me. It sustains me during many periods of self-doubt and discouragement.

THE WAY WE LOOK AT THE WORLD AROUND US DETERMINES WHAT OUR ENERGETIC PATTERNS UNDER THE SKIN ARE

Every Wednesday evening, I spend about three hours with a group of my patients in my autoregulation laboratory. I recommend that all my new patients consider three training sessions with me. In the laboratory, I wire them to various electronic sensors to monitor the energetic patterns of their skin, muscles, arteries and heart. That allows me to study the patterns of electromagnetic energy in their various body organs. It also allows me to help them understand how their body organs cope with stress, and how their energy patterns are normalized when they learn to escape the relentless censor of the thinking mind. At an intellectual level it is all so easy to understand. But healing, as I wrote earlier, is not an intellectual function. We need to enter higher states of energy and consciousness to truly break the chains of the thinking mind.

The way we look at the world around us determines the state of energy we are in. It is when we evade the ceaseless demands of the thinking mind that the body tissues return to their native state of healing energy.

NAMING WITHOUT KNOWING, KNOWING WITHOUT NAMING

The thinking mind thrives on naming things—names are crutches of the cortical monkey. Without names it is disoriented, unable to cope, exposed and vulnerable. In my autoregulation training, I use some time-honored methods of naming things and then letting the names go. In the beginning, my patients often find this very confusing. Unable to latch on to any names, the cortical monkey becomes disoriented, then settles down as the names of things lose their grip. The energy states change and there are limbic periods when perceptions of tissue energy sublimate cortical thoughts. With training, such periods grow longer until a person reaches a state when she recognizes the state she was in only when she comes out of it. Then she *knows* the order of things in human energy dynamics: the relationship of the mind with the body (the mind punishes tissues by its ceaseless chatter), and the relationship of tissue energy with the mind (the energy of living tissues shuts up the thinking mind).

We begin by naming things we do not know and end up knowing things we cannot name.

BREAKING THE CHAINS OF DISEASE MODELS

Many of my patients arrive with thick bundles of medical records, having seen multiple physicians before me. As I thumb through their records, I see the many different diagnoses made by previous physicians. Such patients carry a big burden of uncertainty as to the nature of their illness. Each time they are told that a diagnosis has been firmly established they are expected to respond to the *drug of choice*. And each time, the miracle drug(s) fails them. The dogma of drug medicine holds that precise diagnoses are essential for drug regimens to work. This is, of course, where the real problem starts.

In chronic illness the name of the disease is not important. Recognition and management of the biological burdens that increase oxidant stress on tissues and damage antioxidant and immune defenses are the relevant issues. So my primary task is to help the patient understand the nature of oxidant stresses and the dynamics of the healing phenomenon. I need to help them break free from the disease model of thinking that holds back the healing response. The task of addressing all relevant issues of nutrition, environment, stress and fitness becomes much easier for the patient once those chains are broken.

Autoregulation, with its precise and objective information about biological stresses, is extremely valuable, both for the patient and his physician. It allows both to see the energetic-molecular basis of illness in clear, graphic and unequivocal terms. It underscores the futility of wasting scarce funds for laboratory tests that do not give any useful information. They only help us choose a disease name—a label that hides much and tells little, if anything, about the true nature of the problem.

GIVING THE CORTICAL MONKEY A DOSE OF HIS OWN MEDICINE

Patients often ask me why autoreg is not mind-over-body healing. Don't we use the mind to do autoregulation?

When we *begin* autoregulation, indeed, we use the thinking mind. So the simple sentences that someone in autoregulation training learns may be regarded as a mental activity. However, the purpose of those sentences is not to use the mind to heal the body. Rather, it is to reach a state in which the thinking mind is stilled, and perceptions of tissue energy lead us into deeper energy states that effectively exclude mental chatter.

When I do autoregulation—and I do so frequently during my work in the laboratory and clinic—I do not use the steps I teach my patients in autoregulation classes. I do not follow any technique. After years of training and teaching autoregulation, I have reached a state where perceptions of energy come to me spontaneously, without uttering any sentences or employing any of the other methods I teach others. Almost instantaneously, I perceive the energy in my tissue, then there is nothing more for me to do. The gentle guiding energy does the rest. On rare occasions, when I am extremely rushed or a captive of my thinking mind, the energy perceptions do not arrive readily. At such times, I—like my patients—rely on limbic breathing or simple sentences to quell my screaming mind so that the healing energy can prevail. Many of my patients relate similar personal experiences after long hours of such work. Indeed, all good autoregulators reach that stage when words or techniques are irrelevant to autoregulation.

The essential point here is that autoregulation is not about mind-over-body healing. It is the exact opposite: an energy-over-mind state that brings profound visceral-energetic stillness—a stillness that is too deep for words.

****

Healing is an energy function. I began this chapter by saying that healing is a natural state of energy. I close this chapter now by returning to it. The essence of self-regulation is in achieving a healing energy state—when the energy of body tissue guides us. It is a state in which we banish the thinking mind. Self-regulation with healing energy *is* ending the ceaseless chatter of the mind. *It is surrendering to the guiding energy of the presence that always surrounds each of us.*

None of are victims. All of us are victims. There is a canary within each of us, only the cages look different. Each of us can fly out.

Regret is a thief—it steals life. A life of regret is a life stolen before it arrives.

The Canary and Chronic Fatigue

Time wounds all heels.

Jane Ace

Time heals all wounds.

Anonymous

Chapter 7

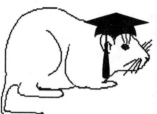

FOURTH INSIGHT

Genes Legislate Life;
the environment interprets the laws set forth by them. Genetic codes are like obscure penal codes - they remain dormant until they are activated by environmental triggers.

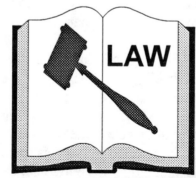

LAW

Heart disease—as everyone knows—runs in families. We are told this is because members of some families are genetically predisposed to heart attacks. A question arose in my mind some years ago: Why didn't people have heart attacks in past centuries? Heart attacks were unknown in the great pathology museums of the world until the beginning of this century. The museum of the Royal College of Surgeons of England displays 18th and 19th century specimens of all sorts of diseases of the heart, lung, kidneys and other body organs. But there are no examples of acute myocardial infarction. Medical texts written before this century do not describe cases of acute heart attacks. So where were the genes that caused heart attacks in the 18th and 19th centuries?

Migraine runs in families. Members of some families are genetically predisposed to such headaches, so goes the party line among physicians. I suffered from frequent and severe migraine attacks that did not respond to pain killers. I needed Demerol and Vistaril injections for relief, even though I knew the addictive potential of the narcotic drug. During my early work with autoregulation, I learned to *dissolve* my headaches without drugs. It has been several years since I took my last Demerol injection for migraine. So what happened to my migraine genes?

Many genetic diseases are incompatible with life, and affected babies die at birth or soon after. It seems that most miscarriages are the result of genetic defects, and abortion is nature's way of reducing the number of people seriously handicapped by genetic deformities. The incidence of chromosomal damage in aborted fetuses is much higher than in newborns. Genetic mutations in aborted fetuses and newborns with defects notwithstanding, it needs to be recognized that most people *are* born with some minor genetic handicaps. They can live their normal life spans unless some nutritional or environmental factors turn those minor handicaps into major ones. *This is a point of crucial importance.*

MICROBES: THE CLEVER GENETICISTS

Microbes think they have as much right to exist on this planet as we do—perhaps more so because they have been around much longer than we have.

In medical school, I was taught that I should be very careful in prescribing antibiotics for bacterial infections because bacteria become resistant to antibiotics. (No one ever told me there were things I could do to avoid using drugs altogether!) I was told that antibiotics kill off the strains of bacteria that are sensitive to them. This is followed by the overgrowth of the strains that are not sensitive to antibiotics. It seemed logical and believable. It was a partial truth—as most medical teaching is in our medical schools. That, of course, is not the only way things work in biology.

Living beings are ingenious energy entities. When facing threats, they sense the threats, realign their energy patterns and respond. The defenses of what we consider low forms of life are, in many ways, as complex and effective as human defenses. Microbes search for and acquire new weapons against threats to their survival. They borrow some DNA sequences from other living beings to cope with the threat of antibiotics. They change their genes.

Thus, the remarkable way in which medically important bacteria have acquired antibiotic resistance in the past 25 years seems to have been by insertion of new genes into existing plasmids rather than by the spread of previously rare plasmids.

Nature 616:306; 1983

At present, there is intense interest in the genetic basis of diseases, yet two serious errors are being made:

First,

we seriously underestimate the importance of oxidative damage to genes in people who do not suffer from classical genetic disorders.

We are ignoring the large-scale oxidative damage to genes inflicted by increasing environmental pollutants and decreasing nutritional antioxidant defenses of the body. The human species is adversely affected by our mindless and relentless assault on our environment and food, just as all other living beings are. The stress of fast-paced modern life takes its toll. Adrenaline—in my view—is the most potent oxidizing molecule in the human body. In clinical medicine, we pay lip service to these factors. I have yet to see an internist in drug medicine address these issues with vigor.

Second,

we grossly exaggerate the importance of research in classic genetic disorders.

At present, the medical research community is intensely interested in mapping out the entire human genome and deciphering genetic codes for various diseases. Some geneticists proclaim that it is only a matter of time before the human genome will be fully decoded, and, presumably we will know all there is to know about human infirmities. Then they will develop genetic manipulative techniques to cure those disorders. Pretty frivolous thinking!

How many sick people have our geneticists helped to date? A few dozens? Or is it a few hundreds? How many hundreds of millions—or should we count in billions—are being injured every day by toxins in our environment and food? How many dozens or hundreds of deformed genes can our geneticists fix? How many hundreds of thousands of genes are being damaged by the assault of oxidants we unleash upon them? What are the track records of our geneticists? What is the track record of man-made oxidants?

Not long ago, only three genes had been linked to cancer. Then there were 13. The last time I heard a geneticist gloat about the successes of his profession, there were 130 genes linked to cancer. I do not doubt that this number will reach 1,300—or perhaps 13,000—in a decade. The tragedy of gene research is this:

We are very successful at identifying an ever-increasing number of genes linked with cancer and other diseases. Yet we have made almost no progress in alleviating the suffering of the sick. How can we? Simply adding to the number of known damaged genes will not alleviate anyone's suffering.

There is an even bigger tragedy in gene research. Literally every month, *Nature* and *Science* magazines publish reports on genes that are being damaged at ever-increasing rates by incremental oxidative damage. The damaged genes include those that regulate key heart functions, indicating the essential role of oxidatively damaged genes in the cause of heart disease. Yet, no great efforts are being made to conduct research in nondrug, natural ways of reducing oxidant stress on human tissues. I do not begrudge our cancer, heart and gene research communities hundreds of billions of research dollars. I only hope that perhaps some day our lawmakers will allocate a few million dollars for research in natural methods of disease reversal.

Once, in Tokyo, I watched Japanese children conduct a program about environmental damage. The Japanese know something about gene damage in ways others do not: The legacy of damaged genes still persists in the cities of Nagasaki and Hiroshima. I was much inspired by the way those children looked at their world. Then my thoughts abruptly shifted to a recent article I read before leaving for Tokyo. The article was written by some drug doctors who pronounced with overriding authority that physicians who practice environmental medicine in the United States are quacks. How ironic! The ecologic awareness of Japanese children juxtaposed with the utter ignorance of American drug doctors.

As a medical student, I learned to recognize cancer in two

colors—eosin-pink for the soup of life in cells and hematoxylin-blue for the genetic material in nuclei. My microscope was an old rusted contraption with a single eyepiece. I learned to squint through my microscope. The slides we studied were faded and badly scratched. The microscope had three lenses that enlarged the images about 10, 40 and 100 times. One thing none of the lenses could do was produce clear, sharp images from the faded and scratched slides. I did as well as I could.

As a boy, I remember seeing fuzzy black and white pictures of a wasteland: charred buildings, heaps of rubble and mutilated bodies strewn across streets. That was Hiroshima and Nagasaki after the atomic bombs were dropped, I was told. Japan was a distant land then. I don't remember being outraged at such a ferocious destruction of human life and property.

As a pathology resident, I was trained to diagnose cancer. My microscope had two eyepieces, with magnification up to 1,000. Sometimes I looked at slides with the double-headed scopes of staff pathologists. The slides were clearer; the microscopic images much sharper. It was exciting to look at cancer that way, mapping out the extent of the tumors, searching for metastasis in blood vessels. I learned to stain cancer cells in more colorful ways—purple, red, brown and black.

At an exhibition in New York City, I saw some pictures of World War II. Someone had juxtaposed old black and white pictures with color pictures, magnified the images and exploded the scale of the horrors of Hiroshima and Nagasaki. The old, fuzzy pictures I had seen as a young boy took on new meaning.

Then came the scanning microscopes that magnified cancer cells by 10,000 times or more, and the electron microscope that pushed the magnifying power to 50,000 times and more. I published my very first paper in *Cancer*. In it, I described a rare type of liver cancer that had not been described previously. I remember the excitement of my first glance at the electron photomicrographs of the tumor showing the tiny granules containing the hormone with insulin-like activity. There was great excitement then. We thought the electron microscope would allow us to understand cancer better.

Pathology literature contains many reports of cancers in the survivors of Hiroshima and Nagasaki. I studied the reports while preparing for some cancer conferences: radiation changes the way tissues look. Cancer that arises in radiated tissues are often atypical and bizarre, and have a tendency to strike early at distant places. Radiation also changes the way cancer cells look. Mutant cancer cells take monstrous shapes that are frightening to a pathologist, even after they have been fixed and killed with formaldehyde.

There is an amusing set of pictures of Linus Pauling and another Nobel laureate physicist that frame a picture of John Kennedy, at the Kennedy Library in Boston. Pauling, of course, was foremost among scientists who warned against the hazards of radiation. The government used the other Nobelist—I do not recall his name—to counterbalance Pauling's influence. How could anyone see the damage in Hiroshima and Nagasaki, yet speak against the possibility of genetic damage? The government obviously persuaded some Nobel Prize-winning scientists to do so.

Then came new techniques for staining molecules with antibodies. In one of my early papers, my co-investigators and I published the first photomicrographs of immunostained IgE antibodies in plasma cells. (IgE antibodies cause a hay-fever-type of allergy.) It was a hot subject then—a quick way to publish papers by staining various molecules in cancer cells—pathologists plying a painter's craft. From the cellular level, we moved to a deeper molecular level. We thought that would allow us to understand cancer better. Alas! It wasn't to be.

Next came the gene research—altogether new ways of looking at cancer cells. There was renewed excitement. This time we *were* going to get to the bottom of things, the geneticists screamed with excitement. We scrambled to find new ways of locating damaged and deranged genes in cancer cells, and we did well. Every month, we published reports of more and more types of gene damage in more and more different types of cancers. More is better, that was the operative mode. Then I thought about a recent cancer meeting. One speaker after another gloated over his findings of damaged, deleted and deranged genes in cancer cells. We thought that would allow us to understand cancer better. Alas! It wasn't to be.

In my pathology work, I came across many reports of increased incidence of childhood cancers (leukemias, lymphomas and others) among the surving children of the two Japanese cities—and among the children of surving adults. There were reports of skin cancers among them. In areas affected by atomic explosions, there were other reports of cancers in other body organs of Japanese children and adults. The photographic skills of the Japanese pathologists did little to prolong their lives.

In the U.S., I saw pictures of cancer in Japanese children, in blazing colors, stupefying magnifications and dizzying details. I knew those children had died the same way children with cancers died in Pakistan.

During the first half of this century, many Americans were exposed to dangerous forms of radiation by their physicians' attempts to treat simple conditions such as acne, tonsillitis, thyroiditis and other disorders. (Oh, the things we physicians do! I wonder if there is another profession so gullible as we physicians. We are ever so eager—as Voltaire would say—to treat diseases we know little about, with therapies we know even less about.) Predictably, many such unfortunate patients developed cancers caused by radiation treatment.

The Japanese fought a different war. They saw the aftermath of atomic explosions, in one light as they happened and in many different lights ever since. But they have not succumbed to the illusion that simply changing the colors of pictures, blowing them up or miniaturizing them, or turning them into giddy images of space-age technology will undo the horror of those events. Instead, they have moved on to *rebuilding*.

We in America are fighting a different cancer war. We are forever inventing and reinventing technologies for viewing newer and newer images of the molecular damage caused by cancer, and examining mutilated tissues, maimed organs, devastated bodies and broken families. But we are adamantly opposed to any effort to repair the environmental damage that causes cancer in the first place. Our environment damages genes at a much faster rate than we can detect such injury, let alone figure out ways of repairing the damage.

Every time I see a pathologist exult at his pretty cancer pictures and every time I hear an oncologist gloat with his new tumor markers, I wonder why they do not see the obvious:

Cancer cannot be controlled by simply classifying it. The war against cancer cannot be won simply by inventing and reinventing new names for old cancers, or by creating still newer technologies for mapping out the genetic damage caused by cancer. The ways and rates with which environmental oxidants injure our genes far exceed the ways and rates with which we can possibly measure them and classify them. If there is any chance of our winning the war on cancer, it is only through looking at our environment. This, sadly, our cancer specialists cannot see.

This is what environmental and nutritional medicines are all about. How ironic that our cancer community is irritated by the principles and practice of two disciplines that are most committed to preserving the internal and external environments of man: nutritional medicine and environmental medicine. And how ironic that our hospital and state licensing boards harass the physicians belonging to these two groups more than any other group.

CHEMICALS: EXPERIMENTS IN BIOLOGY

Every synthetic chemical is an experiment in biology—whether it is prescribed by a physician as a drug, pushed by a drug dealer for a fix, used as an antibiotic to kill disease-causing bacteria (as well as health-promoting microbes), or used deliberately to destroy life as a pesticide. The same holds true when synthetic chemicals are introduced into our tissues unknowingly.

In the United States, it has been estimated that people are regularly exposed to over 65,000 chemicals. Developing countries are rapidly catching up with the U.S. This is a global experiment in biology. Our air is polluted. Our waters are contaminated. Our food is contaminated with fumigants, fungicides, pesticides and other chemicals that we use to "preserve" our food. We are only beginning to know the global devastation of biologic ecosystems brought about by the chemical avalanches that we have unleashed upon ourselves. The thread that binds all these biologic stressors is their essential oxidative nature. Synthetic chemicals are like monkey wrenches thrown into the body's energy and detoxification enzymes—they clog normal biologic pathways.

ECODIS-EASES

"Ecodis-eases" is a term I use to refer to a very large

number of environmentally-induced symptoms that my colleagues in drug medicine glibly dismiss as all-in-the-head problems.

The molecular basis of ecodis-eases is accelerated oxidative molecular damage. I first put forth my theory and furnished evidence for it in a monograph entitled *The Molecular Basis of Environmental Illness* published in the syllabus of the American Academy of Environmental Medicine in the mid-1980s. The body of medical literature documenting the ability of synthetic chemicals to cause ecodis-eases has grown enormously in recent years. It is now possible to support my viewpoint by considering the example of any family of synthetic chemicals.

The pandemic of chronic fatigue that we now witness among our children, adults and the elderly is one face—albeit the most important—of the increasing oxidant stress on planet earth. I discuss the basic chemistry and causes of such oxidant stress at length in *The Canary and Chronic Fatigue*.

In this chapter, I illustrate how progressively deteriorating environment impact on human biology—and cause dis-ease and disease—with discussion of two important areas: the estrogen overdrive and the Gulf War syndrome.

The Age of Estrogenic Overdrive

We live in the age of estrogen overdrive.

I discuss the critical issue of estrogenic overdrive in this chapter dealing with environment for two important reasons:

First,

to show how xenoestrogens—chemicals that have estrogen-like effects—are causing a growing number of ecodis-eases and ecodiseases, including the near-epidemic increase in cancer of the breast and prostate, especially in young women and men.

Second,

to shed some light on the prevailing controversy concerning the clinical value of synthetic estrogens for prevention of heart disease and osteoporosis in women.

NATURE'S PRESCRIPTION
FOR PRESERVING HUMAN SPECIES

Hormones are Nature's molecular messengers. To save the human species from extinction, Nature created a rather simple design: It prepares the uterus for pregnancy each month during the entire reproductive life of the woman. Estrogen peaks during the first half of each menstrual cycle to prepare the soil of the uterus for conception. If conception occurs, estrogen peaks further, but this time estrogen overdrive is balanced with a progesterone peak to protect the beginning of life for the baby from unbalanced estrogen drive. As the fertilized egg develops into an embryo and beyond, there is an outpouring of estrogens from the placenta that also increases its output of progesterone, again to keep the estrogens under surveillance.

Times have changed. There are simply enough of us on the planet now. Women do not need to stay pregnant all the time. The way we live our lives has changed rapidly, but evolution does not work that fast. The result: a fundamental chemical conflict between the needs of 21st-century women and their hormonal clocks. Each month, an estrogen peak goes unbalanced by progesterone. What are the chemical consequences of estrogen overdrive?

Endometriosis—the growth outside the uterus of misplaced cells that normally line the uterine cavity—afflicts 5 million American women. It is a painful, often disabling disorder that can lead to infertility. Endometriosis occurs rarely, if ever, in tribal cultures removed from the rush of modern life.

ESTROGENS AND MOLECULAR MATING

In biologic molecular pathways, molecules compete for "receptor-mates" as aggressively as animals do in the animal kingdom. Such competition among molecules is based upon their structural similarities. This, however, does not always hold, and many synthetic chemicals not belonging to the family of human hormones actively compete for their receptors. This natural phenomenon is well illustrated by the example of competition for receptors among estrogens and estrogen mimics. Following is an incomplete list of estrogen mimics:

> Ingredients in plastics
> Pesticides such as DDT and heptachlor
> Plastic (polycarbonates) breakdown products
> PAHs (polycyclic aromatic hydrocarbons)
> Petroleum byproducts
> Polystyrene
> Marihuana compounds such as tetrahydrocannabinol
> Plant estrogens such as coumestrol, equol and
> zearalenone
> Combustion byproducts
> Electromagnetic fields that boost the concentration
> of estrogens in blood

EXERCISE, ENZYMES AND BREAST CANCER RISK

The body metabolizes its main natural estrogen called estradiol in several ways. Two enzyme systems compete for an opportunity to alter the structure of estradiol molecule, but they do so at two different locations on the molecule: the 2-carbon and 16-carbon regions. The end-products of such reactions are quite different in their biologic roles. For instance, insertion of a hydroxyl radical at the 2-carbon site produces an innocent molecule while that at the 16-carbon location produces a genotoxic and breast cancer-promoting molecule.

Regular and vigorous exercise upregulates conversion at the 2-carbon site and down-regulates that at the 16-carbon location, both changes offering protection against breast cancer. Exercise, of course, has other well established beneficial effects on fat metabolism that reduce cancer risk.

PLASTIC MAKERS AND ESTROGEN MIMICS

Several plastic materials when exposed to high temperatures release BPA (bisphenol-A) that are known xenoestrogen building blocks. Chemical makers of the plastic industry have long claimed that BPA and other plastic breakdown products carry no health risks in small quantities—generally those below the general detection limit of 10 parts per billion. (The old It-Can't-Happen-Because-We-Say-So story.) Recently, researchers at Stanford University exposed the foolishness of such thinking. They clearly showed that BPA exerted hormonal activity at concentrations of just 2 to 5 parts per billion.

BREAST CANCER, ESTROGENS AND XENOESTROGENS

Estrogens drive the rate of proliferation of mammary gland cells. This explains the breast fullness and soreness experienced by many women during menstrual cycles—and less frequently during ovulation—when estrogen levels surge. This seems to be the principal mechanisms by which estrogen therapy increases the risk of breast cancer.

Since 1940, the incidence of breast cancer has increased in the United States and in Western Europe. Thirty years ago during my residency, I remember we saw a very unusual case of breast cancer—unusual because the tumor occurred in a 28-year-old woman. My mentor, Michael Tracht, M.D., asked me to prepare the case for a conference. Some months ago, at our hospital monthly breast conference, I presented three cases of breast cancer—in women who were 21, 26 and 29 years, respectively. No one thought it was that unusual to see breast cancer in such young women.

Two million to six million women in the United States and Europe were prescribed DES—a synthetic estrogen—to prevent miscarriages between 1948 and 1971. DES caused about 10,000 cancers among the daughters of the women given the hormone. Equally distressing is the growing evidence that genital deformities may occur 20 times more frequently in the daughters and sons of such women. During the same period, DES was also fed in massive amounts to cattle to promote growth, thus exposing millions of other Americans to this miracle of synthetic chemistry.

MELATONIN AND ESTROGENIC OVERDRIVE

Melatonin is the primary hormone of the pineal gland located in the center of the brain. It is mainly produced during nighttime darkness. Light and electromagnetic fields suppress melatonin production.

Melatonin is a powerful antioxidant. Among its other important roles is reduction of estrogen production in the body, and probably reduction in the number of estrogen receptors.

Recent studies show that the protective, estrogen-reducing effects of melatonin are significantly reduced by excessive exposure to light (including late night TV viewing), electromagnetic fields (including the power grids in our cities), chemical pollutants, such as pesticides and fungicides, and many commonly prescribed drugs, such as beta blockers for heart disease, high blood pressure and headaches.

Most girls are experiencing puberty at younger ages than in past generations. What people are forgetting is that some girls are menstruating at age 9 now. We've got to instruct them and give them information about what's going on with their bodies.

Dr. John Hobbs, Director of Obstetrics
Rush Prudential Health Plans, Chicago
Quoted in *People* Magazine October 24, 1994

What information do we need to give these girls about what's going on with their bodies? Since the author is not a clinical ecologist nor a nutritionist, what information can he give to young girls, I wonder?

Whenever I see girls watching late night TV, I wonder what changes in their hormonal day-night rhythms it may be causing. Melatonin, as I mention earlier, is a strong anti-estrogenic influence in the body. Light switches off melatonin production in the pineal body, and decreased levels of melatonin almost certainly result in estrogenic overdrive. I strongly suspect that early puberty in girls is due to this and other environmental causes of estrogenic overdrive.

DDT BOOMERANGS

DDT, a highly toxic pesticide, was banned in this country several years ago. So we are told we are safe. In reality, we continue to be regularly exposed to this designer-killer molecule. First, it is produced in large quantities as a byproduct in the manufacture of several chemicals that are legal in the United States. Second, it is legal to export it to developing countries who spray it on their fruits and vegetables before they ship them to us. What goes around comes around.

Higher concentrations of DDE—the breakdown product of DDT—have been found in the fluid of breast cysts in women with breast cancer. DDE is also the prime suspect in reproductive failure in alligators in Lake Apopka, Florida.

The half-life of DDT in a temperate climate is 59 years. That means 10 tons of DDT out of each 40 tons that we unleash on our environment today will still be around our children after 118 years, and five tons will persist for 177 years.

Female-to-female pairing and other changes in reproductive behavior have been reported in gulls exposed to higher amounts of DDT and DDE in Santa Barbara as well as in roseate terns exposed to PCBs in Massachusetts.

Sperm counts in men worldwide have fallen about 50% since 1940. Over the same period, the incidence of testicular cancer has tripled in some countries and that of prostate has doubled...birth defects in the male reproductive tract have increased...alligators on Lake Apopka in Florida are failing to hatch, and the males that do hatch have abnormally small penises...at least part of the reason for the increase in these conditions may be man-made chemicals introduced into the environment since 1940 that mimic or block natural estrogen.

Chemical & Engineering News
January 31, 1994

The biological effects of estrogen come into play when the estrogen receptor in a cell binds to natural estrogen or imposter estrogen-mimics. Next, this receptor-hormone complex binds to specific sites of DNA in the cell nucleus, influences the function of key target genes in that part of the DNA molecule, and so changes the function and structure of cells, tissues and organs.

I have a strong sense that imposter estrogen-mimics

accumulated in the mother and later transferred to the egg or fetus play a detrimental role. For example, I suspect that this is the case when I see little girls with yeast-related vaginal symptoms and other types of immune suppression. I believe it is simply a matter of time before sound scientific evidence for this will be developed.

IF ESTROGEN OVERDRIVE IS REAL, WHY DOES ESTROGEN THERAPY HELP SOME WOMEN?

About eight to ten million American women are prescribed hormonal replacement therapy by their physicians. Of these, about one-half discontinue hormones due to untoward effects of hormones or for fear of developing breast, uterus and other cancers. This means about five million women in the U.S. are taking estrogens and progesterone regularly. If hormonal replacement therapy is all that risky, why do so many women agree to take this?

This question has interested me for some time. On the surface it negates my theory about the estrogen overdrive described above. The answer is that they are not made aware of healthful, natural alternatives to synthetic hormones. I make three important points here.

First, a vast majority of menopausal symptoms can be controlled with sound nutritional therapies, exercise and self-regulation and without estrogen. Indeed, many of the symptoms attributed to inadequate estrogen are in reality symptoms of sugar-insulin-adrenaline roller coasters that respond well to natural, nondrug measures.

Second, for some of my patients who need further relief, I frequently prescribe natural plant-derived progesterone creams. Indeed, it is uncommon for me to have to use estrogen for symptoms that are difficult to control otherwise.

How do I explain the occurrence of hot flashes, fluid retention and related symptoms that seem to respond well to estrogen therapy? An insight into a possible explanation of this phenomenon came to me some time ago as I listened to a patient describe her difficulty with sugar craving and sugar roller coasters. It occurred to me that the need of some women for extra estrogen for hot flashes is similar to the need for sugar in someone craving sugar, or for cocaine in the cocaine addict. These are examples of receptor dysregulation, of energetic-molecular disequilibrium, of molecular responses overshooting their marks. No one recommends that we solve the problem of sugar craving with sugar, or that we treat cocaine addiction by giving the addict regular doses of cocaine. Why do we do so for estrogen? Especially with synthetic estrogens? Because the companies that make estrogen have the money to fly estrogen speakers all over the country extolling the virtues of their drugs.

I include below some brief comments about the synthetic estrogens and progesterones commonly prescribed by physicians.

THE "GOOD" AND "BAD" ESTROGENS

There are three principal estrogens in women: estrone, estradiol and estriol. The first two have been incriminated in the cause of breast and uterus cancers, and possibly cancers of other body organs. The third, estriol, provides a counterbalance to the first two types of estrogens and prevents cancer. Thus, in health the "good" estrogen, estriol, balances the "bad" estrogens, estrone and estradiol. I use the terms *good* and *bad* only to emphasize the differences in their actions. As I write earlier, Nature really does not assign any good or bad roles to its essential molecules.

Premarin, the most commonly used estrogen product derived from pregnant mares' urine, is rich in the first two—those with associated risks of cancer—and low in the third that plays a protective role. Provera, the commonly prescribed progesterone, is also a synthetic molecule that does not fit well with the natural order of hormonal rhythms. Predictably, it has   several side effects.

ESTROGEN AND HEART DISEASE

"Why do you think so many doctors prescribe estrogen for their patients as if it was holy water?" Choua asked one day.

"Most physicians think estrogen protects women against coronary heart disease and prevents osteoporosis," I ignored his sarcasm.

"That's not the *real* reason and you know that," Choua taunted.

"Pray, tell me what is the real reason!" I jested.

"Drug doctors have to give their patients something, and estrogen comes in handy. It gives the patient short-term relief from flushes and creates euphoria. So the patient is satisfied, at least temporarily oblivious to the havoc the hormone plays with her delicate hormonal balance. The doctor is also happy because the hormone helps him get a difficult patient out of the way—at least for some time. The estrogen speakers do well as well—the drugs sell well, and the drug makers reward their hired guns well."

"In cynicism, you are peerless, Choua," I laughed. "It is well established that estrogens lower the risk of heart disease and prevent osteoporosis."

"*Well established!* Let's see." Choua knelt down to shuffle through a pile of journals on the rug in my hospital office and moments later stood up with an opened journal copy in his hand. "Listen to this:

After making certain assumptions, we estimated that the findings, if causal, would translate into a reduction of 42 percent in the risk of coronary heart disease in users of hormones as compared with nonusers.

N Eng J Med 328:1069; 1993

Reduction of 42 percent! Isn't that what estrogen speakers on the payroll of estrogen makers tell everyone?" Choua asked contemptuously.

"It was a major study and physicians do pay heed to what the *Journal* has to say," I replied.

"A major study?" Choua became testy. "I know this study will be quoted by estrogen pushers for decades. But, how many people will bother to read the fine print and find out that the *Journal* arrived at its conclusion in a devious and scientifically invalid way. To begin with:

We did not attempt to address the overall risks and benefits of hormone replacement in postmenopausal women...

N Eng J Med 328:1074; 1993

Did not address the overall risks! Now, tell me how does anyone make a claim of 42 percent reduction in risk if he does not address the overall risk to begin with?"

"Are you quoting the *Journal* accurately?" I asked in disbelief. "If they did not address the overall risk, how could they calculate the risk reduction number?"

"Magic of medical statistics!" Choua grinned broadly.

"No, seriously, Choua, how did they arrive at that 42 percent number?" I coaxed him.

"They did some *elegant* computations! They measured total, LDL and HDL cholesterol levels and found that estrogen users had HDL values 6 to 18 mg/dl higher and LDL values about 16 mg/dl lower than nonusers. Next, they assumed that such changes in cholesterol values indicated reduction in the risk of heart disease—the old hide-incidence-report-risk trick which the Journal is so fond of."

"Oh, that!" I suppressed a smile.

"Cholesterol speakers are magicians. They use complicated, colorful graphs to hide the actual and dismal rate reduction numbers, and fly high banners of made-up risk reduction numbers to sell cholesterol lowering drugs. They keep the drug doctors clinging to the old conviction that such insignificant changes in cholesterol values have any real impact on the true incidence of heart attacks. It continues to amaze me how their brazen deceptions play successfully over and over in our lecture halls. Listen to this:

> *Randomized, controlled clinical trials have failed to offer conclusive proof that a reduction of total plasma cholesterol level is associated with a significant reduction in the clinical incidence and mortality of arteriosclerosis. The specific effects of 13 of these trials have been reviewed.*

N Eng J Med 323:951; 1990

So, they keep playing their silly games of HDL and LDL numbers to sell drugs. It's not that they do not know that the cholesterol story is phony. They arrived at the above conclusion after a careful study of thirteen large clinical trials."

"It is well-known all over the world—and has been so for decades—that the incidence of heart attacks in women increases after menopause, Choua. Are you saying that's not true?" I asked, irritated.

"That's true. But how does that prove that estrogens protect women from heart attacks?" Choua countered sharply.

"If it's not estrogens, what else explains those statistics that show less heart attacks before menopause and a sharp increase in the heart attack rate after menstruation ends?"

"Wow! That's some logic! Especially from an *eminent* pathologist like you," Choua jeered.

"No need to be insolent!" I rebuked him. "Just give me the explanation."

"One good explanation is that women begin to accumulate iron in the body, and iron is a powerful oxidant that causes production of hydroxyl free radicals that are highly toxic. This mechanism appears to be far more important than the phony cholesterol story in the increased incidence of heart attack in postmenopausal women. Here is what some Finnish researchers say about it:

The strongest predictors of AMI (acute myocardial infarction [heart attack], when adjusting only for age (in years) and examination year (covariates for individual years), were pack-years smoked, serum ferritin concentration, maximal oxygen uptake (inversely), serum HDL_2 cholesterol concentration...Our data suggest that a high stored iron level, as assessed by elevated serum ferritin concentration, is a risk factor for coronary artery disease.

Circulation 86:803; 1992

Now, they didn't talk about risk factors. They went by the actual number of heart attacks that occurred." Choua looked up.

"But that's just one study," I contended.

"One study but good one!" Choua smiled. "It's totally consistent with other studies that show an association between high blood levels of copper—another powerful promoter of oxidation and denaturation of body fats—and heart disease. The same holds for selenium, except that selenium protects the heart due to its antioxidant role. It is a cofactor of glutathione peroxidase enzymes that scavenge free radicals and so prevent accelerated oxidative injury to the heart and other body organs."

"You are good at selecting literature that supports your viewpoint and you freely dismiss studies that do not support your concepts," I complained.

"You write about the new EM medicine based on EM dynamics, don't you?" Choua asked. "The EM events that take place *before* the tissues are injured and not on what you can see with a microscope *after* the tissues have been damaged. Right?"

"Right!" I agreed.

"There is no clear energetic-molecular reason that estrogen protects the heart from oxidative injury. Indeed, when a messenger molecule drives a cell to grow and reproduce itself, it has to do so by increasing the oxidative stress on it, for example the respiratory burst that cells show when they are stimulated. In this sense, estrogen might actually do the reverse of what people believe: increase the oxidative stress on the heart."

"You're not serious, are you?" I asked in disbelief.

"Just guessing! Just guessing this once!" Choua laughed and walked out.

Estrogen and Osteoporosis

"The argument of using estrogen to prevent osteoporosis is equally frivolous," Choua continued. "It is illogical from a scientific standpoint, and there are no good long-term studies that prove the value of estrogen for this purpose."

"I think you'll have much disagreement on that," I cautioned.

"Ironically, tamoxifen, a drug used to neutralize estrogen for patients with breast cancer has been reported to increase bone density. Listen to this:

> *In postmenopausal women, treatment with tamoxifen is associated with preservation of the bone mineral density of the lumbar spine. Whether this favorable effect on bone mineral density is accompanied by a decrease in the risk of fractures remains to be determined.*

> *N Eng J Med 326:852; 1992*

Remains to be determined! Risk of fractures has to do with functional strength of the bone, not merely bone density. Resilience is more important than bone mass—brittle bones in many disorders break easily even though their bone density is increased. An excellent example of this is aseptic bone necrosis in which bone density is increased on X-ray studies and yet the bone is at a much higher risk of fracture. In a real sense, this is putting a layer of nonfunctional bone on top of weakened bone spicules—like addressing the problem of a crumbling foundation of a building by adding a heavy floor on top of the building. Would I have been impressed with the benefits of tamoxifen even if this study had shown reduced risk of fracture?" Choua asked.

"Why shouldn't I be?" I asked back.

"Because it makes no sense. The study evaluated the short-term effects of the drug over a period of two years on elderly patients with breast cancer—hardly a suitable group for assessing the efficacy of therapy for promoting the functional integrity of the bone for the entire life span.

"There are yet other important considerations in prevention of osteoporosis. How can a synthetic hormone, that blocks estrogen activity in some ways and promotes it in other ways, have a long-term healthy effect on bone density? Common sense weighs heavily against such a simplistic notion. And, indeed, the clinical experience of nutritionists substantiates my viewpoint.

"Osteoporosis is caused by damage to various receptors in the bone. What causes bone receptor damage? Oxidation, I am sure, though clear scientific evidence for this is not yet forthcoming. The best defense against osteoporosis is reduction of overall oxidative stress with right food choices in the kitchen, meditation, avoidance of oxidizing environmental pollutants, and regular, rebounding exercise."

The use of plant-derived progesterone, used as creams or oils, not only makes theoretical sense, it has been clinically tested and found to be valuable. I discuss this subject at length in the companion volume *What Do Woodpeckers Know About Osteoporosis?*

Estrogen, Environment and Cancer

Choua came over after a few days. A draft of this chapter sat on my desk. He picked it up and started browsing.

"Not a bad piece about genes and environment," he spoke as he put the draft back on the desk.
"Thanks!" I responded.
"Write about estrogens and cancer," he advised. "Use the examples of estrogens and environmental pollutants that mimic estrogen effects to challenge the assumptions drug doctors make for prescribing hormones."
"What assumptions?" I asked, puzzled.
"The most dangerous of all assumptions, of course, is that environmental estrogen mimics are not relevant to their practice of drug medicine. They assume that their synthetic hormone therapies are safe simply because patients can tolerate them for several months or a few years without complaining. Drug medicine has a severely limited attention span—it assumes that the dangers that cannot be readily seen in weeks or months simply do not exist. It is remarkably impervious to insidious and cumulative damage caused by synthetic hormones that do not fit into normal molecular pathways. It is smugly ignorant about slow and sustained cellular and tissue injury caused by environmental pollutants. It is ironic how drug medicine continues to dismiss evidence for links between cancer and synthetic hormones and environmental carcinogens. Hardly a week goes by that I do not see new reports of such evidence."

POURING FUEL ON FLAMES

"Prescribing synthetic estrogens is like pouring fuel on the flames of estrogenic overdrive, isn't it?" Choua resumed.

"It is a serious error," I agreed. "In our clinical work, I am able to avoid the use of estrogens in over 90 percent of women who had been given these hormones previously. It is not my purpose in this book to outline nondrug therapies for hormonal or other disorders. Since I discuss this subject in some detail in this chapter, women readers may feel frustrated to read so much against the clinical use of synthetic estrogens and not be told of anything about the alternatives to cope with problems of menopausal symptoms and prevention of osteoporosis. For my patients, I use liberal amounts of folic acid (10 to 20 mg daily), plant derived natural progesterone products, DHEA in modest doses of 50 to 100 mg on alternate days, and some herbs such as Dong Quai."

"Emphasize for your readers that menopausal symptoms are markedly exaggerated by sugar-insulin-adrenaline," Choua counselled. "And that neurotransmitter roller coasters triggered by them and sensitivity to foods, molds and chemicals are also important. I know you succeed in avoiding the use of synthetic estrogens in a large measure to your total program of preventive medicine that addresses these and other stress- and fitness-related issues."

70-YEAR-OLD BREAST WITH THE ACTIVITY OF A THIRTY-YEAR-OLD WOMAN

"How often do you see breast biopsies of elderly women in their sixties and seventies who show hormonal activities at a level that is expected in young women?" Choua inquired.

"It's not uncommon," I replied.

"How often do you see endometrial biopsies of elderly women who are not taking hormonal replacement therapy and yet show an estrogen effect that suggests a biologic age decades younger than their chronologic age?"

"That's not rare either. As a pathology resident, I was intrigued by such findings. The usual explanation I received from my teachers was that such hormonal changes were secondary to drugs such as digoxin prescribed for other reasons. I don't recall anyone ever suggesting that such effects could be due to estrogenic overload due to the multiple factors I discuss above. Neither do I recall any gynecologist ever speaking about the health hazards of environmental estrogens and xenoestrogens."

"Estrogen enthusiasts don't like to talk about such things, do they?" Choua beamed.

ESTROGENS: THE PUSHER MOLECULES PROGESTERONES: THE PACIFIER MOLECULES

"From an evolutionary standpoint, estrogens are *pusher* molecules—they relentlessly drive the cells in the uterus, breast and many other body organs to prepare them for perpetual pregnancies—to make sure that the species does not become extinct," Choua explained. "Left unto themselves, estrogens are fully capable of pushing the healthy tissues over the edge. Endometriosis, abnormal uterine bleeding caused by endometrial hyperplasia, ovarian cysts, cancer of the uterus and cancer of the breast are examples of the estrogen mischief."

"And progesterones?" I asked.

"Progesterones provide the essential counterbalance," he elaborated. "They pacify the tissues thrown into turbulence by estrogens. It fascinates me when I reflect on the order of things in nature. Estrogen peak during the first half of the period triggers the proliferation of endometrial lining of the uterus and prepares it to receive the fertilized ovum. A similar cellular growth occurs in the breast. When conception takes place, progesterone takes over to protect the developing embryo from the punishing overdrive of estrogen for the entire duration of the pregnancy—the daily progesterone production rises from about 20 milligram (mg) to 400 mg, largely due to its synthesis in the placenta. After the baby is born, maternal progesterone continues its guardian angel role for the suckling baby as well as for the mother. In the natural course of events, estrogen is allowed only a limited freedom of play on the hormonal field."

"What else do progesterones do?"

"Progesterones play many other interesting physiologic roles. This family of hormones serve as precursors to many other major steroid hormones, including cortisone produced in the adrenal glands, aldosterone, testosterone, and estrogens such as estrone, estradiol and estriol.

Some other beneficial roles of progesterones include the following:

1.   They facilitate thyroid gland function.
2.   They promote new bone formation and prevent osteoporosis.
3.   They serve as a natural antidepressants.
4.   They stabilize certain brain functions after a stroke.

PLANTS, LIKE PEOPLE, PROSPER WITH PROGESTERONES

Plants need molecular gofers—hormonal messengers called phytoestrogens and phytoprogesterones—as much as people do. Some plants have more estrogenic affects than progesterones, however, while the opposite holds for others. Under natural conditions, both types of hormones work in a delicate balance to maintain the plant health. Furthermore, in the natural order of things, plant-derived hormones serve similar roles in the food chain.

In their clinical uses, there are two critical differences between natural and synthetic hormones:

1.   Natural hormones have a broad range of safety due to their mild, slow and sustained effects, while synthetic hormones work rapidly and are much more potent.

2.   Natural hormones slide easily on and off on the cell membrane receptors, while the synthetic hormones cling tenaciously to such receptors and often disrupt the physiologic hormonal pathways for long periods of time.

Those are the two principal reasons why phytohormones used in experienced hands do not produce any of the serious side effects of synthetic hormones.

Following is an incomplete list of plants best known as sources of natural phytohormones.

Estrogens:

Alfalfa   Black Cohosh
Black Haw   Chaste Tree (Vitex)
Hops   Licorice
Sage leaves   Sweet Briar

Progesterones

Sarsaparille   Wild Yam
Yarrow Flowers and root

A Synthetic Hormone
for Breast Cancer Prevention

"Just when I think that I have heard about all the silly notions of drug medicine, something else comes along that tops everything," Choua said as he entered my office.

"What is it now?" I asked, looking up from my microscope.

"The National Cancer Institute has decided to spend millions of dollars to pour a synthetic hormone into the bodies of thousands of women to prevent breast cancer."

"Breast cancer is a growing problem. It is spreading like an epidemic. It used to be rare among young women—and now we see it in women in their twenties and thirties. A bad problem! By some estimates, 180,000 women develop breast cancer each year and about 60,000 lose their lives to this tumor. Tamoxifen is helpful for some breast cancer."

"Since estrogen overdrive is a major causative factor, it makes perfect sense to pour more estrogen in women to prevent cancer, doesn't it?" Choua asked impishly.

"Tamoxifen is used to treat breast cancer because of its antiestrogen effects," I explained. "That's how..."

"Huh! If tamoxifen is really antiestrogen, how is it that it causes cancer of the uterus?" Choua rudely interrupted me. "The drug doctors can't see something that simple, can they?" Choua asked tartly.

"It's not that simple. Tamoxifen is well-known for the complexity of its biologic effects on women. It plays both sides of the field—exerts mixed antiestrogen and estrogen-agonist activity,"

I explained.

"Are you trying to defend the sheer stupidity of using a synthetic hormone to prevent breast cancer?" Choua jeered.

"No, I'm not defending it. But, your vitriol is belated. NCI ordered the researchers of the University of Pittsburgh to halt the tamoxifen trial last April."

"You don't know drug doctors, do you?" Choua asked churlishly. "Synthetic cancer-causing hormone for cancer prevention! The idea is alive and thriving. How could it die? There is simply too much money behind it—$68 million, to be precise. That much money always assures the continuity of drug regimens no matter how many innocent women get serious disruptions of their delicate hormonal pathways—no matter how many get cancer of the uterus. We *know* synthetic estrogens cause cancer. So why would anyone dream up such a preposterous notion? The very idea is an abomination. But, does that stop the drug doctors? No! Listen to this:

The National Cancer Institute broke new ground 2 years ago when it launched a large-scale test of a synthetic hormone in healthy women. The $68 million trial is designed to see whether tamoxifen can cut the incidence of breast cancer.

Science News 146:268; 1994

Broke new ground! In what? Sheer stupidity?" Choua asked, visibly angry.

"The case against the use of tamoxifen for prevention of

breast cancer is far from proven, Choua. In any case, women who volunteer for such experimentation are well-informed and are required to sign full-disclosure consent forms mandated by the study."

"Full disclosure? You have such faith in drug doctors," Choua chastised me. "How can you make full disclosure of the risks of such therapy when they simply are not known. Listen to this:

Finally, Goebel's memo says NSABP (National Surgical Adjuvant Breast and Bowel Project) can't claim it provided recruits full disclosure of their risks when "no mention is made that determination of the safety of tamoxifen for this study is one of the purposes of the study.

Science News 146:269; 1994

Full disclosure, my foot!" Choua waved one hand contemptuously. "How can anyone disclose the risks of a drug during the duration of the study when the study is undertaken to do exactly that—determine the risk?"

"Medical research has its problems," I confessed.

"And the biggest problem is dishonesty," Choua added.

"You are entitled to your opinion."

"If the tamoxifen trial was all that NCI touts it to be, why did Canada's Hamilton Regional Cancer Centre pull out of it?"

"I didn't know they withdrew from the trial. I suppose

because they might be concerned about tamoxifen toxicity and the risk of cancer of the uterus," I replied.

"When the Canadian physicians explained the risks, 70 of 80 volunteers opted out. But, American drug doctors are more determined. Watch, what happens. There is that $68 million and they have already signed up 11,111 women to take tamoxifen for a period of five years. Do you know what will happen when the drug doctors are finished with those gullible women?"

"What?"

"Something akin to women who took DES hormone in the 1960s and their daughters had cancer of the cervix. Many of their male offspring suffered from genital malformations. But, the researchers made out well, didn't they?"

"How do you mean?" I asked, surprised.

"The first group of drug doctors who administered the hormone earned their professorships writing papers about their wondrous hormone, and the second group became professors writing papers about the cancers they discovered among the daughters of women who received the hormone. Now we will see a similar play: Some doctors will make a name for themselves pushing the hormone and some years from now another group will bask in the glory of the cancers they will discover in study subjects and their daughters," Choua stopped and winked.

"No one has a crystal ball, Choua," I said in the defense of the study. "Medicine moves on with missteps."

"Missteps, huh!" he mumbled, walked over to the window and gazed out.

Choua stood by the window motionless for several moments, staring at some distant clouds. I wondered what subject he was going to hit next and who he was going to lash out at when he returned. I braced myself.

"Misstep?" Choua growled as he turned and looked at me with intense eyes. "What misstep? Giving large quantities of a synthetic hormone to thousands of healthy women—woman without any symptoms and without any disease? Pushing a drug on unsuspecting women for years and years? A drug that causes a cancer—a cancer that kills? You know women have died of cancer of the uterus caused by tamoxifen, don't you? Did you ever look at the side effects of this drug listed in Physician's Desk Reference? It causes fatigue, depression, anorexia, water retention and edema, menstrual irregularities including total loss of this essential physiologic function, nausea, abdominal cramps, flushes, cough and ovarian cysts. Tell me, what do you think is the common thread among these adverse effects?" Choua heaved as he glared at me.

"They all seem to be related to female hormonal derangements," I replied timidly. "Not surprising because tamoxifen exerts both antiestrogen and pro-estrogenic effects."

"Tamoxifen also causes blood clots in vessels, hepatitis, retina damage and risk of liver cancer. The consent form used by drug doctors to push tamoxifen on poorly-informed women trivializes the risks and grossly exaggerates the potential benefits," Choua went on.

"Those potential risks must be low because I don't think too many people know about that."

"Drug doctors don't like to be told about the toxic effects of drugs. Listen to this:

...reported earlier that 48 percent of the tamoxifen-treated women had persistent vasomotor and gynecologic symptoms (hot flashes and vaginal dryness), as compared with 21 percent of the placebo-controlled women, and that 10 percent of the women receiving tamoxifen and 3 percent of those receiving placebos discontinued treatment during the first year because of unacceptable side effects.

N Eng J Med 326:886; 1992

Now, you don't think drug doctors tell all that to women who *volunteer* for drug trials, do you?"

"That *is* a problem. But, tell me, why did women who took the placebo suffer symptoms?" I asked.

"If you were a healthy woman and someone was pumping a synthetic hormone into you—or you thought he was doing that—you would have had some symptoms too. Drug doctors usually recognize that their drug studies do cause stress. At some intuitive-visceral level, the victims of such studies know they are being wronged."

"Now you're distorting! You make it sound like those studies were designed to be a deliberate deception," I rebuked him.

"Deliberate deception! If that is not deliberate deception, I don't know what deliberate deception is!" Choua snarled.

"How else do you conduct studies to prove that..."

"Do you think all tamoxifen does is protect women from

estrogenic overdrive?" Choua bluntly cut me off. "Does that mean every woman should take the drug to counter the estrogen avalanche that is disrupting the delicate hormonal pathways? Don't you see the sheer stupidity of it?" Choua gored.

"I didn't say that," I protested. "Clearly, you cannot alter the estrogen status of a woman without affecting her progesterone activity—and that means a lot of other hormonal pathways."

"Aha! Progesterone!" Choua shouted. "You *do* have some common sense, don't you?"

"And you *don't* have to insult me," I groaned.

"Progesterone! Natural plant progesterone! That's the answer silly," Choua's voice suddenly dropped.

TAMOXIFEN OR WILD YAM

"Are you saying the National Cancer Institute should redirect that $68 million to research on the protective effects of plant progesterone for women with high risk of cancer?" I asked, relieved at Choua's softened tone.

"Estrogen increases the risk of breast cancer, and most likely, of prostate and testicular cancer as well. How does that fit in with your oxidative theory of cancer?" choua sidestepped my question.

"It's consistent! At least I think it fits in. Estrogen drives the breast tissue—makes it grow actively—and, of course, actively growing tissues are more vulnerable to DNA injury caused by oxidant stress. Do you agree?"

"Yes, I do!" Choua snapped. "But that's not why I asked you the question."

"Then, why did you ask me the question?" I asked, baffled.

"How do you care for patients with chronic fatigue? And for those with asthma and other environmental disorders?" Choua asked, then began to answer his own question. "Empirically and holistically—always keeping the whole person in the center stage, not letting mere symptoms distract you from your global view of oxidative stresses that injure DNA beyond its ability to repair. Right?"

"Right!" I agreed, then asked, "But what does that have to do with estrogens and cancer?"

"When DNA is oxidatively damaged, there are DNA-repair enzymes that clip away the damaged part of the threadlike DNA molecule and insert healthy bits of DNA to complete the repair process. As we grow old—or prematurely age because of unrelenting stress on our antioxidant defenses—our DNA-repair capacity declines. Our DNA-repair enzymes lose efficiency and fail to perform their repair function in a timely manner. Qingyi Wei and colleagues, of the Johns Hopkins University School of Medicine, showed that nicely in their paper published in the February, 1993 issue of the *Proceedings of National Academy of Sciences.*"

"So, you agree with my oxidative theory of cancer?" I asked with satisfaction.

"There are two central issues in cancer prevention and selecting therapies for cancer," Choua continued without directly answering my question. "First, there is the matter of cumulative oxidative injury sustained by DNA, DNA-repair enzymes and other energy molecules in the cell. And, second, the health and functional integrity of the molecular repair mechanisms. Right?" Choua smiled a little.

"Right! Go on, you're describing my theory pretty well." I nudged him on.

"*Injury and repair! Injury and repair! That's the energy equation of life.* Spontaneity of oxidation—as you put it—is

Nature's grand design to make sure that nothing lives forever. So DNA, DNA-repair enzymes and other living molecules are constantly hit—up to 10,000 hits a day for DNA in each cell according to *Science*. That's the simple scheme of life. And cancer is nothing more than oxidatively injured DNA, DNA-repair enzymes and their companion molecules in the cells. Right?"

"Go on, Choua, make your point," I urged.

"So, why don't they use that simple model in the management of cancer? Look for accelerated oxidative stress in choices in the kitchen and in environment! And reduce adrenaline stress by meditation! Why don't those wizards at the National Cancer Institute see something *that* simple?" Choua charged, his voice abruptly becoming shrill with emotion. "It's about money, isn't it? Women's hormonal health be damned! The hormonal health of their unborn daughters be damned! Disrupt their delicate hormonal pathways! Ruin their normal menstrual cycles! Give them bloated bellies and swollen hands! Drug them out of their wits! Haze them with estrogenic fog!"

"Choua, you're getting carried away. Can't you ever argue your case without such emotional tirades?" I vented my frustration.

"*Long live drugs!*" Choua contemptuously waved me into silence. "Long live blinded drug research! Sixty-eight million dollars worth! Ten years from now, another generation of drug geniuses at the Cancer Institute will fund another sixty-eight million dollar study to detect—and treat with yet newer synthetic hormones—cancers in their daughters caused by tamoxifen. Or, perhaps by that time the financial needs of those drug researchers would have grown to three or five times as much," Choua thumped the desk in uncontrollable anger, looked at me with piercing eyes for a few moments, then walked to the window and looked out.

I waited in silence. Some minutes passed.

"Why do you think the folks at the National Cancer Institute cannot see the obvious?" I asked. "If estrogenic overdrive is setting the stage for breast and ovarian cancer, why not provide a natural counterbalance? Why not use natural plant-derived progesterone?"

"There is no money in wild yam progesterones!" Choua answered impassively, without turning. "With $100,000, NCI could buy all the plant-derived progesterones those 11,111 women will need for the study period of five years. That would help reduce the risk of cancer much more than tamoxifen. But what would NCI do with a mere $100,000? It wouldn't be enough just to buy them pencils and pads. Profits are not in plants—patents are where the real money is. The fat chemotherapy cats know that. So they pay their chemists to keep twisting and distorting natural molecules until they come up with some potent and patentable synthetic hormone that will bring them riches. The chemotherapy cats know *that*!" Choua finished scornfully and briskly walked out.

IS MALE MENOPAUSE REAL?

"Are males immune to environmental estrogenic overdrive?" I asked Choua when he returned.

"Can xenoestrogens mess up male hormonal equilibrium? Why not?" Choua responded.

Midlife crisis in men ia not a menopausal analogue...it is not related to hormonal changes. Some people would rather blame their behavior on hormones rather than psychological problems...there is no convincing evidence that the gradual decline in testosterone levels experienced by most men results in any symptoms...

Journal of Medical Association 268:2486; 1992

Blame behavior on hormones rather than psychological problems!" Choua remarked acidly.

"There is no clear scientific proof yet that male menopause exists," I responded.

"Right now the Olympian N^2D^2 medicine dismisses the notion of male menopause because no drug company yet has an FDA approved drug for treating hormonal symptoms in men. Watch what happens when a drug company is rewarded by the FDA," Choua chuckled gleefully.

"Oh, you never cease to amaze me. Your cynicism has no limit," I laughed.

"I know that as soon as a skin patch delivery system for prescribing testosterone to men is approved by FDA, all this will change," Choua smiled. "Then we will see hordes of "testosterone experts" paid in N2D^2 dollars roaming about our hospital conference rooms, preaching their gospel of synthetic testosterone."

"So, you think male menopause *is real?"* I overlooked his

scorn.

"Male menopause is real in the sense that if testosterone level drops sharply—as after castration—men may suffer many of the menopausal symptoms, including hot flashes, persistent fatigue and loss of sexual interest or function. Testosterone levels may decrease 30% to 40% in men from late 1940s to early 1970s. In general, however, men do not suffer from sudden drops in testosterone levels at any time as women do during menopause."

"But all this is conjecture on your part, isn't it?" I expressed doubt.

"The assumption of the *Journal*, that there is no evidence that changes in male hormone levels are associated with functional loss, is not based on any actual studies," Choua chugged along. "It is simply an assumption that I believe the *Journal* will readily dismiss when the FDA approves some synthetic male hormone for clinical use. It always works that way, doesn't it?"

"You can't help yourself. You have to make snide remarks at every step," I chided Choua.

"The real issue here is altogether different," Choua was unimpressed by my protest. "It is the issue of how the male-female hormone balance in health is disrupted by synthetic hormones and by xenoestrogens that clog up the testosterone receptors.

"Nature gives both female estrogenic and male androgenic hormones to men and women—estrogens dominate the field in females and androgens in the male. In health, there is a delicate balance between the two types of hormones in both sexes. Estrogenic overdrive can be expected to—and indeed does—disrupt such balance in both sexes.

"There is an alarming increase in rates of cancer of the prostate gland in recent decades—especially of the kind that grows quickly and strikes at distant sites. This trend is certainly related to estrogen overdrive and hormonal disruptions caused by xenoestrogens. A similar rise in the incidence of cancer of the testes has been observed in recent decades. The sperm count in men have been steadily declining during the past several decades so that some studies show a near 50 percent drop in some European communities. Biologists have observed similar changes in wildlife so that the frog and butterfly populations reportedly have been halved in some regions due to pesticide and other types of chemical contaminations of their natural habitats. Is drug medicine interested in any of that? No. They are quite happy with their chemotherapy drugs. More cancer means more money."

"Oh God!" I threw my arms up in the air. "You can't..."

"I strongly suspect that xenoestrogen molecular mimicry contributes to the pandemic of immune diseases, chronic fatigue and related ecodisorders that you now see among previously healthy children, adults and the elderly. You claim there is no scientific proof of that. Watch what happens as soon as drugs are approved for estrogenic ecodisorders. Suddenly the proof will be all over—in living colors, it will be splashed on the screens of conference rooms everywhere in the U.S. It never fails, does it?"

I yawned. Choua broke out in a loud laughter and left my office.

Oxidative Storms in Desert Storm:
Lessons not learned from the Gulf War

"War is a hell of oxidative fires," Choua said one day, his head buried in a journal. "And Desert Storm was a hell of oxidative storms, wasn't it?"

"Yes," I replied.

"It's interesting how your predictions about Operation Desert Storm and Desert Shield came true."

"You mean the Gulf War syndrome?" I asked, without leaving my microscope. "That was easy to predict."

"In *The Canary and Chronic Fatigue,* you included brief comments about lessons not learned from the Gulf War. You made five predictions," Choua continued, putting the journal back on my desk:

"First, you foresaw that a large number of men and women in the service in the Persian Gulf region would return with a variety of chronic environmental, immune and stress-related problems.

"Second, you predicted that disabling fatigue would be a dominant clinical feature—other symptoms would be those seen in chronic fatigue states and will include skin rashes, malaise, low-grade fever, breathing disorders, recurrent viral and bacterial infections, swollen glands, chemical sensitivity, worsening of mold and food allergy reactions, abdominal problems, menstrual difficulties, and disorders of mood, memory and mentation.

"Third, you stated that the sick veterans would be initially dismissed as malingerers. Many of them would be labeled with various psychiatric diagnoses including obsessional psychopathology—the all-time favorite of many immunology professors. Next, such veterans would be prescribed large doses of mind-numbing drugs—the favorite trick of the N^2D^2 docs for fogging out the complainers.

"Fourth, you said that the chronic health disorders of the sick veterans would worsen with multiple drug therapies. As the pressure would build, the maestros of N^2D^2 medicine would hold conferences to come up with a diagnostic label—"a working definition" as they like to call such labels. For assistance, they would invite experts from medical schools and some from the Centers for Disease Control. A suitable label would be invented to serve as a basis for N^2D^2 docs to administer the sick veterans with some experimental drug protocols.

"Fifth, you predicted that when everything else failed, some N^2D2 wizards would embark upon long-term broad-spectrum antibiotic therapy that might give some temporary relief but would play havoc with the injured bowel ecosystems of sick veterans. When the N^2D^2 researchers would finish with their ground-breaking research studies, the unfortunate veterans would be declared permanently disabled. Those were your predictions, right?" Choua chirped.

"In essence, yes!" I laughed at the way he embellished my words.

"What led you to make those predictions?"

"I simply knew them," I answered.

"*You simply knew them!*" Choua raised his eyebrows. "How did you know more than 40,000 veterans would develop the Gulf

War syndrome?"

**THE FIRST PREDICTION:
MANY GULF WAR VETERANS WILL DEVELOP
CHRONIC ECOLOGIC AND IMMUNE DISORDERS**

"It was obvious," I answered. "The Gulf War was to be a grand experiment in human biology and it was simple to foresee its results. War is a hell of oxidative fires. Anyone could have seen the shape of things to come. Two factors were involved:

> **1.** *Genetic predisposition to oxidative injury, and*
> **2.** *Cumulative oxidative injury to energy and detoxification enzymes.*

"Wartime environment exposes soldiers to intense oxidative stress," I continued. "First, fear of mutilation and death sparks a Fourth-of-July chemistry, which in turn generates oxidative flames. Long hours of hard physical work, sleeplessness, crowded and unsanitary conditions fan the flames. Diesel exhaust and toxic fumes of military operations further fuel the oxidative fires that burn energy and detoxification enzymes. Exposure to pesticides and toxic paints increase oxidative injury to delicate enzymes. The list of pesticides used in the Gulf War is long and includes d-phenothrin, chlorpyrifos, resmethrin, malathion, methomyl, DEET and many others. Military personnel were given vaccines against infectious diseases that caused flu-like illnesses, adding yet more fuel to oxidative fires."

"So the stage was set," Choua remarked.

POISONS USED FOR PREVENTING WAR POISONS

"There was yet more trouble to come before the fighting broke out," I replied. "All military personnel were given a supply of the drug pyridostigmine and were advised to take it for at least seven days as "pretreatment" against anticipated exposure to nerve gas and other war chemicals. Pyridostigmine blocks an essential enzyme called acetylcholinerase, and is known to cause adverse effects such as abdominal cramping, nausea, vomiting, tingling in limbs and genitourinary symptoms. Reports of such side effects among treated troops ranged from 5% to 50%. The enzyme acetylcholinestrase plays a pivotal role in neurotransmitter function and—like other *neuroenzymes* is especially vulnerable to oxidative injury. The use of the drug was a necessary evil. Clearly it added to the total neurotransmitter stress, causing respiratory, gastrointestinal and muscle symptoms in many personnel during the troop buildup—before the conflict began. And then..."

"The war broke out," Choua completed my sentence.

"Yes." I resumed. "Then come the avalanches of toxic fumes and the smoke of military operations. The Gulf War, I knew, was to be a different war from any the United States had ever fought, and..."

"A different war?" Choua asked eagerly. "Why? I mean how was it going to be different from the Vietnam War, Korean War and other major engagements?" Choua asked.

A TV WAR,
A BRAND-NEW EXPERIMENT IN HUMAN BIOLOGY

"Anyone could have foreseen that Operation Desert Storm was going to be a brand-new experiment in human biology for two reasons," I explained. "First, Sadam threatened to unleash massive quantities of unknown war chemicals and put Kuwaiti oil fields to fire. This was sure to generate oxidative hurricanes for the fighting men and women. Second, this was to be the first full-scale TV war. Soldiers would learn, in virtual reality, the full dangers facing them in minute-by-minute blood-curdling details. The Czechs reported detection of war chemicals such as sarin and mustard gas. Others reported numerous sightings of dead animals. I knew there would be massive problems. There would be showers of erosive acids such as sulfuric and nitric acids, and looming clouds of toxic, oxidizing fumes of gases such as nitric oxide, sulfur dioxide, carbon monoxide, ammonia compounds and related compounds. Anyone with any ecologic sense of human biology would have known that."

THE SECOND PREDICTION:
FATIGUE WILL BE A DOMINANT PROBLEM

"Tell me, how did you know chronic fatigue was to be a dominant symptom among Gulf War veterans?"
"That was equally simple," I replied. "The energy level in

human biology is a function of energy enzymes, and as you know, enzymes are delicate proteins that are quickly damaged by oxidative injury. I knew the enzymes of the thyroid, adrenal and pancreas glands—the troubled trio in all major ecologic and immune injuries—are especially vulnerable to oxidative stress. I learned that from my research and clinical work with chronic fatigue sufferers."

"The human canaries," Choua interrupted me.

"Yes!" I continued. "Injury to thyroid enzymes results in lower body temperature—cold hands and cold feet that human canaries almost always complain of. Oxidative injury to adrenal enzymes causes chronic stress states, and that to pancreatic enzymes causes problems of sugar-insulin-adrenaline-neurotransmitter roller coasters. And oxidative injury to all three major endocrine enzyme systems causes chronic fatigue, individually as well as in combination. I also knew the oxidative storms in Desert Storm would injure the energy enzymes of mitochondria—the cellular powerhouses. It was quite evident to me that the enzyme pathways of the military personnel were not different from those of civilians—*the ecologic-immune disorders among the military personnel could not be different from chronic fatigue states that I observe every day in my civilian human canaries.*"

"Why can't N^2D^2 docs see something that simple?" Choua asked, then answered his own question, "because they can't think ecologically. They don't understand the two basic issues of genetic predisposition and cumulative oxidative enzyme injury. If they don't see the cause-and-effect relationship between the trigger and tissue response within a few hours, they can't understand it, right? Unless they see fields littered with bodies, they can't see toxicity in anything, can they?" Choua frowned.

"That *is* a problem," I agreed.

"You called that one right," Choua grinned. "Here is a

quote from the NIH statement that concerns your second prediction:

Data on the symptom profile reported in the Gulf War Registry were also compared with those reported for Vietnam veterans in the Agent Orange Registry. Fatigue, muscle and joint pain, headache, and shortness of breath were more frequent among those serving in the Persian Gulf area; skin rash was less frequent.

JAMA 272:392; 1994

Let's move to the third prediction," Choua said, putting the *Journal* down. "How did you know N^2D^2 docs would deny the problems of Gulf veterans existed?"

THE THIRD PREDICTION:
THE GULF WAR PROBLEM DOESN'T EXIST

"That was simple too! Because I knew mainstream physicians did not recognize the two essential issues of accelerated oxidative injury: the *genetic* predisposition of tissues to progressive oxidative stress and *the cumulative* oxidative injury to energy and detoxification enzyme pathways. It was so predictable that army physicians would ignore these two essential issues and deny that the problem existed at all—just as mainstream physicians do for environmental illness among civilians. Since they don't understand genetic vulnerability and cumulative oxidant stress, the problem of chronic illness in veterans simply did not exist for the mainstream physicians in the military."

"Right again!" Choua turned his eyes to the pages of the journal he was holding, "Here, listen to this:

> *What is the evidence for an increased incidence of unexpected illness attributable to service in the Persian Gulf War?...The available data are too limited to draw any conclusions.*
>
> *JAMA* 272:391; 1994

Data are too limited!" Choua joshed. "Never fails, does it? Do you think N^2D^2 docs ever worry about limited data when they prescribe psychotropic drugs?"

"You do have a point," I replied.

"Here's another quote from the statement prepared by NIH Technology Assessment Workshop Panel. The NIH experts asked themselves four questions when they held a two-day public session. Funny stuff, isn't it? The experts proclaim that the data are too limited—a polite euphemism for saying that the problem actually does not exist."

> *If unexpected illnesses have occurred, what are the components of the most practical working case definition(s) based on existing data?...it is impossible at this time to establish a single case definition.*
>
> *JAMA* 272:392; 1994

Impossible to establish! You know why that is so, don't you?"
Choua winked.

"Why?"

"Because the veterans complain of fatigue, muscle and joint pains, and memory loss—and N^2D^2 docs don't have "fatigometers," "painometers" and "memorymeters" to put the suffering of the veterans into some numerical model. What cannot be measured, the N^2D^2 experts reason, is not scientific enough for them—or worth serious inquiry."

"The mainstream physicians are baffled by symptoms caused by accelerated oxidative stress," I explained.

"They try to determine the component(s) of an illness they don't believe exists. Funny stuff, isn't it?"

THE FOURTH PREDICTION:
THE GULF ALL-IN-THE-HEAD SYNDROME

"Your fourth prediction siad that N^2D^2 experts would declare the Gulf War-related health disorder to be an imagined problem—a malingerers' syndrome. How did you figure that one out?"

"Nothing to figure out, Choua," I explained. "Whenever we physicians cannot understand a patient's suffering, the easiest way for us to solve the problem is to dismiss the patient as a malingerer, a shirker. If our drugs do not work, we assert the problem must be with the patient."

"Drugs can never *not* work, right?" Choua sneered. "The veterans are too stupid to know that, right? How could our Star Wars medical technology fail?"

"Stick to the point, Choua," I admonished.

"Long live the label of obsessional psychopathology! Long live N^2D^2 medicine!" Choua chimed.

"You're impossible today," I moaned.

"You were right with your fourth prediction." Choua cheered me. "You called that one out right too. Here is what the NIH panel says about your third prediction:

If unexpected illnesses have occurred, what are the plausible etiologies and biological explanations for these unexpected illnesses?...We are not suggesting that there is no physical basis for the reported symptoms, but that expression of the reported symptoms of posttraumatic stress disorder represents a psychophysiological response that needs to be evaluated.

JAMA 272: 394, 1994

Dead right again!" Choua chirped cheerily. "Long live all-in-the-head syndrome! Zeus bless N^2D^2 medicine!"

"These are complex biological issues of the 21st century that are difficult to adapt to 19th-century notions of diseases and drugs," I gave my usual explanation.

THE CDC GETS INTO THE ACT

"Then you predicted that the military N^2D^2 docs would

address this problem the same way civilian N^2D^2 docs addressed the so-called chronic fatigue syndrome—they would look toward delphic oracles at the CDC for answers. How did you know that?"

"What else could the army physicians do? They do not understand the core issues of genetic predisposition and cumulative oxidant injury. They do not comprehend the cumulative impact of environmental agents on human biology any better than their civilian colleagues. They were as ill-equiped to deal with ecologic injury as were mainstream physicians in patients with chronic fatigue. Drugs are chemicals, and chemicals cannot revive delicate energy enzymes injured by chemicals. Drugs cannot undo the damage done by accelerated oxidative molecular injury, can they?"

"Well, you called that one right too!" Choua laughed. "Here is what the NIH panel said about that prediction:

> *What future research is necessary? ...An assessment strategy modeled after the Centers for Disease Control and Prevention for chronic fatigue syndrome is recommended.*
>
> *JAMA* 272:394; 1994

Isn't that a riot?" Choua erupted sarcastically. "The experts at the CDC recommend that no one should diagnose chronic fatigue syndrome if an organic or psychiatric cause for fatigue exist. They believe that the chronic fatigue syndrome descends from Mount Olympus. Now the NIH panel takes its lead from the CDC. It tells us that the Gulf War syndrome also descends from Mount Olympus. It does not want any N^2D^2 docs to look for the causes of veterans' health disorders in cumulative oxidative injury to enzymes, do they? Answers in environmental, nutritional and stress-related factors? Nay!" Choua mocked. "They have no concepts of bowel, blood and liver ecosystems."

"The NIH Panel's conclusions truly surprise me. What do you think is the reason?" I asked.

"Don't you see the reason?" Choua pouted. "What could be simpler to figure out than that? Just look at the list of people who made up the NIH Panel. Then look at the list of speakers who addressed that panel, and you will understand the reason why the panel thinks the problems of the Gulf War veterans actually do not exist," Choua jeered.

POURING SALT ON WOUNDS

"Here, look at the lists," Choua thrust the journal pages at me. "You will not see the name of a single clinical ecologist. N^2D^2 docs want to keep their medicine pure and pristine! Why dirty it up with ideas of quacks who don't use their blessed drugs? There minds were made up. Why let anyone confuse them with facts? Why ask physicians who practice environmental medicine?"

"That's awful!" I responded, in frustration.

"In that list, all you see are names of people who hate ecologists and those who think enviromental illness is psychopathology—a belief system, obsessional psychopathology as they are fond of calling it. If that is not pouring salt on the wounds of the sick veterans, I don't know what is?"

"I'm sure things will change this time around," I replied. "It took the government almost fifteen years to acknowledge that Dioxins in Agent Orange sprayed in the Vietnam War caused serious chronic health disorders among some Air Force personnel who sprayed the chemical. I don't think that will be the case with the Gulf War syndrome. I think the plight of the sick veterans will be understood much sooner."

"Not if those epidemiology professors from prestigious medical schools can have their way," Choua countered.

THE FIFTH PREDICTION: DESTROYING ECOSYSTEMS WITH ANTIBIOTICS

"Finally you predicted that when everything else failed—as it is bound to fail—N^2D^2 docs would prescribe mega doses of broad spectrum antibiotics to cure this fell disorder. What was the basis of that prediction?" Choua asked.

"Simple! The mainstream physicians are trianed only to use drug therapies. They are not taught nondrug restorative therapies needed by people with inhjured energy and detoxification enzymes. I knew when antidepressants, antianxiety and other drugs fail, mainstream physicians will resort to long-term—and very destructive—broad-spectrum antibiotic therapy."

"Antibioticists will take over," Choua sneered. "And..."

"Wha...t? An antibioticist?" I interrupted Choua. "What is an antibioticist? Did you just make that word up?"

"An antibioticist is an N^2D^2 doctor who believes:

Where there is a disease,
There is a bug.
Where there is a bug,
There is a drug.

Antibioticists are super specialists who are very skillful in destroying microbes—and the delicate bowel, vaginal, urinary and blood ecosystems," Choua grinned broadly." *Long live antibioticists!* You have anesthesiologists, podiatrists, pathologists and chemotherapists! Why not antibioticists?" Choua chirped. "What do you think will happen to those poor veterans when that antibioticist is finished with them?"

"I shudder to think," I expressed my alarm at the proposed large-dose antibiotic therapy. "Their bowel ecosystems will be battered," Choua went on. "Their antioxidant defenses will be shattered. They will be more and more vulnerable to yeast infections and parasitic infestations. Old viral infections will be reactivated. Food amd mold allergy symptoms will become more intense. New chemical sensitivities will develop. Their hands and feet will become cold—and so will their brains as the delicate neuroenzymes are injured. They will deteriorate mentally. Their fatigue will be unrelenting and paralyzing."

"Well, you called that one right too!" Choua shook his head. "Listen to this how it validates your last prediction:

So far, the odd array of symptoms associated with the syndrome (Gulf War), including debilitating fatigue, diarrhea and sensitivity to chemicals, has defied diagnosis... Legislators direct that the remaining $3.4 million support ongoing research on an "antibacterial treatment method"...He prescribes large doses of antibiotics to his patients and recommends that they take the drug for at least a year after they feel better.

Science News 146:252; 1994

"Take the drug for at least a year after they feel better!" Choua repeated. "These N^2D^2 docs are really sure of themselves, aren't they? How many veterans are going to survive that kind of assault by antibioticists?"

"A poor strategy! A tragic error!" I responded.

SOMALIA SYNDROME, BOSNIA SYNDROME, ANY-WAR SYNDROME AND WAR CANARIES

"It's fortunate that we got out of Somalia quickly," Choua continued. "What do you think would have happened if there had been an extended war, and if Somalis had been vicious enough to unleash toxic chemicals on us, I'm sure there would have been a *Somalia War Syndrome,"* Choua resumed.

"Somalia is a poor, little country. They couldn't have done significant damage," I refuted Choua's assertion.

"And, if the situation deteriorates in Bosnia and we get pulled into that war," Choua went on, "we would have to invent *Bosnia War syndrome* because it is utterly predictable that some soldiers will return with injured antioxidant and immune defenses. They will go on to develop the N^2D^2 docs' vague, ill-defined symptoms associated with chronic fatigue. The military doctors would have a problem: They wouldn't be able to call their illness Gulf War syndrome because obviously there is no Gulf in Somalia or in Bosnia," Choua grinned impishly.

"Are you saying that we Americans will never be able to fight a war in the future without coining a term for a syndrome for war veterans who develop chronic illness?"

"Right! Right! That's the idea. You see the problem is that all wars are hells of oxidative fires—of lives in danger, sights of mutilated and dead bodies, fumes of war technology, sleeplessness and the fear of nerve gases and other war chemicals. War is an unrelenting oxidative storm. So some veterans who go to war with damaged body ecosystems will turn out to be war canaries—they will return sick with multiple organ disorders. None of those people will ever fit the neat disease classifications of N^2D^2 doctors."

"So what's the answer?" I asked, disheartened.

"There is no answer! There is no need for any. N^2D^2 docs in the armed forces will have no difficulty inventing new names for old afflictions—after all that's what professors do in your medical schools. Finally someone will wake up and create a generic all-encompassing term *Any War Syndrome*. Everyone will live happily ever after," Choua muttered, fell silent and looked out the window.

It was late afternoon. I looked at my watch. It was time to leave the laboratory for evening hours with my patients. I stuffed papers in my briefcase and reached for my jacket in the closet. Choua turned to face me, his face grim and distraught.

"What do you think will happen to those sick veterans?" he asked.

"Many will get better in spite of onging biologic insults of drugs used by their physicians. The human body has an enormous capacity to recover," I said hopefully.

"Even after those N^2D^2 antibiotists are through with their massive doses of killer antibiotics?" Choua pressed.

"That's a mistake! "A bad, bad mistake!" I sighed. "I have no doubt that a vast majority of disabled veterans can revive their damaged energy enzymes and return to their pre-war jobs if only funds were available for them to receive comprehensive, integrated nondrug therapies from physicians experienced in restorative enzyme work. What these sick veterans need are effective nutritional, herbals and environmental therapies. They need someone to teach them things about hope and spirituality."

"You're a dreamer," Choua smiled, then somberly continued. "the Gulf War should have taught N^2D^2 docs many lessons about the delicate human ecosystems and their vulnerability to environmental oxidative stresses of the war," Choua spoke softly then. "But that wasn't in the cards! They are smug with their high-powered expert panels, their elegant diagnostic labels, their stupid notions of diseases and drugs. Meanwhile, the sick veterans will get sicker—many will be permanently disabled. The oxidative storms of Operation Desert Storm blew over. But the simmering oxidative coals of denial and drug therapies of N^2D^2 docs will continue to cook whatever is left of the energy and detoxification enzymes of the poor sick veterans! Every war will produce its war canaries. But that won't change anything. The Olympian remedies will forever flourish for Olympian maladies! And Prince Chaullahs of N^2D^2 medicine will forever..."

Choua left his sentence unfinished and walked out.

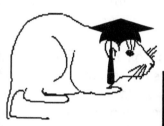

Chapter 8

FIFTH INSIGHT

The Bowel and Blood are Open Ecosystems

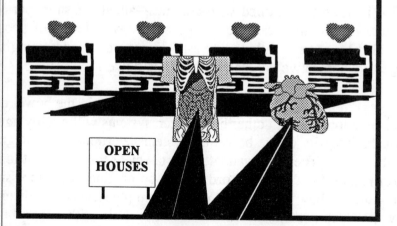

OPEN
HOUSES

The bowel is an ecosystem—as diverse, dynamic and delicate as any other on planet Earth.

The most remarkable phenomenon in the field of human biology is this: A great many disorders are spontaneously resolved when clinical management turns its focus to the bowel ecosystem. This is true even for disorders that seem unrelated to the bowel.

How often do headaches, mood swings and concentration difficulties clear up when a damaged bowel ecosystem is restored to health? How often are symptoms of sugar craving and sugar roller coasters relieved when clinical management is directed at the bowel? How often are symptoms of PMS and menstrual irregularities controlled by nondrug therapies that reduce the bowel transit time and normalize the bowel's internal environment? How often does acne in the face and skin rashes on other parts of the body disappear when yeast overgrowth in the bowel is brought under control? How often are joint pains in young patients with immune disorders relieved with herbs that act on the bowel? How often is asthma controlled with colonics—albeit for short periods of time? How often can the energy and activity levels of people disabled by chronic fatigue be vastly improved by addressing the digestive-absorptive derangements in the bowel?

Physicians who reflect on the happenings in the bowel and their relationship with other body organ systems will readily agree that the integrity of the bowel ecosystem determines the integrity of the bowel. They will validate my statement that excellent long-term results for diverse disorders can be obtained by addressing the issues of bowel ecology. Conventional physicians will dismiss my statement, skeptical of the bowel's link with other body organs. They will be quick to point out that none of these conclusions have been drawn as a result of double-blind cross-over studies. They will regard empirical methods of bowel management as quackery and will identify the physicians who practice empirical medicine as charlatans.

The ancients believed that death begins in the colon. It took me a long time—25 years of study of immunology, examination of over 12,000 bowel biopsies and long hours of listening to patients with chronic bowel disorders—to appreciate their wisdom. Now, every working day I see patients who bear out this enduring ancient truth.

In my clinical practice, I consider the bowel ecosystem as the centerpiece of my management strategy for *all* chronic immune and degenerative disorders. I discuss this subject at length in the companion volume *Battered Bowel Ecosystem—Waving Away A Wandering Wolf.* Here, I include some brief comments.

In medical school I was taught much about the diseases of the bowel but nothing at all about bowel health. That, of course, was consistent with my learning about other body organs—I learned about disease names and names of drugs to treat them. But there was never any mention of health—what it is, and how it can be preserved.

In classrooms, we learned about typhoid dysentery and colitis caused by *Shigella* microbes. We were taught how much chloromycetin should be administered to a patient to kill typhoid microbes and how much tetracycline should be prescribed for controlling *Shigella* organisms. (*C. difficile* was not recognized as a significant problem yet.) Then came a long list of other pathogenic microbes. The emphasis was always the same: search-and-destroy missions, identify the bug and zap it with a drug of choice. So I grew up to be a drug doctor—as did all my classmates—believing that the bowel was a dirty drainage tube that should be kept free of all disease-causing microbes. Not an irrational belief on the surface!

THE GREEK, HAKIMS AND THE BOWEL

Our professors regularly railed against *hakims*—the physicians who used natural remedies based on the Greek philosophy of medicine as preserved by the Arabs. Their practices were dismissed as sheer quackery—willful and dangerous neglect of the scientific principles of modern medicine. I remember that the *hakims'* clinical approaches almost always focused on the bowel. We scoffed at their ideas. How could headaches, skin problems, joint pains, respiratory and other disorders be treated effectively with remedies directed to the bowel? Still, people went to *hakims* in droves. That seemed to irk my professors even more. I don't recall any professor ever seriously discussing the reasons why a large number of sick people might prefer *hakims* to them. Sometimes they would mumble something about the superstitious beliefs of the ignorant. (What could be better than nontoxic superstition if it could really help? At that time, this question had never crossed my mind.) Now, the *New England Journal of Medicine* tells us that Americans also prefer nondrug therapies to drug regimens. I suppose, at heart, we Americans today are as superstitious as the illiterate masses in Pakistan were then—and still are now.

THE BOWEL: A DARK, DIRTY DRAINAGE TUBE

During my surgical training, I saw a large number of bloated, constricted, inflamed, ulcerated and bleeding bowels on the operating tables. A surgeon is usually occupied with two questions: what to cut out and how to put back what is left behind. The imperatives of a surgical schedule do not leave much room for ecologic thinking. I remember we were obsessed with the danger of spillage of the bowel contents into the abdominal cavity and the risk of peritonitis, but that was about the extent of our concern about the bowel during abdominal surgery.

Gastroenterologists were fond of classifying colitis in many different ways. Ulcerative colitis was supposed to bleed more often. Crohn's colitis was considered to cause obstruction more often. Elderly persons suffered from ischemic colitis due to poor blood supply, and those receiving antibiotics developed pseudomembranous colitis, in which layers of the bowel lining sloughed off to make membranes of tissue debris. But for us surgeons-in-training, an inflamed bowel was an inflamed bowel. We were not given to much speculation about why things happened in the bowel—let alone fuss about ecologic relationships within the gurgling, dark, dirty drainage tube that was the gut.

BOWEL THROUGH THE MICROSCOPE

During my early years of pathology residency training, I

was obsessed with microscopic images. I wanted my biopsy slides to speak to me immediately and clearly. I had little patience with the diagnostic criteria that I was required to learn. A favorite pastime of pathology residents is to show each other slides without clinical information and to try to stump the opponents. That is when I got into the habit of looking at slides "blindly" and not asking for clinical data—a habit I keep to this day. I discovered something interesting about the bowel: With very high magnification, I could play games with the slides of colon biopsies of a patient suffering from ulcerative colitis—I could convince my peers that the slide was actually taken from colitis of any other type. The type of the cell in acute inflammation was the same whether the patients had ulcerative colitis, Crohn's colitis, ischemic colitis or any other type of colitis.

I accumulated a huge library of slides of various diseases—as almost all pathology residents do. It didn't take me long to collect examples of all sorts of gut lesions, including all known types of colitis. When we residents reviewed colon biopsies, I often pulled out slides from my collections and tricked them into making wrong diagnoses—all in fun and games. Somewhere along the way, doubts began to grow in my mind about the validity of microscopic classification of various types of colitis. I began to recognize that what I was being taught were discrete colon diseases in reality were not discrete after all—they were points along a continuum, forever changing patterns of tissue injury and healing.

QUACKS AND THE BOWEL

Then one day quacks—physicians who *really* believed that

food allergy can cause colitis and environmental pollutants can trigger immune responses in the gut—came into my life. These quacks regaled me with their tales of patients with advanced immune and degenerative disorders who improved with unscientific treatment methods, and got better with their *clearly* unscientific concepts of disease and methods of treatment. I listened to their accounts with a grain of salt, but what shook my belief system was when I began to accept their invitations to see for myself some of their clinical results. (Why were these quacks so intent on winning me over? I don't know. Perhaps they try to win everyone over and I just happened to be there.) I patiently listened to them for long periods of time. I began to see with as much objectivity as I could muster how many chronic, unremitting health disorders—clearly unrelated to the bowel according to the prevailing pathology precepts—are resolved with natural therapies directed to the bowel.

When I returned to the clinical practice of environmental and nutritional medicine after years of pathology work, I began carefully testing the claims made by those quacks. To my great surprise, I found the quacks were right after all. My patients responded well to the *unscientific* therapies vehemently rejected by my colleagues in drug medicine. In my practice, I focused on bowel transit time and on symptoms such as abdominal bloating, cramps, flatulence, and episodes of diarrhea and/or constipation. I began to document predictable clinical patterns. It didn't take long to establish clear, unmistakable relationships between events taking place in the bowel and symptoms manifested by other body organs. It took several months before I concluded that all patients with chronic immune and degenerative disorders respond in some degree to therapies directed at the bowel. In fact, the results became quite predictable—though some were very slow in coming—when I holistically addressed food allergy and other incompatibilities, digestion, absorption, bowel transit time, yeast overgrowth, intestinal parasites and other types of altered bowel flora.

In my hospital pathology work, I began to examine bowel biopsies with a renewed interest, focusing on events that might have occurred before the bowel wall was damaged rather than simply recording how bad the damage was. Still, I continued to subscribe to the prevailing view that the bowel is well protected from our external environment—and is, in essence, a closed system.

THE BOWEL IS AN OPEN ECOSYSTEM

Very slowly, I realized that, in fact, the bowel is an open ecosystem.

Physicians are not ecologic thinkers. Most are essentially Oslerian in thinking. Sir William Osler, the American physician eminent at the turn of the century, taught that a physician must think of one disease for a given patient, strive to fit all clinical and laboratory data into one diagnosis, and use one drug of choice to treat the disease. Sometime ago, Choua dubbed this model of one-Disease-one-Diagnosis-one-Drug thinking as D^3 medicine. I am not sure that Oslerian medical thought was ever a valid philosophy, but I am certain it is irrelevant to 21st-century problems related to nutrition, the environment and stress which clearly feed upon each other and lead to nutritional, environmental and stress-related disorders.

Life comprises many ecorelationships—the bowel ecosystem

interfaces with the outside world as well as with the blood ecosystem, which, in turn, interfaces with body organ ecosystems. The cellular ecosystems within the body organ interface with those in the neighboring cells. Within the cells are microcosms of cellular organelles that, in their own right, are complete ecosystems that interact dynamically among themselves and with others in close vicinity.

Ecosystems in nature are diverse and dynamic systems that are in constant flux—they sense change within and without the system and actively respond to it. This is as true of human ecosystems as it is of marine or marsh ecologies.

The events that occur in the stomach cannot be regarded as isolated, separable from those that occur in the small bowel—and those taking shape in the small bowel must be viewed in connection with the happenings in the colon. Chemical events taking place in one body organ cannot be separated from biologic interrelationships in other body organs. Digestive enzymes cannot be understood except within the context of food substances they act upon. Acid and enzymes in the stomach chew up the unwanted, toxic agent-producing microbes which I call TAPs. Yet, in the colon the friendly lactic acid-producer microbes—LAPs in my language—complete the digestion of food microparticles that digestive enzymes leave behind. Serious injury to TAPs cannot be inflicted with broad-spectrum antibiotics without injuring the LAPs at the same time—hence the enormous dangers of antibiotic abuse, especially in children in whom the bowel ecosystems have not matured and in whom the LAPs have not yet gotten their stronghold.

THE NAKED, MUTANT MICROBES MATE PRECOCIOUSLY IN THE BOWEL

Microbes injured by antibiotics act like rabid dogs—barking, biting and damaging the delicate bowel ecosystem. In scientific jargon they are called L-forms or cell wall-deficient microbes. Often, these naked microbes mate precociously—like the Greek god, Zeus, they make love to anything that moves. And like the Greek Titans, they produce mutant offsprings, spawning generations of wild microbes that dare all our antibiotics. We call this phenomenon drug resistance.

In biology, when we change one thing in one way, we change everything in some way.

Many disruptive cascades of chemical and microbial events can be cited to illustrate disruptions of the bowel ecosystem. I cite one example:

Many disease-causing bacteria reduce the level of taurine in white blood cells—the first line of immune defense against invading bacteria. Taurine is a powerful antioxidant that protects the cell wall against oxidant injury. Its deficiency weakens white blood cells. As a result, bacteria multiply freely. We use antibiotics to check bacterial growth. Antibiotics damage the bowel flora and spawn mutant microbes that destroy the P-450 system of enzymes that immune cells use against toxins. The result is impaired ability to detoxify waste and increased potential for development of chemical sensitivity. This, in turn, interferes with the digestive-absorptive functions in the bowel. Partially digested food substances—what I alluded to earlier as macromolecules—overwhelm the immune system leading to autoimmune reactions. Weakened immune defenses allow the bacteria to multiply freely which, in turn, reduces the taurine level in the white blood cells. A vicious cycle is thus set up in motion—more infections, more antibiotics, weakened antioxidant defenses in immune cells, more chemical sensitivity, greater vulnerability to infections.

Food sensitivity reactions disrupt normal digestive-absorptive functions in the bowel and damage the bowel lining—quite literally poking holes in the gut mucosa. Undigested macromolecules of foods now flood the lymph and blood ecosystems, lighting up tiny oxidative fires along the way. When the first-line chemical defense systems fail to cope with such macromolecule overloads, second-line immune defenses are called into action. The immune defense mechanisms have an enormous—yet finite—capacity for enduring such assaults. Overwhelmed and confused, the immune system turns on the body's own molecules, producing autoantibodies that damage a person's own cells and so cause autoimmune disorders. Autoimmunity hits the vulnerable organs most. Genes determine who comes down with an underactive adrenal gland and who develops an overactive thyroid gland.

In my pathology work, I searched for answers with my microscope and soon discovered the primary limitation of the microscope: It only shows damage *after* it's been done. In spite of the many classifications of colitis that have been proposed, there are only so many patterns of bowel injury. It became impossible for me to look at chronic bowel diseases as specific diseases. Instead, I came to regard bowel diseases as altered states of bowel ecology that eventually affected even distant organs. Immune disorders turned into patterns of bowel injury expressing themselves in the various arms of the immune system.

I became aware how physicians in alternative medicine were utterly committed to the notion that the yeast *Candida albicans* was the dragon that caused all clinical problems. They look at nystatin and Diflucan as the dragon killers. How could a yeast that is almost always present in the bowel ecosystem be the main villain? I wondered. At the same time, gastroenterologists searched for the microbe *Clostridium (C) difficile* whenever their patients suffered from any abdominal symptoms—even though they knew that reports indicated that 10 to 15 percent of all hospitalized persons acquired *C. difficile* organisms as a hospital-acquired colonization of the bowel. Those colon specialists then prescribed Flagyl and other powerful antibiotics to banish the microbe from the gut. How could *C. difficile* become such an important invader of the bowel ecosystem overnight? I wondered.

I realized that there are three essentials of the bowel ecosystem:

First,

our immunologic—and at a more fundamental level, antioxidant—defenses are implanted in the soil of the bowel contents.

Second,

acute and chronic bowel disorders cannot be fully understood and well managed without ecologic thinking—both from chemical and biologic perspectives. In N^2D^2 medicine, a patient is labeled with a disease name and then his symptoms are suppressed with a drug of choice. While this one-disease-one-diagnosis-one-drug approach—Choua's D^3 medicine—provides the physician with the comfort of a reimbursable diagnosis and the patient some symptom relief, it does nothing to help any of them gain any insights into the true nature of suffering caused by the events in the bowel.

Third,

the bowel is an *open* ecosystem. Many life forms—viruses, mycoplasma, bacteria, yeasts and parasites—freely wander in and out of this ecosystem. In a healthy bowel ecosystem, these organisms do not gain a foothold and cause disease. In a damaged state, however, the bowel is unable to weed out these wandering microbes. The notion that these living beings can be permanently banished from the bowel is as simplistic as the notion of eliminating all butterflies, insects and birds from our towns and cities. We cannot destroy these living beings without doing permanent damage to ourselves, and especially our children.

It has become commonplace for me to see little children who live on antibiotics. They catch new infections of the throat, ear and bronchi before they have even rid themselves of the preceding infection. Each course of antibiotics adds to the devastation of the bowel ecosystem just as industrial pollutants lead to defoliation of forests.

KILLING THE CANDIDA DRAGON

Many patients consult me for a *yeast problem*. They vehemently plead with me to cure their yeast. In *The Battered Bowel Ecology—Waving Away a Wandering Wolf*, I discuss this issue at length. Here is an example of a conversation I have had with innumerable patients who were told that all their clinical problems could be resolved only if their yeast problem could be cured.

"Dr. Ali, will I ever be cured of my Candida problem?" the patient asks.

"I hope not!" I respond.

"No?" the patient looks puzzled. "You mean you cannot cure my *Candida* yeast infection? Oh, I have had so much hope you were going to solve that problem forever—rid me of yeast for good!" she pleads her case earnestly.

"No!"

"Why not?" she looks disappointed.

"Because the only way I can eradicate all yeast from your bowel ecosystem is if I were to sterilize it. If I did that, I'm afraid, you would not live for long," I explain.

"You're not serious, are you?" she expresses doubt gravely.

"Of course, I am!" I reassure her. "What you need is not eradication of Candida but restoration of the full integrity of the bowel ecosystem. Everyone has *Candida* species in her or his bowel. Women begin to have vaginal yeast infections when the yeast overgrows in the bowel and spills over into the vaginal tract. Women and men have systemic problems when yeast—*Candida, Aspergillus* and *Alternaria* species and others less commonly—begin to slip into the tissue. So, that's how we'll approach the problem."

LARGE STOOLS, SMALL HOSPITALS
SMALL STOOLS, LARGE HOSPITALS

I began this section about the bowel ecosystem with the ancient Indian and Chinese wisdom that death begins in the colon. Now, I end it with another observation the ancients made about the the bowel transit time and human health. They were very sensitive to patterns of systemic toxicity that resulted from stasis of fecal matter in the gut. They considered proper elimination of the bowel contents as essential for good long-term health.

If we were to paraphrase the ancients, we could say we have a choice:

We can keep our stools large and bulky that are effortlessly eliminated, maintain good health, and so keep our hospitals small.

Or, we can retain small, dried and shrunken stools in the bowel for long periods, and allow the waste products to seep into the lymph and blood and cause chronic disorders in various body organs. If so, we most assuredly will need to build large hospitals.

The Bloodstream: An Open Ecosystem

Although the concept of the bowel as an open ecosystem evolved slowly in my mind, the idea of the bloodstream as an equally open ecosystem came as a flash.

On the morning of January 14, 1994, two Canadian physicians, Paul Drouin, M.D., and Louise Comeau, M.D., visited me with their attorney. Their licenses were in jeopardy because of several charges brought against them by some of their peers. The Corporation des Medecins & Chirurgiens du Quebec—the medical licensing board of the province of Quebec—was conducting hearings of their case. They flew down to discuss their case with me and see if I could testify on their behalf.

Drs. Drouin and Comeau faced several charges. Major charges against them included inaccurate diagnoses of oxidative cellular injury, *Candida* yeast organisms and parasites established by an examination of blood smears with the use of a high-resolution microscope developed by my friend, Dr. Robert Bradford. Their accusers, among them a local retired surgeon appointed by the Corporation to investigate the case, took the position that none of this work was scientifically valid, and that their diagnoses based upon microscopic observations were incorrect. Indeed, it was believed that these two physicians were guilty of gross professional misconduct in diagnosing conditions that didn't exist and administering therapies that were unnecessary.

The Corporation brought before the disciplinary committee experts from the local university who testified that they had examined the blood slides of 10 patients in question and were unable to find any of the yeast organisms or parasites that Drs. Drouin and Comeau claimed to have seen. The university experts seemed irked by the fact that Drs. Drouin and Comeau, two general practitioners, were making diagnoses with a Bradford microscope, an instrument about which they, the university experts, knew nothing about.

Two weeks earlier, Bob Bradford, Ph.D., a former physicist at Stanford University who developed the high-resolution microscope that bears his name, had asked me to review the case of these two Canadian physicians and go up to Montreal to appear before the Corporation panel in their defense. In a letter to me some days later, Dr. Drouin wrote me that the case was "in fact a Canadian test to have Dr. Bradford's work known and respected in this country (Canada)." Bob evidently had a strong interest in the case and in validation of his technology.

Bradford was with me when our Canadian visitors arrived. Paul Drouin, a tall, thin man in his early forties entered first, and awkwardly shook my hand, a vexed smile on his face. His smile did little to hide the anguish in his blue-gray eyes. I knew this anguish—it is always there when holistic physicians are inquisitioned by the disease doctors of drug medicine. Drouin's face was one that could tell long hurtful stories in a fleeting moment. His hair was receding and wind-blown. He wore a wrinkled, blue shirt, one or two sizes too large for him and a brightly colored, green, red and mustard neck tie, dazzlingly mismatched with his shirt and with his faded brown leather jacket. He carried a denim sack, the kind that boys carry on their backs to schools. "Thank you, Dr. Ali, for agreeing to help us," Drouin spoke slowly and hesitantly, obviously unable to hide his discomfort with the position he was in.

Oh, no! Not him, I muttered under my breath. A sharp image of a holistic physician—gentle, vulnerable and wholly unprepared for dodging the killer instinct of his inquisitors sitting on a disciplinary committee—took form before my eyes. Strange how such events turn out—physicians who wear dark pinstripe suits with fitted, white dress shirts and expensive silk ties are never investigated for their philosophic views about medicine. (Sometimes they are hauled before medical disciplinary committees for charges of substance abuse or sexual misconduct.) It seems that docs who have difficulty dressing well tend to be the docs who have difficulty steering clear of medical disciplinary committees. I shook Dr. Drouin's hand warmly, trying to put him at ease.

Louise Comeau, an attractive blonde, somewhat younger than Drouin in age, entered next, her shoulders tilting back and her tummy bulging forward with the pride of pregnancy. She wore a pink blouse with large flowers, a dark skirt, and carried a glistening red leather briefcase. She grinned broadly, extended her hand in a self-assured way. She is the fighter of the two, I thought. She seemed in no hurry to assess me or to judge my competence as a witness.

The attorney, a handsome man in his mid-fifties with well-groomed silver-gray hair, was last to enter the room. He was clearly a no nonsense lawyer, and looked his part—immaculately dressed, a buttoned-down white shirt, a dark suit, a woolen overcoat, the requisite leather bag, the air of a seasoned attorney that he obviously relished. He shook my hand and looked around at the shelves brimming over with medical books in my office, heaps of papers on my desk and some piles of journals on the rug.

Moments later, he looked at me, smiled again and sat down on a corner chair. Drouin flopped onto the couch facing my desk. I waited for Comeau to find a seat between the two, and then sat on a high stool by my double-headed microscope, closer to them rather than on my swivel chair across my desk. Then the attorney began in slow, measured sentences, taking command of the meeting.

After some introductory remarks about my curriculum vitae, the attorney asked me the expected question:

"Have you ever seen *Candida* organisms in an unstained blood smear with the Bradford microscope?"

"No," I replied.

"No?" he asked, taken by surprise.

"No," I repeated calmly.

"Oh!" He glared at me in silence for some moments, as if deciding whether there was any point to pursuing this subject anymore. "Is it possible to see *Candida* in such smears?" he continued after a while.

"Probably, if I can develop a sufficiently sensitive immunostaining method," I replied.

"What is immunostaining?" he inquired.

"A procedure in which specific antibodies are used to stain the organisms."

"But you have never done so before, have you?"

"No, I haven't, but Dr. Bradford and I have talked about it."

The attorney then asked many other questions. I explained my views on oxidative injury and my observations about direct oxidative damage to blood cells and blood plasma.

A WITNESS FOR THE DEFENSE

I have been asked to testify in defense of holistic doctors in similar cases both in the United States and Canada. Though specific details of the cases varied from case to case, the core issue is always the same: The drug doctors who preside over disciplinary committees—and who, by their admission, never practiced nutritional nor environmental medicine—are always eager to punish, often severely, holistic physicians accused of practicing "unscientific" methods.

I understood that the case of Drs. Drouin and Comeau was not about oxidative injury, yeast or parasites. This case was but one skirmish in the raging war between practitioners of N^2D^2 medicine and those who seek nondrug alternatives for their patients. Investigations of professional misconduct of holistic physicians are always a farce. Drug doctors who conduct such inquiries always come to the same conclusions: That the testimony of experts against holistic doctors is always scientifically valid, while that of experts for holistic physicians is not.

Therefore, I had no illusions about the investigating committee sitting in judgment of the clinical work of Drs. Drouin and Comeau. The system never fails. For holistic physicians charged with professional misconduct, justice almost always means punishment. I knew the witnesses for the prosecution were to be considered eminent scientists; that for the defense, misguided charlatans. On the rare occasions when the accused holistic physicians are eventually exonerated, the proceedings usually leave them bankrupt, both financially and emotionally. The predators succeed in decimating the prey.

"THIS BATTLE COST ME TWO YEARS OF MY LIFE"

Holistic physicians facing disciplinary committees always feel isolated. Some years earlier, a Canadian clinical ecologist, Marion Zazula, M.D., had described to me his experience with a disciplinary committee of drug doctors that investigated him. I quote:

> *"It's awful! They know nothing about our work—nothing about environment, nothing about nutrition, nothing about time-proven nondrug therapies. They do not understand us. They never see our clinical results. And yet they pounce at us no matter what we say. I felt so isolated! This battle cost me two years of my life."*

Practitioners of drug medicine are hard task masters when they investigate vulnerable holistic physicians.

On January 21, 1994, a little over a fortnight after Dr. Drouin visited me, I received this letter from him:

19 January, 1994

Dear Dr. Ali,

I am still overwhelmed by the meeting we had with you, Dr. Bradford, and the lawyer, Maitre Andre Payeur. Believe it or not, I feel it is the most important encounter that I have witnessed in nineteen years of my professional career.

In fact it was comforting to discover such eloquent support for holistic medicine principles coming from a man with such a high level of medical authority and scientific competence. I must admit to you that these last months we have been pathetically alone and isolated in our combat. Personally, I consider this to be THE battle of my professional life. I have ten years of positive holistic medical experience yet have so few arguments articulated in a language that could convince official and traditionally formed medical doctors. Thank you for your brilliant communication.

I will never forget the panache with which you replied to Maitre Andre Payeur's questioning! You are truly a son of a judge! In your expose I heard some of the most beautiful arguments for holistic medicine principles that I have ever heard and I regret only that I did not have a tape recorder with me! The ease with which you were able to put this debate in a global perspective was very impressive. It has given a formidable momentum to our case in particular...and will wake up many others besides our conservative lawyer. Before meeting with you, he looked at us with all the disdain worthy of quacks and charlatans! The day after our meeting with you, he was no longer the same man! Magically, we had regained the respect and dignity, which is our due. You shook him for good! And every day since, he is beginning to sound more like a holistic medicine advocate.

Needless to say, Doctor Louise Comeau and I are jubilant with regard to the confirmation through strictly controlled scientific experimentation of Candida in the Lab. It is indeed extremely exciting and positive news.

*I am presently reading your books
and find them very interesting. As vice-
president of the Association of Holistic
Doctors in Quebec, I believe that my
colleagues will certainly be very happy to
discover your works. This is why I have
taken the initiative to order other copies of
your books so that we can make known
your ideas and have exchanges with regard
to them, and thereby enrich our collective
medical experience.*

Gratefully Yours,

Paul Drouin, M.D.

The above letter obviously sounds self-congratulatory. Still,
I take that risk and reproduce it in full to illuminate how deep the
anguish of holistic physicians is when they are hounded by Prince
Chaullahs of N^2D^2 medicine.

Pathetically alone and isolated in our combat. Drouin's
words dropped like stones in my stomach. *I have ten years of
positive holistic medical experience yet have so few arguments
articulated in a language that could convince...*I knew Drouin's

anguish, his helplessness, his sense of personal inadequacy, in *"the battle of my professional life."* The stones turned within me.

Drs. Drouin and Comeau, of course, are not the only physicians pathetically alone and isolated in this combat. This sad play—the battle of life for holistic physicians—is relished by drug medicine in every state, every month. The stage is the same, and so is the plot. Only the victims change.

BLOOD: A STREAM OF COMMERCE

Circulating blood, I thought in medical school, is the stream of commerce in the body.

In my high-school science class, I had learned that blood carries oxygen from the lungs to the tissues, nutrients from the gut to the liver and beyond, hormones from endocrine glands to their target organs, and waste products from tissues to the kidneys. Blood must be a conveyer belt, I remember thinking—a red stream in which float the round red and white blood corpuscles and the odd-shaped bits of colorless life called platelets. The blood circulation also maintains body temperature, my science teacher had told me.

BLOOD IS STERILE

The *fact* that blood is sterile was burned deep into my

professional consciousness in physiology classes, in microbiology courses, in pathology laboratories, and finally in the operating rooms of Pakistan, England and the U.S.

Medical school years were a dazed time for me—the need for rote-learning was absolute, and the amount of information we were required to remember would have numbed anyone. As I look back now, I wonder why they thought it was necessary to enforce sterility of blood upon us in so many different ways. After long, long hours of memorizing numbers, figures, diagrams and formulas, I wasn't—none of us were—in any condition to question anything they fed to us.

Sometimes the bloodstream *is* invaded by microbes. When this happens, the invaders are efficiently removed from the circulating blood. An example that almost every teacher relished was the temporary presence of bacteria in the blood after brushing teeth—the toothbrush bacteremia. The teachers took pains to assert that this was very different from septicemia—a life-threatening condition in which bacteria actively replicate in circulating blood and make the patient very ill and toxic and cause death unless the condition is expeditiously reversed.

For about 20 years after I left medical school, I taught my students and pathology residents the party line—that the blood is sterile. Actually, I never had any reason to reflect on the issue of blood sterility. Blood is sterile. Physiologists knew that. Microbiologists knew that. Pathologists knew that. What was there to think about anyway?

CANDIDA FLOATING IN THE BLOODSTREAM

I acquired a Bradford microscope and published the results of my studies of oxidative injury to red blood cells in patients with autoimmune disorders and chronic fatigue (Ali M. *Am J Clin Pathol* 94:515; 1990). Bradford thought that the fact that I had conducted some research with his microscope would be very helpful to the case of the beleaguered Canadian physicians and his Bradford Institute in Montreal. Specifically, he asked if I would describe my experience with oxidative injury as seen through his microscope. He also asked if it would be possible for me to prove that *Candida* yeast organisms could indeed be seen in blood smears using his microscope.

l had seen structures in the blood of such patients that looked like yeast organisms but knew that no one had ever used specific immunologic methods to prove that those were *Candida* organisms. Bradford, of course, was aware that my research colleague, Madhava Ramanarayanan, Ph.D., and I had used such immunodiagnostic methods extensively to detect anti-*Candida* antibodies in blood. I listened to Bradford and then expressed considerable reservations about the feasibility of performing such a task on such short notice. I knew I would be required to testify within a few weeks if I were to be of some help to the Canadian physicians. Vagaries of immune responses defy schedules set by investigators.

THE MICROSCOPE: A TOOL OF DECEPTION?

A Canadian hematologist, brought in as an expert by the Corporation investigators had testified before the disciplinary committee that blood is sterile, and that Drs. Drouin and Comeau couldn't possibly have seen *Candida* organisms in smears made with circulating blood. He maintained that the presence of *Candida* organisms—fungemia in the common medical terms—is a fulminant condition that threatens life rapidly unless it is aggressively treated. Evidently, people who walked into the offices of Drs. Drouin and Comeau couldn't have been acutely sick. Hence, he concluded that the doctors were treating a disease that really didn't exist. The Bradford microscope in their hands was clearly a tool of deception.

The task of the disciplinary committee now, the experts advised, was to protect the unsuspecting public from medical charlatans who concoct diseases and then dare to treat them with unproven natural and homeopathic remedies. The committee regarded the case as a proverbial open-and-shut case of professional misconduct that justified revoking their licenses. The Corporation-appointed conservative attorney seemed to agree.

A RAGING CONTROVERSY

Candida is the subject of a raging controversy in the

Western world today. On one side are many physicians in alternative medicine who believe *Candida* overgrowth and infection are the most frequent causes of chronic symptom-complexes involving multiple body organs. On the other side are mainstream doctors who believe that *Candida* infections are quite uncommon, and that physicians who treat so-called yeast problems are treating imaginary diseases—the favored all-in-the-head theory.

Many of my colleagues in holistic medicine think *Candida* anywhere is a dragon that must be slain. They hold it responsible for everything: bloating; flatulence and bowel cramps; muscle aches and joint stiffness; recurrent sore throats and ear infections; vaginal symptoms and prostatic pain; headache and PMS; mood, memory and mentation difficulties; anxiety and depression; and hyperactivity and autism in children.

My colleagues in mainstream medicine think *Candida* in the bloodstream means imminent death. Not difficult to understand at all! After all, we regularly see *Candida* invasion of tissues and blood in patients dying with AIDS and those dying after chemotherapy for cancer. Pathologists frequently see *Candida* overgrowth and tissue infections when performing autopsies on AIDS patients or those who have had extensive chemotherapy. Thus, mainstream physicians believe fungemia must be eradicated with potent (and, of necessity, toxic) antifungal drugs. They steadfastly maintain that *Candida* problems among people who walk about and complain of multiple symptoms *is nothing but* an all-in-the-head nuisance perpetuated by medical miscreants. They scoff at the idea, even as their patients regularly complain of yeast-induced vaginal symptoms after taking antibiotics.

The Centers for Disease Control in Atlanta have made some dire predictions about *Candida*. They project that by the year

2000, *Candida* species will be the most frequently encountered and dangerous organism to threaten hospitalized patients. Furthermore, they forecast that this yeast will invade the bloodstream of patients more frequently than any other organism.

Candidus in Latin means white, pure or sincere. *Candere* means white or hot. *Candida* fungus was probably so named because it grows in white-colored colonies. It is possible that its name had something to do with its toxicity—a single milliliter of one percent suspension of *Candida albicans* species in sterile salt solution injected into the veins of a rabbit will kill the animal within a week.

Candida is not a single organism. There are over 200 species of this yeast, and the best-known species, *Candida albicans,* has over 100 strains. Many members of *Candida* species have been used for commercial purposes. Specifically, strains 752, 20032 and 20308 are used to produce citric acid, and strains 20402 and 20408 are used to produce yeast biomass.

Although *Candida* species have received much attention among researchers and clinicians alike, little, if any, attention is paid to the role it plays in preserving the integrity of the bowel ecosystem in health.

Strain 10231 of *Candida* produces some substances that act as naturally produced antibiotics and guard the bowel ecosystem against virulent strains of many bacteria such as *Pseudomonas, Proteus* and disease-causing forms of *E. coli* bacteria. Specifically, phenethyl alcohol and tryptophol produced by this strain serve the bowel as autoantibiotics (*Science* 163:192-4; 1969).

Among the other benefits of *Candida* in the bowel is digestion of food substances in the large bowel that have not been broken down by the digestive enzymes in the small bowel.

Candida: THE GREAT WHITE GHOST

If *Candida* is such a villain, why did Nature put it in the human gut? This question arose in my mind during a recent trip from Dezhou to Jinan to catch a flight to Shanghai. In Dezhou, my co-researcher, Dr. Robert Bradford, and I gave a three-day seminar to a large group of Chinese physicians. The Chinese seemed fascinated by my concept of the open bowel ecosystem—largely because the bowel is regarded as the centerpiece of traditional Chinese medicine. During one of the breaks in the seminar, a Chinese physician asked, "Dr. Ali, you seem to think Nature has a reason for doing everything. Why do you think it put *Candida* in the bowel?" I told him it was an interesting question, but I had never really reflected on it.

During the van ride on our way to Shanghai later that afternoon, the question returned to me. Notwithstanding the limited chemical dividends of *Candida* listed above, Nature couldn't have given such prominence to this yeast in the bowel ecosystem just for those reasons. Or, at least that's the way it seemed to me. There are close to 50,000 yeast species on planet Earth. Why bestow a high status to *Candida?*

Nature has its own sense of economy—it abhors waste. Nature is discrete in its energy transactions. It is not given to undue or prolonged commitment of its resources in preserving the injured. Rather, it favors new beginnings. When confronted with a choice between the badly damaged and dying or the young and unborn, it chooses young and unborn. With a fraction of the energy required to rebuild the badly damaged or dying, it can bring forth large groups of the yet unborn of that species. Why not simply let the badly damaged and dying perish?

So far, but no farther.

During the van ride I saw *Candida* as a great white ghost. I saw this yeast as a white monster that Nature unleashes when it wants to warn physicians who are infatuated with broad-spectrum antibiotics and other toxic drugs. *Candida* is Nature's ultimatum to chemotherapists and radiotherapists: So far, but no farther. If you persist in your destructive pursuits—Nature proclaims with its *Candida* hand—I'll dispense with the whole being and unleash the yeast to expeditiously carry out the mopping up operation. I'll disintegrate the person's immune defenses and so expedite the end of life so I may redirect my energy toward bringing forth new babies.

A harsh, harsh reminder of Nature's economy! Perhaps too cruel a way of revealing Nature's master plan! But is it too far-fetched? I don't believe so. I have cared for patients—too numerous to count—who were told their yeast problem was too far gone. That's sheer nonsense. *Candida* overgrowth and infections can be successfully managed with holistic, integrated therapies in most patients, albeit after many months in some cases. The only exceptions are patients with advanced cancer given massive doses of chemotherapy, patients with advanced stages of AIDS treated with toxic antiviral drugs and other patients in similar clinical states.

THE IRON CURTAIN OF DOUBLE-BLIND CROSS-OVER JUSTICE

Early on the cold morning of February 4, 1994, I flew up to Montreal to testify before the disciplinary committee of the Corporation des Medecins & Chirurgiens du Quebec in the case of Drs. Drouin and Comeau. They met me in their attorney's office and were very eager to review several details of the case. I listened to them politely but knew that this case was not about details of medical care provided to some patients. It was a turf battle. The drug doctors of disease medicine spoil for a kill when they have cornered some holistic doctors. The details in the patient chart are ammunition—bullets with which to blast the holistic physicians away. I was preoccupied with how best to deal with the ignorance of drug doctors regarding nondrug therapies.

How was I going to argue the case of Drs. Drouin and Comeau before the panel of investigators? How would I break through the iron curtain of the double-blind cross-over? The tyranny of drug medicine? The logic of drug doctors? The banner of science under which drug doctors wage war against holistic physicians? The only chance I had was with the lay people on the panels. How was I going to talk about my insight from Mount Washburn? How was I going to explain the global threat of incremental oxidative injury? The pollutants in the air, the contaminants in the water, the pesticides and insecticides in the food! Antibiotics are designer killer molecules—we design them to kill life. Would the committee have the patience to listen to me describe how each course of antibiotics batters the delicate bowel ecosystem of the baby? How was I going to make a case for recognition and management of the state of absence of disease when people are not well despite negative CAT scans and blood tests? How would I expound upon the principles and practices of empirical medicine—of my energetic-molecular medicine? How would I convince them that they should award Drs. Drouin and Comeau trophies for resisting the false promise of a drug cure for immune and degenerative disorders? How would I defend the use of nutrients as agents of healing before doctors who only know drugs?

It was clear to me that the defense attorney wanted me to succeed, notwithstanding any difficulties he might have had with my rather radical views on health and healing. He briefed me about some aspects of giving expert testimony. "I'm going to give you a lot of latitude," he spoke reassuringly. "You can take time to explain your ideas of oxidation, bowel ecology and the *Candida* story."

At the hearing, the president of the committee, an attorney, sat in the middle, and was flanked by two other physician members. I didn't know anything about their background. In the past that didn't seem to make any difference—I didn't think it would this time either.

Drs. Drouin and Comeau were also charged for practicing oxidology—a medical discipline that focuses on oxidative injury to cells as observed with a microscope.

FREE RADICAL INJURY IS A LOCAL TISSUE PHENOMENON AND CANNOT BE OBSERVED IN BLOOD SMEARS

I quote below from one of Dr. Drouin's letter:

First of all, Dr. XYZ (one of the Corporation's expert witnesses testifying against Drs. Drouin and Comeau and medical research director of one of the major drug companies) wished to impress the court by presenting a lecture on free radical activity, demonstrating the sheer impossibility of detecting such activity from one simple drop of blood. Dr. XYZ wished to demonstrate that the free radical phenomenon is rather a local activity that is part of the defense or compensatory mechanisms of an individual, and that this local reaction cannot be proven on the level of a whole individual and can certainly not be measured by the observation of a single drop of blood of any such individual.

Ignaz Philipp Semmelweis (1818-1865), a Hungarian

physician who practiced in Vienna, proved that fatal childbirth fever is septicemia, thus becoming the pioneer of antisepsis in obstetrics. The mainstream physicians of his day were outraged by his idea and viciously persecuted him. He died insane. I read the above lines in Dr. Drouin's letter and understood how persecution by peers could drive a physician insane. I also understood how the great medical experts of the Academy of Science in Paris could have sworn Pasteur was an imposter, a delusional chemist blaming human diseases on microbes. Or more recently, how the editors of *The New England Journal of Medicine* could have decreed that Linus Pauling, another chemist, was all wet about the efficacy of vitamin C for preventing the common cold. Drs. Drouin and Comeau are in good company—and so, I'm afraid, is Dr. XYZ.

I decided to begin with the first contentious issue of the role of oxidation and free radicals in health and disease. The Corporation's expert witness had categorically stated that free radicals were a *local* tissue phenomenon, and couldn't possibly have caused the cell damage Drs. Drouin and Comeau claimed to have seen with their Bradford microscope.

I briefly described my understanding of the molecular Dr. Jekyll and Mr. Hyde role of oxygen in nature. Oxygen, I told them, ushers life in. It also terminates life. Oxygen is the spark that revs up all engines in living beings. It can also cause instantaneous combustion of all life-forms unless it is held in abeyance by cellular carburetors. Oxidation is a spontaneous phenomenon—it requires no outside cues. Nor does it require any expenditure of energy. Reduction—the chemical counterpart of oxidation in Nature—requires energy expenditure.

Did you ever wonder how much energy a matchstick contains? I asked the panel members. And yet, a single carelessly thrown lighted matchstick in a park can ignite fires that consume hundreds of thousands of acres. How does a *local* phenomenon, such as a lighted matchstick, trigger the *general* fires in a park? The park burns, and continues to burn, not because the energy in the tiny phosphorus head of the match stick is sufficient, but because it *initiates* a process of burning. Free radicals in injured tissues work the same—tiny matchstick heads that can blow up the whole body.

I wanted to ask the panel if they thought the drug doctors who testified before them prior to my testimony had ever reflected on such things. I decided not to. Those experts arrogantly, and ignorantly, had testified that oxidation is a local tissue phenomenon and couldn't be seen in a smear of circulating blood, thus convincing the panel that Drs. Drouin and Comeau had been utterly wrong.

Oxygen, I wanted to explain to the panel, is a molecular Dr. Jekyll and Mr. Hyde. Oxygen is the initial spark of life. Oxygen is also the life terminator. Oxygen is a molecular Dr. Jekyll at every level—at the electron transfer level, at a molecular level, at a cellular level, at a tissue level, at an organ level, and at the level of the whole human organism. Where, on God's green earth, did Dr. XYZ (one of Drouin's accusers) get the idea that oxidation was only a local phenomenon? How can anyone who has ever reflected on the redox reaction—the fundamental reaction of life on planet earth—ever conclude that oxidation is a local reaction? Every week, my copies of *Nature* and *Science* carry reports about biology and medicine that, in one way or another, validate this basic concept of oxidation as the essential reaction in life.

I could only conclude that Dr. XYZ, like his colleagues in

drug medicine, had never conducted any research experiments about the role of oxidation in nature, nor had he ever reflected on the observations made by others in this area. Poor Drs. Drouin and Comeau! They were hapless against the experts of drug medicine who clearly had no understanding of oxidative stress in nature.

THE SURGEON-ACCUSER

I thought about the surgeon-accuser of Drs. Drouin and Comeau. A surgical mind—I write earlier—looks at problems differently. I know that because once I was a surgeon myself. Surgical imperatives call for a sharp focus on only two issues: what to cut out and how to restore what is left behind. I remember those were the only two essential questions that concerned me when I performed surgery. How is the surgeon-accuser going to take my concerns about the larger issues of the environmental impact on human biology—the matters of increasing oxidative stress and diminishing antioxidant defenses? Would he buy into our concepts of host defenses—the ideas of total burden of biologic stressors on human healing responses that determines whether we remain healthy or get sick? In an hour or so of the time allotted to me, would I be able to explain to the retired surgeon what it took me 35 years of diligent study to learn? If he never tried to examine those issues before he retired, how was he going to do so now? What chance did Drs. Drouin and Comeau have with him?

Briefly, slowly, and in as measured a way as I could, I began to present the scientific knowledge that formed the basis of the diagnostic and therapeutic approaches of Drs. Drouin and Comeau. The nonphysician president of the disciplinary panel listened to me intently. The two physician members of the committee sitting on two sides thumbed through copies of my curriculum vitae and infrequently raised their heads to look at me impassively—giving me a sense that a polite silence was all that they were willing to accord to my views in defense of Drs. Drouin and Comeau.

(Mr. Pierre D'Esormeau, an attorney who was present there later said, "Dr. Ali, there were tears in my eyes when you talked about how we are systematically destroying our ecosystems, and how we are hurting our children and those who are not yet born." My editor asked me to delete Mr. D'Esormeau's comment because 'it sounds too much like bragging'. I don't delete this quote to show how passionately people feel about chemical injury to children and to unborn babies—the subject that drug medicine arrogantly dismisses as a phantom issue because such injury has not yet been proven by controlled studies.)

After my testimony I learned that the committee was expected to render its decision after several months. Would they remember any of what I'd said then? I wondered. "You did well, but I'm afraid they will still lose their licenses," D'Esormeau told me later at lunch.

THE NIH SYNDROME

When I first came to the United States in the mid 1960s, I was amused by what I thought was a peculiar American phenomenon: Medical researchers in America readily reject whatever they think was not discovered right here in America.

Sometime later, I learned that there is a name for it: the NIH (not invented here) syndrome. Now I know that Canadians do not like to be left behind. I quote again from Dr. Drouin's letter:

"Another point that comes forth continually in this debate is the fact that no university organism and no private laboratory (apart from ours) uses this screening method of blood analysis. "

The surgeon-accuser appointed by the court appeared to have been highly irritated by the fact that Drs. Drouin and Comeau had the audacity to use a technology that his hematology experts from the local university knew nothing about. The idea of two holistic physicians using a high-resolution, phase-contrast microscope with capability for dark-field examination irked him. His university hematology experts were also chagrined that some nonhematologist could know more about blood than they. They took pains to point out to the committee that a magnification power of 400—presumably the highest that they had access to—was all that was necessary, and that Drs. Drouin and Comeau couldn't possibly see anything more with their 12,000-magnification microscope.

How could a man who had never worked with a highly advanced technology as the Bradford microscope make an absurd statement like that? I wondered. How can anyone act that irrationally?

HEMATOLOGICAL OUTLAWS

Dr. Drouin wrote in another brief he sent me:

"Because we call it the Bradford test and the scientific literature does not...this makes us medical and hematological outlaws worthy of having our licenses revoked!"

This frivolous argument—that scientific literature does not contain the therapies of holistic physicians—is often thrown at us regularly by the disease doctors of drug medicine. Little do people know how readily the editors of drug journals reject articles concerning nondrug therapies.

There are two medical literatures: one that publishes drug studies and the other that publishes clinical outcome studies of nondrug therapies. The drug doctors, in general, are totally ignorant about the literature of nutritional medicine, environmental medicine and the medicine of self-regulation. The drug doctors' argument is based on the assumption that what is unknown to them cannot be true—and, hence, of any value to anyone else. If the principles and practice of holistic medicine had any validity, the argument holds, why wouldn't the professors in medical schools adopt them? It never occurs to them that the professors in medical schools do not know nondrug therapies because they never tried to learn them. *Long live the NIH syndrome!*

OUR CELLS BELONG AS MUCH TO US AS THEY DO TO MICROBES THAT VISIT OUR BODIES

Next in my testimony, I addressed the contentious subject of the presence of *Candida* yeast organisms in blood smears.

The HIV virus, I told the panel, has taught us an essential lesson in human biology: When the virus invades a human cell, its RNA mates with the DNA of the host cell—the DNA of its daughter cells is as much the progeny of the virus as that of the parent cell. We cannot destroy the viral DNA without destroying our own. Virologists have known this for several decades.

It amazes me how slow the general physician community has been to recognize an obvious corollary: When a microbe invades a cell, its molecules also mate with the molecules of the host cell. A part of the host cell changes forever. We can stem the growth of the microbe sometimes with antibiotics—sometimes even kill them—but what can we do with those mated (and permutated) molecules? They become alien molecules in the immune system, which now struggles to subdue the foreigners. And often it fails. This is the beginning of autoimmune injury. This is how all these hundreds of autoimmune disorders begin that we treat by suppressing the immune system with steroids and other immune suppressants.

There are no drugs—and there will never be—that only

destroy life around us without destroying parts of us. I wondered if the Canadian surgeon-accuser and the two other physicians on the disciplinary committee, who so relentlessly prosecuted Drs. Drouin and Comeau, had ever reflected on such matters.

IMMUNOSTAINING OF *Candida* IN BLOOD

On January 20, 1994, my research colleagues, Drs. Robert Bradford and Madhava Ramanarayanan (Ram), and I met early in the morning to finalize our experiment that sought to find if *Candida* organisms in circulating blood could be definitively identified. We reviewed in detail the composition of the reagents for immunostaining and the procedural steps that we were going to employ in our first attempts. Dr. Ram retains a very large library of sera, collected and catalogued over a period of many years. The specificity of the detecting antibody that we planned to use had been defined with meticulous absorption experiments several years earlier. We decided to use smears prepared with fresh blood obtained from three patients with chronic immune disorders and three volunteers from among the staff at the Institute of Preventive Medicine, Denville, New Jersey. The experiment design was to recognize the *Candida* organisms, or parts of such organisms, using a serum containing high titers of anti-*Candida* antibody. The steps of the immunostaining methods are summarized below:

1. Preparation of fresh smears with a single drop of blood
2. Addition of two drops of human serum with high levels of anti-*Candida* IgG antibodies
3. Washing step

4. Addition of two drops of a reagent containing rabbit anti-human IgG antibodies linked with horseradish peroxidase enzyme
5. Washing step
6. Addition of two drops of DAB solution (a color developer)
7. Examination of smears with a 18,000 magnification Bradford microscope with accessories for phase-contrast and dark-field microscopy

It took us about 17 hours to complete the first set of experiments. At about 1:00 AM, Bob Bradford and I began to look at the stained blood smears with a Bradford dark-field and phase-contrast microscope. We expected to see the positively stained *Candida* organisms as dark brown to black bodies, about one-half the size of red blood cells. There were no such bodies to be seen in all the smears we examined. We were not particularly disappointed. We were used to numerous failures before finally succeeding in our previous experiments. At 1:52 AM, about 18 hours after we started our experiment, I looked at my watch and realized that not many hours were left before I had to return to the Institute the same morning to conduct a chronic fatigue workshop. Taking out the commuting time, that left me about four hours of sleep time. I told Bob that we had to stop. The experiment was a failure. There were no positively staining organisms on the smear. We would have to stop and start all over again.

On the drive back, Bob suddenly sat up in his seat, shook his head with dismay and exclaimed, "Majid, I don't think I added the DAB!" The DAB solution, as I indicate above, was the "ink" in the experiment, a color developer. Without color developer, of course, there couldn't have been any staining. "How could I have forgotten that?" Bob said, still shaking his head. I found the whole event amusing. This is how real science works. This is how science is.

I knew that peroxidase enzyme once incorporated in the *Candida* complex remains viable and functional for about 24 hours. Next morning, I confirmed that with Ram. We still had time. We returned to the office earlier than we had originally planned. Bob wanted to attend my conference, but that was clearly out of the question because Bob had to finish the staining step. At the mid-morning break in the workshop, I rushed to the microscopy room. Bob looked at me and said, "I think we have something!" I took a quick peek through the lens and had no doubt that our first experiment had proved, with unassailable immunologic proof, that *Candida* organisms can indeed be detected in the circulating blood of people who are not acutely sick. "Ram, your chemistry is great!" I exclaimed.

Then I thought what this experiment's outcome meant to the Drouin-Comeau case and to thousands of holistic physicians all over the world. I wondered how the doctors who had a hand in revoking the licenses of their holistic counterparts on this very issue would react. Then the words of Marx Planck came to me:

A new scientific truth does not triumph by convincing its opponents and making them see the light, but, rather, because its opponents die and a new generation grows up that is familiar with it.

Holistic physicians were not going to have an easier time just because we had successfully identified the *Candida* organisms with a highly sensitive and specific immunostaining method.

We presented our observations at the Spring 1995 Meeting of the American Academy of Otolaryngic Allergy at Palm Desert. Below I reproduce the first (to our knowledge) photomicrographs of immunostained *Candida* organisms in the blood—identified with arrows as two dark bodies in the upper picture, while the organisms disappear in the lower dark-field picture (sugar in the yeast wall does not reflect light). The two bright bodies in the two pictures are red blood cells that do not take the immunostain. See color plates after page 210.

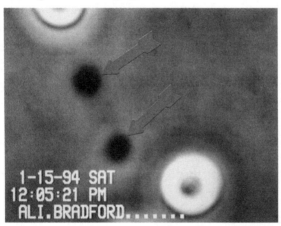

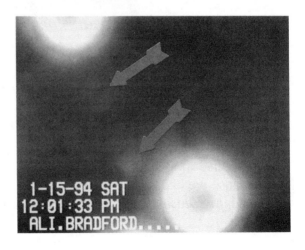

NAKED BACTERIA, NAKED YEAST

Why do holistic physicians see *Candida* in blood smears of their patients with their dark-field microscopes so frequently while microbiologists fail to grow the yeast on their culture plates in their laboratories? The answer to this riddle, which has preoccupied me for so long, may lie in the story of naked bacteria and naked yeast.

It has been known for many years that when the bacterial wall is injured by antibiotics or is damaged under certain conditions, bacteria survive but cannot grow as they do under optimal conditions. The cell wall-damaged bacteria are called L-forms—other terms used for such microbial variants include cell wall-deficient (CWD) bacteria, transitional forms, or simply naked bacteria. Several such bacterial forms are known to be highly toxic, presumably because they lack the cell wall that contains the poisons within the cells. Naked bacteria are naked killers.

Fusion of wall-deprived microbes among themselves and with similarly damaged microbes belonging to other species occurs readily. Naked bacteria, like naked people, are more prone to experiments in DNA sharing. Such fusions create triton forms with new and unique characteristics—the partial or complete lack of a rigid bacterial wall results in endless variations in size, shape and growth patterns. The variant growth patterns have been called spheroplast, protoplast and L-phase. They usually do not conform to the established patterns of growth by which bacteria are recognized and classified in microbiology laboratories.

As a young surgeon, I was often surprised by a negative bacterial culture report from the laboratory for a sample of pus I had obtained from the abdominal cavity of a patient with peritonitis. I had wondered if the culture had failed to grow any bacteria because I had administered heavy doses of antibiotics to the patient before surgery. At that time, I was not interested in experiments in biology that I conducted inadvertently by hitting microbes with massive doses of antibiotics. I had little, if any, understanding of how injured but not dead bacteria may not grow in culture plates and yet be very dangerous to my patients. In Pakistan, and later in England, I never understood why some people died after surgery who shouldn't have. Now I have no difficulty speculating about the role naked—but live and rabidly destructive—microbes might have played in those deaths.

Naked bacteria are crucially important in many cases of meningitis, pneumonia, heart valve infections, difficult-to-eradicate urinary infections, septicemia and many other life-threatening infections. In many such cases, the only microbial forms isolated are the naked bacteria. There are yet other unrecognized roles played by naked bacteria in all aspects of life.

Pseudomonas aeruginosa is a bacterial species that requires a rich organic medium in the laboratory for its growth. What is not commonly known that in its cell wall-deficient form, it can grow in distilled water, utilizing carbon dioxide from the air and the few molecules that diffuse from glass (Susan, S., Thesis, Wayne State University, Detroit, 1972). It is also known that water, "sterile" by routine tests, may contain wall-deficient forms of this bacterial species, and that this microbe may attain the critical number necessary for reversion to the classical pathogenic form (Mattman, L., *Cell Wall Deficient Forms,* CRC Press, Boca Raton, Florida, 1992).

I believe the discrepancy between the views of holistic physicians and drug doctors about the presence or absence of *Candida* in circulating blood arises from failure to understand the phenomenon of "naked yeast". The yeast cell walls, like the bacterial cell walls—are also damaged under certain conditions, and naked yeast (or otherwise damaged yeast organisms) may be expected to behave in as many unpredictable ways as do naked bacteria.

Strong support for my viewpoint is provided by the fact that in one study a *Candida* enzyme called enolase was dectected in forty-two percent of patients who had proven invasive tissue candidiasis and who showed negative blood cultures for yeast (*N Eng J Med* 324:1026; 1991). I have a strong sense that future research will provide additional evidence for my hypothesis. I know of no valid reason why cell wall-damaged yeast cannot behave the way naked bacteria do.

What is clear—since Drs. Bradford and Ram and I unequivocally identified *Candida* organisms in circulating blood of chronically ill outpatients—is that this yeast finds its way into the bloodstream with impunity. And that the burden of proof that what Drs. Drouin and Comeau saw with their dark-field microscopes were not yeast organisms rests on the disciplinary panel. Mere failure to grow damaged, naked yeast on the culture plate is not a valid argument that such yeast forms cannot be seen with a suitable microscope.

Dr. Drouin wrote in his second letter to me:

Dr. ABC (a professor in microbiology testifying against Drs. Drouin and Comeau) says this is not so... To him the veritable **Candida** *syndrome is extremely rare and he is profoundly astonished that we can observe* **Candida** *so frequently in live blood analysis.*

Candida gets around. If it didn't, how would it colonize the heart, liver and other body organs in AIDS patients and in those severely damaged by chemotherapy? Don't we culture *Candida* in the blood routinely in hospitalized patients? If *Candida* can get into the bloodstream of hospitalized patients, why can't it do so in nonhospitalized patients whose immune systems have been severely damaged with excessive antibiotics, environmental injury and unremitting stress? When I read about Dr. ABC's opinion I was amazed at the extent to which drug doctors will go to discredit holistic physicians. Doesn't Dr. ABC know that the CDC has predicted that *Candida* will be the most frequently cultured organisms from blood samples *in the United States by the year 2000?*

Dr. Drouin's letter continued:

It is brushed aside as being squarely against all present scientific knowledge and experimentation ... concerning the possibility of the presence of **Candida** *as being a frequent condition in asymptomatic individuals and a frequent result in the Bradford analysis. Dr. ABC is in complete disaccord with such a possibility...with Giemsa (a type of stain used in hematology laboratories) one can see* **Candida** *in live blood without phase contrast...*

What could be unscientific about the presence of *Candida* organisms in blood smears? How can anyone take such an indefensible position? I wondered if I was missing something. I read the letter a second time and then a third time. *In asymptomatic individuals*! Perhaps that was the catch. But, then, Drs. Drouin and Comeau were not treating asymptomatic individuals, were they? They were caring for chronically ill patients whose immune and antioxidant defenses had been shattered by drug medicine during the years before they became disillusioned with multiple drug therapies and sought out holistic physicians for nondrug therapies.

Then Dr. ABC reverses himself. He agrees that *Candida* organisms can be seen in live blood. So why such anger about the work of two holistic practitioners! Now the question of rarity of the *candida* syndrome. There is a truism in pathology: The less you recognize a particular lesion, the more rare it becomes. The *candida* syndrome—in the sense that it represents yeast overgrowth within a battered bowel ecosystem—is a very common clinical condition. I have stated on several previous occasions, however, that candidiasis must not be considered as the primary lesion in anyone.

One only sees what one looks for,
one only looks for what one knows.

Goethe

BLOOD: AN OPEN ECOSYSTEM

Blood fascinates me.

Blood is an ecosystem—as diverse, dynamic and delicate as any other on planet earth. Blood is not simply a running stream of commerce—a conveyer belt to carry molecules to and fro—as I had imagined it in my high-school science class. It is a living, sensing, responding system, in delicate equilibrium with bowel ecology and other cellular ecosystems in the body. It is a hospitable ecosystem. It invites, recognizes and sustains some living beings—some others it rejects and expels. It has its own intelligence system and its own surveillance monitors.

A mere presence of an alien microbe in the blood is just that—a visitor in transit. This is a biologist's view.

Candida, a single-celled yeast species, also fascinates me. It is a vagrant, forever insinuating itself among the sentinel cells lining the bowel, forever wanting to float in the bloodstream. And succeed it does.

I began this section on blood ecology by writing that the idea that the blood was an open ecosystem came to me as a flash. Now, I close this chapter by returning to that subject.

In setting up the experiments for immunostaining of *Candida* organisms in a blood smear, I included blood smears from four of our staff as controls for the experiments. After the initial excitement of a successful experiment died, we began to study the blood samples volunteered by some of my staff at the Institute. To our great surprise, we saw positively stained *Candida* organisms in all of them with one important difference: While the blood smears of some of our patients with persistent, disabling fatigue showed *Candida* organisms in most microscopic fields, we had to search for those organisms in several fields in the blood of control subjects. *The conclusion was obvious:* Candida is present in the circulating blood of many people; however, it occurs in a significant number of patients with weakened immunity.

Evidently, *Candida* does not always cause the mischief that we think it does. If it were the demon we physicians believe it to be, why would Nature provide it with such a luxuriant abode in the human gut? It thrives on sugar. (Little do we realize that when we crave sugar, we feed *Candida* before we attend to the sugar needs of other cells.) In health, it is a playful microbe, always on the look, always smarting for trouble. The problems begin when its ecologic relationships in the open bowel and blood ecosystems are disrupted.

This is what drug medicine does not understand. This is what the accusers of Drs. Drouin and Comeau do not understand. I have seen patients die of toxicity of amphotericin B, a drug used in drug medicine for yeast infections. I do not know of any drug doctor who lost his license for such a death. This is the true nature of the conflict.

At the time of this writing, the fates of Paul Drouin, M.D. and Louise Comeau M.D. hang in balance. The Corporation des Medecins & Chirurgiens du Quebec—the medical licensing of the province of Quebec—has not made its decision.

A MEDICINE OF ECORELATIONSHIPS

As our concepts of biologic ecorelationships change, so will our notions of caring for the sick. I believe such changes are inevitable. The dogma of drug medicine has serious flaws when it addresses ecologic illness. Most immune and chronic infectious diseases essentially begin as ecologic disorders—immune injury is the consequence rather the cause. Degenerative disorders also begin as ecologic aberrations, albeit with dominance of some chemical ecorelationships in some instances.

The bowel ecosystem interfaces with the world outside and with the blood and lymph ecosystems within the body. The blood ecosystem interfaces with the various body organ ecosystems within which exist tissue and cellular ecosystems. All these are living, breathing and dynamic ecosystems. The idea of chronic diseases as discrete entities to be cured with drugs is obsolete. When we physicians cling to the 19th-century notions of diseases and drugs—in defiance of scientifically sound precepts of ecorelationships, our patients pay the price. The price often is exorbitant.

Chapter 9

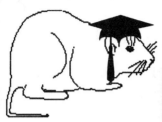

SIXTH INSIGHT

Science
has not failed
medicine
Medicine
has failed
science

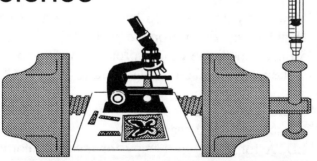

"What is the purpose of science in medicine?" Choua
asked me one day.

"To make medicine scientific," I replied.

"What does that mean?"

"To make therapies effective," I gave the standard answer.

"And?"

"To make therapies safe."

"And?"

"To make the results of therapies more predictable, less
random."

"What is the basic purpose of medicine?"

"To cure diseases."

"Cure diseases!" Choua frowned. "How often do you cure
degenerative, ecologic or immune disorders?"

"Well, we really do not cure those diseases," I retracted
my statement."

"What else?"

"To alleviate suffering."

"And?"

"To prevent diseases."

"And?"

"To promote health."

"How many drugs do you know that promote health?"

"None! Drugs don't promote health."

"So drug medicine cannot promote health no matter how
scientific they claim their drug studies are," Choua said
emphatically.

"There *are* some exceptions to that," I disputed him.

"Name one," he demanded.

"EDTA for chelation therapy for reversing coronary heart
disease." It's not common for me to so clearly win an argument
with Choua, but I knew Choua had no answer for that.

"What is a physician's calling?" Choua changed the

subject.

"Pray, tell me what is a physician's calling?" I replied sarcastically. "I have often wondered about that question myself."

"What are the major chronic problems you face today?"

"Cancer, heart disease and other degenerative disorders. But I thought you were going to tell me what a physician's calling is," I returned to his earlier question.

"How are those disorders caused? I mean, what is their root?" Choua again dodged my question.

"Well, you know my viewpoint on that. All diseases are caused by accelerated molecular oxidative stress."

"What causes oxidative molecular damage to become accelerated?"

"Factors related to nutrition, environment, stress and lack of physical fitness."

"What is a physician's calling?" Choua asked, and then began to answer his own question. "A physician's calling is to relieve suffering, reverse disease and promote health, right?"

"Right!" I agreed.

"If disease is caused by accelerated oxidative injury, and if such damage is caused by factors related to nutrition, environment and stress, then it follows that a physician's calling must be to address issues of nutrition, environment, stress and fitness. Right?"

"Right!" I agreed.

"How many pediatricians practice nutritional medicine?"

"I don't know, but there must be some."

"How many internists practice environmental medicine?"

"There are several in the Academy of Environmental Medicine."

"That doesn't count," Choua countered.

"Why?" I challenged.

"Everyone knows those are quacks. How many family

practitioners teach self-regulation to their patients?"

"I don't know any," I admitted. "But, Choua, you don't understand."

"Understand what?" Choua scowled.

"That's not what is done in doctors' offices. Doctors are not set up to do those things," I asserted.

"So, what are doctors set up to do? Push pills?" Choua wrenched one hand contemptuously.

"Oh, shut up, Choua. Do your doctor-bashing someplace else," I lost my temper and scolded him bitterly. "What bottomless pit do you draw your venom against us from?"

"I...I..." Choua stammered at my sudden outburst.

"You...You what?" I interrupted him, trying to control the surge of anger rising within me. "Physicians are hard-working people. They train for many years and sacrifice much during their studies. They care deeply for their patients and put in long hours—working late into the night and on Saturdays and Sundays. They know there is not much room for error in their work. When people are sick and in pain, they require immediate attention. What's routine work for them is a crisis for their patients. You walk around the hospital a lot. Don't you ever see the dying being pulled out of the jaws of death? Don't you ever see patients coming in with heart attacks, blue and gasping for breath? Don't you ever see people brought in with smashed faces and torn bellies and limbs hanging on their sides with shreds of tissues? Don't you see how untiringly and desperately physicians work to support those failing hearts, repair those gaping wounds? Don't you see how tenderly and compassionately nurses care for them? Don't you see how grateful and happy their faces are when they leave the hospital days and weeks—and sometimes months—later? Doesn't any of that mean anything to you? You brim with hate. Your pail of venom has no bottom."

Choua stood frozen. I realized my hands trembled with anger. Choua stared at me impassively. I stared back at him. It is not common for me to be carried away by the passion of the argument that way. We were quiet for several moments. Then Choua slowly stepped away from my desk, moved closer to the window and escaped into his favorite place—the distant horizon. Choua is a strange blend. His attacks on my profession are often vitriolic and unrelenting. I usually take them in good stride. On rare occasions when I erupt, he undergoes a sudden metamorphosis—and sheepishly crawls back to his own space, leaving me to cool off on my own. As calm returned to me, I wondered how he was going to retreat. I suppressed a smile. I wasn't going to let Choua off the hook that easily.

"How does the science of drug medicine address the problems of nutrition, environment, stress and fitness?" Choua asked as he moved back from the window and lingered.

"You alone can do *that*, Choua," I shook my head and couldn't hold back my laughter anymore. "I don't know anyone who can change subjects like that."

"How does your Star Wars technology help people who cannot sleep due to heart palpitations caused by stress? What does Star Wars medicine do for young women disabled by PMS?"

"You are a master!" I said sarcastically. "Did you hear anything I said?"

"What do you doctors do for men who walk around with bloated bellies and confused minds?" Choua continued in a shrill tone. "And for children who live with sugar roller coasters and daily face the indignity of a hyperactivity label or the brilliant diagnosis of attention deficit disorder?"

"It's impossible!" I nearly shrieked at him. "It's impossible to have an intelligent conversation with you."

"Diseases are not sudden departures from health," Choua taunted me with my own words. "Diseases begin with accelerated oxidative damage. Drugs and scalpels cannot undamage the cells and tissues damaged by oxidized, denatured foods, pollutants, Fourth-of-July chemistry and relentless muscle spasms in the neck, shoulders and back, can they?"

"No," I conceded.

"How well does drug medicine care for people troubled by such problems?" Choua pressed.

"Not well," I conceded.

"You doctors worship at the altar of the gods of the double-blind cross-over and dole out drugs that make your sick patients sicker. Do you ever reflect on the true purpose of a physician's work?" Choua abraded me.

"Drugs *do* work in acute illnesses!" I contested his position.

"Oh, so a physician's calling is limited to treatment of acute disease. I thought you doctors were committed to disease prevention and health promotion. How awkward of me!" Choua rubbed in.

"You can't blame us physicians for everything that is wrong with medicine, Choua," I objected. "Most people are not interested in disease prevention."

"How do you know?" Choua shot back.

"It's common knowledge," I insisted.

"What is common knowledge is that no internist's office is organized to provide proper nutritional guidance and support. No family practitioner makes the effort to look into environmental causes of illness. You fellows pay lip service to stress but never lift a finger to do anything about it."

"No, that's not true. Most clinical ecologists dig deeply into the nutritional aspect of chronic illness, and, of course, they all rigorously investigate the environmental factors that make their patients sick."

"Clinical ecologists are quacks. C'mon, everyone knows

that. Disease doctors of drug medicine pronounced that decades ago. Everyone knows ecologists' methods of diagnosis and treatment of environmental illness are unscientific. Even *Science* said that, didn't it?"

"That was most disappointing!" I replied, remembering the piece in *Science.*

"Who do you think wrote that piece? A drug doctor!" he answered his own question and then continued. "What do people with degenerative diseases need, drugs or nutrients?"

"Both!" I answered emphatically.

Choua shifted uneasily on his feet, stretched his back and walked over to the window—not unusual for him whenever he thinks he has not made his case decisively. I looked on with satisfaction.

"What questions do you ask your patients on follow-up visits?" he asked as he moved away from the window.

"You know all that! Why do you ask what you already know?" I replied angrily.

"Don't be angry," he replied in a conciliatory tone. "I want to make a simple but important point. I'll list those questions if you don't want to. You tell me if you disagree. Questions you ask patients concern stress, sleep, choices in the kitchen, bowel discomfort and transit time, patterns of energy, mold and environmental sensitivities, exercise and autoregulation. Right?" Choua coaxed.

"Right!" I agreed grudgingly.

"Now, let's consider how the Prince Chaullahs of N^2D^2 medicine—the practitioners of scientific drug medicine, as they proclaim themselves—approach the problems of stress, sleep, nutrition, environment and fitness. You do your work with your microscope and I'll fetch some journals," Choua didn't wait for my response and momentarily disappeared into the hallway.

A Mounting Concern:
Not Enough Americans Are Taking Drugs for Anxiety

"I am very concerned about Americans," Choua declared when he returned with a thick pile of journals.

"What troubles you now?" I asked.

"Not enough Americans are taking drugs."

"Uh! Back to drugs, are we?"

"I'm serious," Choua spoke solemnly. "I am terribly worried about Americans who live a drug-deprived existence."

"Drug-deprived existence," I repeated Choua's words.

"Yup! Drug-deprived existence. It's a pretty bad problem. And there is no visible solution. Even the great *New England Journal of Medicine* is helpless. It can only tell us how bad the problem is, but it has no answers."

"So, tell me how bad is it?" I asked, my curiosity kindled.

"The *Journal* thinks forty-four percent of adult Americans should be taking drugs for anxiety," Choua answered in a matter-of-fact way.

"That's absurd! Ludicrous! It simply can't be." I couldn't let Choua go unchallenged.

"Are you saying the great *Journal* erred?" Choua winked.

"No!" I screamed. "You are distorting things badly."

"Distorting? Me? I don't distort things. Before you jump to the conclusion that I succumb to cheap sensationalism," Choua added hurriedly, "I call the *Journal* to my defense:

Data on the use of psychotropic drugs do not support the popular perception of Americans as excessive and inappropriate users of anxiolytic medications. Only about one in four adults in the United States identified as having severe symptoms that might warrant anxiolytic therapy is actually receiving such therapy.

N Eng J Med 328:1399; 1993

Clearly the *Journal* is concerned about the fact that *only* one in four adults in the U.S. who should take drugs for anxiety is actually taking any drugs."

"Go on, Choua. What's the catch?"

"There is no catch here. The *Journal* obviously believes that free access to drugs is an inalienable right of all Americans. It champions the cause of the Valium- and Ativan-deprived individuals in the U.S—people who are regularly denied adequate daily rations of the drug of their choice. Health care, in an advanced, civilized country is a basic right of all citizens, isn't it?"

"Life is hard. Many people who suffer from anxiety states do need help. But, where did you get the forty-four percent number from?" I asked, ignoring all his sarcasm.

"The *New England Journal of Medicine,* of course. Where else? Now, everyone knows that the *Journal* cannot be wrong. It is by far the most prestigious medical journal in the United States. It holds itself to the highest standards of 'scientific vigor.' Where would American medicine be were it not for the unfailing devotion of the *Journal* to excellence in medical science?"

"Come to the point, Choua," I rebuked him mildly. "Where does the *Journal* say forty-four percent Americans should take drugs for anxiety? That's an absurd number."

"Here, listen to what the *Journal* writes a few sentences later:

The overall prevalence of the use of any anxiolytic drug during a one-year period among adults in the United States, regardless of the frequency or duration of use, is estimated to be 11 percent.

J N Eng J Med 328:1399; 1993

The *Journal* tells us that eleven percent took the drug and it tells us that only one in four who should take drugs actually takes them. Now, if my grade school math doesn't fail me, putting the two *Journal* quotes together gives us the number of forty-four percent. If you don't believe me, why don't you calculate the percentage yourself?"

"If you are quoting the *Journal* correctly, that's the percentage," I agreed. "But..."

"Hard to believe!" Choua interrupted. "Who would have guessed that two out of every five Americans live a Valium-deprived life? But then who among us has the courage to question the wisdom of the *Journal?* Then the *Journal* moves to rescue other drugs from the unsavory critics of drug medicine," Choua winked. "Here, I quote some more:

*Like many other classes of drugs that are
extensively prescribed, the benzodiazepines
have also been the focus of intermittent
criticism by the lay media, much of it
sensationalistic and without adequate
scientific basis.*

N Eng J Medicine 328:1399; 1993

Scientific basis! Clearly that is what the lay public doesn't understand to the chagrin of the *Journal*. Isn't it a shame?" Choua
asked scornfully.

"It does surprise me. I wouldn't have expected the *Journal*
to publish such articles."

"Americans have such irrational phobias against drugs?"
Choua spoke in a mock tone of sadness. "And they are not
paying any attention to the rigors of science of the great
Journal."

"Who wrote that article for the *Journal*?" I inquired. "Did
they write about nondrug approaches to anxiety and panic
attacks? About the role of self-regulation, meditation and spiritual
work? About the value of slow, sustained exercise?"

"Nah! The *Journal* won't write about such frivolous
notions. It likes *hard* scientific data. Take a guess who wrote that
article," Choua asked impishly.

"Some professors of medicine?"

"Nope! The authors are pharmacists—two men of the drug
constituency."

"You made your point, Choua," I conceded.

"*Science has not failed medicine,*" Choua suddenly

became somber and spoke softly. "*The medicine of the Prince Chaullahs of N^2D^2 medicine has failed science.*"

A Crying Shame:
So Many Americans Sleep Without Nose Machines

"I'm also very concerned about the quality of sleep of Americans," Choua resumed, putting the issue of the *Journal* down and picking another.

"From stress to sleep!" I remarked, amused.

"The *New England Journal of Medicine* also published a *scientific* study conclusively proving that too many Americans sleep without machines stuck up their noses."

"What? Sleeping with machines stuck up their noses?"

"Yes, the machines that whir like refrigerators and push air into the patient's nose."

"How many Americans need to sleep with such machines?" I asked.

"One out of every four American men," Choua replied matter-of-factly.

"And you happen to have a direct quote from the *Journal* that supports your contention, do you?" I asked, eyeing the issue of the *Journal* in his hand.

"The *Journal* advises us that *one of four* American males should sleep with a machine hooked up to his nose." Choua spoke with relish.

"Does it really say that? What nose machine?"

"The one that makes whirring noises like a bad refrigerator and keeps everyone wondering about the great advances of Star Wars medicine." Choua grinned.

"One of four American males. Is that what you said?" I expressed doubt.

"I didn't say that. The great *New England Journal of Medicine* said that," Choua shrugged. "I don't make things up about the *Journal*, do I?" Choua crowed haughtily. "Here, I'll read you a piece:

> *"The estimated prevalence of sleep-disordered breathing, defined as an apnea-hypopnea score of 5 or higher, was 9 percent for women and 24 percent for men...Undiagnosed sleep-disordered breathing is associated with daytime hypersomnolence.*

> *N Eng J Med* 328:1230; 1993

Now, do you see the *Journal's* science? Twenty-four percent—one of four American males—have sleep-disordered breathing."

"That really stretches the imagination."

"Do you know what people would have said if the *National Enquirer* had ever made such a statement?"

"What?"

"That the editors of *National Enquirer* had been bribed by the makers of the sleep machine to publish such ludicrous numbers."

"Surely, you don't think the editors of the *New England Journal of Medicine* would have done something like that?" I asked hesitantly.

"The *Journal* stooping to such low levels. Nah! It would never do such a thing," Choua swung his arm widely and winked naughtily.

"What else does the article say?"

"The scientists of the *Journal* studied a random sample of six-hundred and two persons and made an important discovery—that when people don't sleep well at night, they're sleepy the next day. Now isn't that a rare insight? But, let's not stop here. The *Journal* has some more stuff. Listen to this:

Evaluation by current standards includes full-night polysomnography, at a cost per procedure of approximately $1,100. Sleep-disordered breathing can usually be eliminated by the nightly use of a nasal device that delivers continuous positive pressure to the upper airway. Since patients must continue to receive this therapy throughout their lives, it is often viewed as a hardship.

N Eng J Med 328:1230; 1993

A nasal machine to wear for a lifetime! Interesting, isn't it?" Choua chortled.

"Sleeplessness is a growing problem, and is the subject of intense research these days," I said, without really wanting to make any statement.

"Oh yes! The medical researchers are at it, aren't they?"

"Do I sense some sarcasm?" I asked in jest.

"Sarcastic? Nah! Not me!" Choua replied calmly and leaned to shuffle through some journals. Having found one to his liking, he resumed, "Here is something else that *Science News* published:

Much controversy surrounds the definition of sleep disorders...Many sleep-disorder specialists criticize DSM for ignoring physical ailments linked to sleep problems, and some prefer an alternative classification system that lists nearly 70 sleep disorders.

How many sleep disorders did the folks in Kirto suffer from?" Choua asked.

NO SLEEP-DISORDER SPECIALISTS, NO SLEEP DISORDERS

Kirto is my ancestral village in Pakistan. I don't know what it's like there now, but back then during my boyhood, people slept soundly on the bare cots, on dirt under the trees, in the fields. Choua's words carried me back to those years. I remembered many things. I don't remember anyone complaining about sleep. No one ever said they woke up tired. No one was ever tired except after hard manual labor. I don't recall anyone taking sleeping pills. Darkness brought all the sleeping pills they ever needed, the light of the eastern sky all the pick-me-uppers. It was a different time. I wondered how things might be there now.

The villagers now have TV, and they probably stay up late watching American reruns. Do they have problems with their sleep now? I wondered.

"So, how many different sleep disorders do they have in Kirto now?" Choua's voice startled me.

"How do I know? I haven't been there in years," I answered wistfully.

"How many sleep-disorder specialists do you think Kirto has?" Choua didn't seem to notice my irritation.

"Kirto is a poor village, Choua. It can't afford any sleep-disorder specialists," I replied.

"Aha! No sleep-disorder specialists and no sleep disorders," Choua chuckled.

"Sleep-disorder specialists do not create sleep disorders, Choua," I protested vehemently. "They only diagnose and manage those disorders. Sleep problems are increasing because the stress of modern life is increasing and the standard American diet doesn't help. Too many coffee and sugar roller coasters."

"Sleep disorder specialists are quite inventive, aren't they? They've racked up seventy different sleep disorders now." Choua didn't acknowledge my comment.

"Sleep affects different people differently," I added lamely.

"It's not about sleep problems. It's about the money needs of sleep specialists and the people who build sleep centers," Choua countered sharply.

"Sleep physiology is complex," I ignored Choua's attack on sleep centers.

"How complex?" Choua blinked and frowned.

"I don't know how complex. Choua, you know I don't specialize in sleep disorders and..."

"Oh yes you do! You just don't know that you do. You ask every patient about the quality of his sleep and you hammer at this theme on every visit. You search for causes of poor sleep in every patient. You talk and write about it all the time. You just don't care for those loathsome machines," Choua interrupted me. "So tell me how complex it really is."

"Choua, you don't..."

"Don't understand," Choua rudely interrupted me. "One separate sleep disorder for each person! Is that it? Two hundred and sixty million sleep disorders for two hundred and sixty million Americans! Is that it?" Choua's eyes narrowed.

"Now that's absurd," I protested.

"Absurd! You think that's absurd? I don't. Watch how much your sleep specialists milk gullible Americans with their gadgets! Watch how they gouge innocent sufferers from poor sleep with creative diagnostic labels—all in the name of great science," Choua spoke venomously.

"It isn't the fault of sleep-disorder specialists that there are so many disorders in sleep medicine," I replied sternly.

"Sleep medicine? It's not sleep medicine. It's sleep business." Choua was unrelenting.

"Choua, your cyclopean eye sees things only one way," I said bitterly.

"Watch how far these merchants of sleep business carry their craft—how cleverly these money-men of medicine market their machines. Watch how they prevail on insurance companies to reimburse them for their machines, and how they manipulate the Prince Chaullahs of N^2D^2 medicine to prescribe the awful machines for their unsuspecting patients."

Choua's words brought back a conversation I had had with a patient some months earlier. When evaluating clinical outcome in follow-up visits, I always ask about sleeping patterns. One woman replied to the routine question with visible anger. I asked her if my question offended her. She quickly regained her composure and told me about a $1,300 bill she had paid for a test at a famous sleep-disorder clinic. "Can you imagine, Dr. Ali, I paid them thirteen-hundred dollars to rent a sleep machine for one night. Then, they had the gall to ask me to pay another thirteen-hundred dollars for another machine they wanted me to stick up my nose at night. I just ran out." I understood why my innocent question provoked such vehemence.

"We Americans are an ingenious people," Choua's words brought me back from my flashback.

"That we are," I agreed.

"Do you know where we really excel?" he asked.

"Hard to say where we are most ingenious," I replied tentatively. "Space? Quantum physics? Genetic engineering?"

"No, it is in medicine!"

"Medicine? Not space? Not quantum physics?" I asked, incredulous.

"Yes, it is in medicine that our ingenuity finds its most florid expression. We invent medical gadgets to make money. The problem is that medical gadgets don't sell unless we have some disease to cure with those gadgets. So we invent diseases to fit our mechanical inventions," Choua poured on his vitriol.

"Choua, I don't know why you are so wired about the *Journal* article. Medical technology is expensive in this country. Everyone knows that," I tried to calm him down.

"Why don't sleep experts try to find out why one-quarter of American men cannot sleep well? Why don't they try to find out what keeps people restless during their sleep hours? Why is sleep so often interrupted for most people? Why do people wake up tired and stale? Don't these sleep experts know that sleep is just a continuation of the waking hours? I mean when we sleep, we aren't dead! Didn't their moms and dads ever tell them about food reactions that interrupt sleep, bowel problems—what you call battered bowel ecology—problems of aches and pains in muscles that disturb deep sleep, and stress and anger that keep people awake? Why are your sleep experts so impervious to common sense?"

"I don't know why," I replied.

PEOPLE VISIT THEIR DOCTORS TO BE DRUGGED, DON'T THEY?

"Why don't sleep experts teach their patients things about stress, metabolic roller coasters and environmental triggers? Why don't they teach them how they can extinguish the oxidative flames of Fourth-of-July chemistry with self-regulation—with your limbic breathing and directed pulses? Teach them how to meditate and reflect on the order of things in nature? Something about your limbic language of silence? Something about spirituality!"

"Get serious, Choua! People don't go to their physicians for spirituality," I answered testily.

"Oh yes!" Choua recoiled with evident sarcasm. "I forgot why people see their doctors. People go to their doctors so they can be drugged."

"That's preposterous! What's wrong with you today anyway? I mean what set you off like that?" I controlled my growing frustration.

"Your sleep experts estimate that five to twenty percent of Americans suffer from bruxism—teeth grinding while sleeping," Choua resumed. "Now, if you add this number to the number of people with sleep-disordered breathing reported by the *Journal*, it comes to half the population of American males."

"Poor quality of sleep is a common problem, but I don't think percentages can be simply added that way," I commented.

"Of course when we add all the other sixty-eight remaining types of sleep disorders, it may turn out that very few Americans sleep well according to the criteria developed by sleep experts. You know every health problem doesn't require an electronic gizmo," Choua resumed. "Some *loathsome* device that is stuck up the gullible patient's nose! Does it make sense? Why don't the folks at the *Journal* show some common sense? I mean, don't they forever preach excellence in standards of care? How about some standards of common sense in medicine?"

Choua stopped, his gentle frame heaving with each breath. He peered hard into my eyes. There was no protest there. There was nothing there for me to refute. We were silent for a few moments. Then he spoke.

"This is the journal that champions the cause of the underprivileged, the rights of the poor who cannot afford health care. These self-appointed gods of N^2D^2 medicine! These gurus of Star Wars medicine! It is sick! And it is sickening. Do you know what the truth is?"

"Pray, tell me what the truth is. I have always wanted to know," I goaded him.

"The truth is this whole thing is about money. It's about the gadgets of Star Wars medicine that bring riches to those who make them and those who push them. It's about therapies that enrich the medical-industrial complex, which the *Journal* is so fond of ridiculing. It's about therapies that impoverish folks who are already impoverished by ill health. It's about Star Wars technology in search of diseases."

"You see conspiracy in everything, don't you?" I laughed.

"*Science has not failed medicine,*" Choua spoke solemnly, "*The Prince Chaullahs of N^2D^2 medicine have failed science.*"

A Self Deception:
Americans Worry Needlessly About Nutrition

"I'm concerned that far too many Americans ask frivolous questions about SAD," Choua spoke somberly.

"What is SAD?"

"The standard American diet."

"Oh, that! What troubles you there?"

"There is a growing cult of food fascists that think foods cause medical conditions. They are blaming common foods for various diseases."

"What is this cult of food fascism?"

"They are nutrition charlatans—ignorant people who know nothing about nutrition science. Still, they persist in their belief that foods can cause illness. Many of them also believe that foods and nutrients can reverse legitimate diseases. The frightening thing is that many of them now have the initials M.D. after their names. It's awful! These M.D.s who attempt to legitimize food fascism as a medical science."

"Whose case are you on now, Choua?" I asked.

"The quacks! If only those quacks would read the *New England Journal of Medicine*. Then they would understand how unfounded their claims are, and how badly they are misguiding the innocent folks who ask for their advice. Do you know that many of them actually advise their patients to change their eating habits and to stop taking drugs prescribed by good drug doctors. Awful! Isn't it?"

"Who are you railing against, the *Journal* or nutritionists?"

"I'm not railing against anyone. I am just exposing the follies and frauds of food fascists. The *Journal* has warned us against them so many times. Those quacks perform tests of dubious value, and diagnose food allergies. Then they eliminate several foods and create nutritional deficiencies. They concoct fancy rotation diets that compound the problems. Do you know they actually believe that colitis can be caused by food allergy and that food allergy can induce wheezing and lead to asthma. A little knowledge is a dangerous thing. And you cannot reason with them. If only they would heed the *New England Journal of Medicine*. Here, I'll read something:

Food Sensitivity or Self-Deception?

Self-deception affects doctors as well as patients, and through kindness and enthusiasm many of us may be doing a great disservice to ill patients anxiously seeking a nonpsychiatric diagnosis. If we apply the wrong label with conviction, and then treat the symptoms with suggestion and placebo, relief is likely to be only transient, and psychopathology will probably reemerge.

N Eng J Med 323:478; 1990

Treat the symptoms with suggestion and placebo! Do you see the problem now?" Choua lifted his eyebrows. "If only quacks would read the *Journal*. They would learn that what they consider food sensitivity is nothing more than deception. Then they would not fall into the trap of treating symptoms with suggestion and placebo."

"The *Journal* slipped that time. Food sensitivity is very common in patients with immune and ecologic disorders. It deserves your cynicism," I remarked.

"Those people for whom the quacks diagnose food sensitivity are really sick," Choua dug in. "They suffer from psychiatric disorders for which they need legitimate psychiatric diagnoses—not self-deception of food allergy, not suggestion or placebo. With proper psychiatric diagnoses, psychiatrists can put them on effective psychotropic drugs that will numb their minds and keep them from asking disturbing questions about food sensitivity."

"You are too much, Choua," I laughed.

"Not really! I'm serious. I'm only following the advice of the great *Journal.* "

"Why give drugs when you can relieve symptoms by avoiding incompatible foods?"

"Who cares what is fair? You see, psychiatric diagnoses offer freedom from the burden of thinking! Freedom from the need to search for the true cause of a patient's suffering. Above all, freedom from having to answer silly questions. One neat psychiatric diagnosis and one choice prescription clears up the problem—and the unsavory, difficult patient—like a magic wand. And that holds for the patient's lifetime. The more he fights the psychiatric diagnosis, the more certain the psychiatrist can be of the validity of his diagnosis."

"That's disgusting!" I cried out.

"Disgusting? Maybe! But does it work? Of course, it does.

Wake up, Dr. Gullible. Do you really think the *New England Journal of Medicine* can ever be wrong? Here, I'll read some more:

> *When the provocation of symptoms to identify food sensitivities is evaluated under double-blind conditions, this type of testing, as well as treatments based on "neutralizing" such reactions, appear to lack scientific validity. The frequency of positive responses to the injected extracts appears to be the result of suggestion and chance.*

> *N Eng J Med* 323:429; 1990

The result of suggestion and chance! The quacks are creating food sensitivity with their suggestions. Awful! Isn't it?"

"The *Journal* talks about chance. How does chance cause food allergy?" I asked, amazed at the *Journal*'s statement.

"The *Journal*'s wisdom escapes me sometimes," Choua pouted.

"Who wrote that paper?" I asked.

"Two orthopedic surgeons and a psychiatrist," Choua replied with a wink.

"*Wha...at!*" I nearly screamed. "Why would two orthopedic surgeons write a foolish thing like that?"

"It's not foolish," Choua contradicted me. "Why would the *Journal* take such a position unless it was sure of its

Science?"

"You're not serious, are you?" I expressed doubt.

"Read it yourself. The paper was from the Departments of Orthopedic Surgery and Psychiatry, School of Medicine, University of California."

"Amazing! Absolutely amazing!"

"I'm not surprised that the poor psychiatrist acted so flippantly, but what got into the orthopedists? Since when have the bone-setters become so interested in food sensitivity?"

"But, Choua, they must have some basis for making such a statement. They must have done some studies, they must have some data."

"Of course, they had data. Didn't they say they evaluated food sensitivities under double-blind controlled studies. That's the magic of the double-blind!" Choua grinned.

"So, the *Journal* published what the investigators found. Perhaps there were methodological errors," I ventured a guess.

"Everything is wrong with it, Dr. Gullible. Plumbers can do a better job evaluating the work of clinical ecologists than the maestros of N^2D^2 medicine," Choua groused.

"Don't be silly! I wouldn't go that far."

"There is nothing silly in that. If you were to ask some plumbers or masons to assess the adequacy of clinical ecology methods, they would begin by admitting that they don't have any knowledge of the subject. If required to proceed, they would keep their minds open and let the experts in the field guide them—as intelligent persons serving on a jury do. They would not jump helter-skelter at ecologists and do a brazen hatchet job on diagnostic methods that they don't know anything about. They would not besmirch a medical specialty the way the *Journal* did. Would they?" Choua looked at me askance.

"Probably not," I yielded. "The *Journal* seems to have goofed that time. I'm disappointed with the *Journal*."

"And, can you imagine a psychiatrist sitting in judgment of clinical ecology? Since when have the psychiatrists tried to understand the environmental causes of human suffering? Since when have they searched for answers in nutrition? As far as they are concerned, suffering of the mind descends from Mount Olympus. Their job is simply to classify the mental problems into neat psychiatric disorders, then find ways to drug their subjects out of their wits so they are no longer able to question the folly of their care-givers," Choua heaved as he finished.

"That's going too far, Choua," I cautioned.

"Is it?" Choua frowned. "Here, listen to this. This is John H. Boyles, Jr., M.D. Chairman, Practice Standards Committee of the American Academy of Otolaryngic Allergy, writing to the editor of the *Journal* in response to the article in the *New England Journal of Medicine*.

The list of inaccuracies and poor scientific protocol involved in this study is so long I hesitate to list them...We, in the world of environmental medicine, tried to explain to him that testing patients who are on special diets or receiving immunotherapy would not produce accurate results and that the test only works on patients whose diets or immune systems have not been tampered with.

Tried to explain! Experienced ecologists did try to save the *Journal* from its folly. Did they get anywhere?"

"Amazing! Did the *Journal* publish his letter?" I asked.

"Nah! It wasn't scientific enough for the *Journal*," Choua wailed.

"That's grossly unfair," I complained. "The *Journal* shouldn't smear other people's work without giving them a chance to defend themselves."

"I wonder if the *Journal* would print an article by clinical ecologists that declared useless an orthopedic procedure considered valuable by all orthopedic surgeons," Choua said harshly.

"No! I don't think it would accept such a paper," I replied.

"The orthopedic community would be up in arms, wouldn't it? And there would be many letters of protest."

"I think so."

"Science has not failed medicine..."

"I know! I know! The Prince Chaullahs of N^2D^2 medicine have failed science," I completed Choua's sentence.

An Appalling Ignorance:
Americans Have Irrational Fears of Chemicals

"I'm very concerned about clinical ecology crusades," Choua continued.

"What crusades?" I asked.

"Crusades against chemicals. There is a fertile social environment today for antichemical crusades—a result of a strong environmental movement in the country."

"Are you speaking for or against chemicals?" I asked, amused.

"I'm very perturbed by irrational fears of chemicals that your friends in clinical ecology foster among the lay public."

"You are?" I feigned surprise, then went along with the gag. "Since when?"

"Here, I'll read an excerpt:

That the field of clinical ecology may have developed disease and treatment concepts based on placebo responses is suggested by the increase in the number of placebo responses that are considered to be symptoms of disease.

N Eng J Med 323:429; 1990

Placebo responses! Tell me," Choua shrugged after he

read the excerpt, "why do clinical ecologists insist on basing their disease and treatment concepts on placebo responses?"

"First, you have to tell me what a placebo response is," I replied. "All I know is that clinical ecology is about searching for the cause of illness in the environment."

"How do you know pollutants can cause illness?" Choua asked.

"Because I see patients every day who react to environmental agents and who gradually begin to feel better when they reduce the total burden of adverse food reactions, chemical detergents and disinfectants at home, and whatever pollutants they can reduce in their work environments. I'm at a loss as to why the *Journal* took such an untenable position."

"Could it be that the *Journal* likes drugs and clinical ecologists teach their patients how to avoid drugs?" Choua asked mischievously. "Here, I want to read something else:

Clinical ecology lacks scientific validation, and the practice of "environmental medicine" cannot be considered harmless. Severe constraints are placed on patient's lives, and, in many cases, invalidism is reinforced as patients develop increasing iatrogenic disability. Treatment by clinical ecologists frequently creates severe financial burden for patients and imposes significant costs on health insurers and worker's compensation.

J All Clin Immun 85: 437; 1990

Iatrogenic disability-problem caused by doctors! Now, do you see the problem?"

"I read that article a long time ago. They are entitled to their opinions."

"It's not that simple. The *Journal* is terribly concerned that you are enforcing invalidism—increasing iatrogenic disability."

"That's absurd. The exact opposite is true. The clinical ecologists that I know are committed to returning their disabled patients to work—as soon as possible."

"The *Journal* holds that you make up things. Pollutants have not been proven to be bad for humans."

"Who says environmental pollutants do not cause disease?"

"Pro-pollution docs!" Choua sneered. "Here is some stuff:

Of at least 60,000 chemicals in use in the United States, no health research data exist on some 50,000 substances. And nothing is known about the synergistic mixes of these substances in the air, soil and water. In 1984, The National Research Council found toxicity health data nonexistent or incomplete on 81 percent of food additives, 84 percent of cosmetic ingredients, 66 percent of pesticides and herbicides, 64 percent of pharmaceutical drugs and 88 to 90 percent of commercial chemicals.

Minneapolis Star, July 8, 1990

"That's what the National Research Council says. Let's see what folks at Johns Hopkins say about chemical toxicity and sensitivity:

> ..., *head of the Johns Hopkins allergy clinic, said...the case of C.D. is "tragic," not only because of her self-imposed withdrawal from normal life, but most assuredly because of the complicity of so-called clinical ecologists who have given birth to and continually reinforce C.D.'s unrealistic and distorted belief system.*

Minneapolis Star, July 22, 1990

"*Belief system!*" Choua winked. "Pay heed to what Johns Hopkins says."

"Belief system, my foot," I said bitterly.

"Dr. Braun, your associate pathologist, gets migraine headaches when she is exposed to formaldehyde in the gross pathology laboratory two days in a row. Right?"

"Right!" I replied.

"Next time she talks about her migraine provoked by formaldehyde, you tell her what she suffers from is not migraine but a distorted belief system—invented by clinical ecologists," Choua chuckled.

"Preposterous!" I shook my head in disgust.

"Don't lose your temper," Choua counseled with a smile. "Here, listen to this..."

"How can those allergists from Johns Hopkins believe that

chemical sensitivity is a distorted belief system? Don't they read relevant literature?" I expressed surprise.

"Your problem is this," Choua became serious. "You have tightly held beliefs and are not open to alternative interpretation. I'll read some more:

Other allergists relate environmental illness to a cult. Dr. John Yuninger of the Mayo Clinic, said, "My personal opinion is that it is more of a religion or a cult than a science. These people have very tightly held belief systems and are not particularly open to alternative interpretation.

Minneapolis Star, July 22, 1990

More of a religion! Or a cult! Clinical ecology is not science. Drugging people who react to foods and pollutants is science," Choua beamed.

"Alternative interpretation! What might that be?" I asked, puzzled.

"Psychopathology! That's what they mean by alternative interpretation. When people like Dr. Braun react to chemicals, you should make an alternative interpretation of a psychiatric illness. That will make everyone's life simple, wouldn't it?" Choua chuckled again.

"How?" I asked.
"Here, listen to this:

According to the National Academy of Science, 15 percent of Americans suffer from increased chemical sensitivity and are at increased risk for illness due to exposure to synthetic materials.

Minneapolis Star, July 8, 1990

That's one in six Americans," Choua finished reading and looked up. "It will make the life of all those millions of people simple."

"Why would that make life simple?" I asked.

"If we were to refer people who react to chemicals to psychiatrists, they could be diagnosed with correct psychiatric diseases, then they could be appropriately drugged out of their distorted belief systems," Choua jeered, and continued, "*Science has not failed medicine, the Prince Chaullahs of N²D² medicine have failed science.*"

A Despicable Action:
Quacks Are Mistreating Psychiatric Disorders
With Nystatin

"I'm very troubled by the despicable actions of quacks who mistreat psychiatric disorders," Choua announced the next day.

"What do they do?" I asked, raising my head from my microscope and putting the slide of a breast cancer biopsy back in the slide tray.

"They mismanage psychiatric illness with nystatin."

"Oh, that!" I shrugged.

"Why do clinical ecologists and nutritionists do such dumb things? Treat *legitimate* psychiatric disorders with nystatin—an antiyeast drug?"

"So, now you are taking on the holistic docs. Does that mean you are finished with mainstream medicine?" I asked with amusement.

"Are those ecologists and nutritionists really that stupid that they think *Candida* yeast can cause psychiatric disorders? And that nystatin can cure such disorders?"

"*Candida* is but one type of yeast found in the bowel—there are many other species of yeast that often inhabit the bowel. And I don't think those holistic doctors are that simple-minded. The happenings in the bowel ecosystem, however, do affect the workings of the mind," I explained.

"Oh, you also believe nystatin can help troubled minds!" Choua leaned forward and grimaced.

"Nystatin, which reduces the yeast burden in the bowel,

seems to relieve many symptoms of confusion, concentration and memory. It also reduces emotional stress. I have seen examples of dramatic behavior improvements in children with serious hyperactivity associated with emotional outbursts. Such responses are of short duration unless the underlying problems of food and mold allergy are addressed," I described some of my clinical observations.

"Is *Candida* always present in the gut?" Choua asked.

"*Candida* yeast is a part of the normal bowel flora, so it may be considered to be present in everyone," I replied.

"Does that mean everyone has a yeast problem? Does that mean every psychiatric patient's illness can be blamed on *Candida*?"

"No!"

"Why not?"

"Because Candida rarely creates problems in healthy subjects. It's only when the immune defenses are shattered that yeast grows and causes problems."

"Do you have any idea how many women are duped into thinking Candida is their problem?"

"I know it is a problem."

"The charlatans in medicine! Now they are out to convince women with psychiatric problems that they suffer from the *Candida* yeast problem."

"How do you know they have psychiatric problems, Choua?"

"If they didn't have psychiatric problems, why would a starch placebo cure them?"

"Nonsense! That's absurd. Placebos do not cure any problems," I countered with irritation.

"Don't carp on me. I'm only reporting what I read in the *New England Journal of Medicine*," Choua said with a grin.

"Oh, the *Journal* again!" I laughed out loud. "Okay, let's

see what you have now."

"Just a simple quote," Choua leered while shuffling through some *Journal* copies. "Here is a piece:

In women with presumed candidiasis hypersensitivity syndrome, nystatin does not reduce systemic or psychological symptoms significantly more than placebo.

N Eng J Med 323:1717; 1990

See, the *Journal* is very clear. Nystatin doesn't work for psychological problems," Choua finished with a smirk.

"The *Journal* is wrong," I responded emphatically.

"Are you disputing the *Journal?*" Choua raised his eyebrows.

"Yes, I am! With good reasons."

"Wow! For once, you have the courage to stand up against the *Journal*," Choua chirped. "Let's hear your reasons."

"I've hundreds of valid reasons. Hundreds of patients who suffered from symptoms of neurosis, psychosis and schizoid perceptions obtained clinical relief with therapies that restore battered bowel ecosystem. Nystatin and other antifungal drugs such as diflucan are very helpful, if given for short periods of time as a part of a holistic plan to support the bowel ecology."

"Are you saying you hold your empirical observations higher than the scientific data of the *Journal?*"

"Yes, I do! Didn't the *Journal* contradict itself in that article, Choua? It's been a long time since I read that report, but that's the way I remember it."

"Not a bad memory for an old man!" Choua flashed a smile. "Here, I'll read some more:

> *The only nystatin-containing regimen that exerted any appreciable influence on systemic symptoms was regimen A, and its benefit was significant for only 4 of the 15 systemic symptoms.*

N Eng J Med 323:1721; 1990

Regimen A, of course, comprised oral as well as vaginal nystatin."

"I was right. I also recall there is a bar graph included in this report clearly showing that all three nystatin-containing regimens had greater clinical improvement in overall vaginal and systemic symptoms than did the placebo."

"Hey, you're doing fine. I'm impressed. That's exactly what Figure 1 on page 1,720 shows." Choua smiled broadly and put the opened page of the *Journal* right under my nose.

"That perplexes me. Why did the *Journal* make the statement that nystatin showed no benefit?" I asked.

"The magic of medical statistics! For one thing, the authors used an inappropriate statistical method. They employed a two-tail probability curve, while the correct method should have been a one-tail curve because the observed changes were unidirectional."

"Wow! Only someone like you would have caught a mistake like that, Choua," I exclaimed. "I mean how many people do I know who would appreciate the subtle but essential difference between the proper use of two-tail and one-tail statistical methods for a study like that? Certainly, the *Journal* didn't in this instance. Now I'm impressed. But, I am still baffled. Quite apart from the matter of employing an inappropriate statistical test, the bar graph shown in the article made the conclusion quite obvious. Didn't it? Tell me, Choua, what could the reason be for such a misstatement by the *Journal*?"

"Remember, the *Journal* said it wasn't statistically significant." Choua winked.

"That's outrageous!" I protested vigorously. "Any child can take one look at the bar graph and know that regimen A, including oral and vaginal nystatin, gave the best results. And, regimen A was followed by regimen B, which included oral nystatin and a vaginal placebo, and finally, by regimen C which included oral placebo and vaginal nystatin. All three gave better symptom relief than the placebo."

"A bad error! The *Journal* made a bad error," Choua flashed another smile. "There are other more serious problems with this report. When drug doctors design studies to evaluate the efficacy of therapies recommended by holistic physicians, they always mess things up, don't they?"

"How do you mean?"

"Drug doctors cannot seem to understand an elementary fact of holistic medicine: The ill individual must be looked at as a whole person, and not as shreds of tissue. A holistic plan of management must address the total clinical picture—all the relevant aspects of a patient's illness—and not simply push this or that drug. This was a badly designed study in the first place because it did just that—push a drug and neglect all other essential clinical issues," Choua spoke scornfully.

"A badly designed study! Inappropriate use of a statistical test! Erroneous conclusions! I agree, Choua, the *Journal* really slipped that time."

"*Candida* is a villain, isn't it?"

"If *Candida* were all bad, why would Nature put it there? This yeast, like its cousin yeasts in the bowel, performs several useful functions. It completes the digestion of food matter not digested by other mechanisms. It produces autoantibiotics that inhibit the growth of some disease-causing bacteria."

"So, you don't buy the Truss-Crook yeast connection theory, do you? You don't think *Candida* is the real culprit?"

"Not all of it."

"Why not?"

"Because I think *Candida* overgrowth and infections occur when the bowel ecosystem is badly battered. The bowel ecology is far too delicate, diverse and dynamic to be addressed simplistically as chronic candidiasis, candida hypersensitivity syndrome, candida-related complex or—as it goes around these days—the yeast problem. There are the essential issues of bowel parasites, microbes such as *Proteus* and *Pseudomonas*, bowel transit time, absorptive-digestive functions and acid-alkali changes."

"So you don't agree that antiyeast drugs such as nystatin or diflucan should be used for women who suffer from recurrent yeast infections and bloating, fatigue, headache, PMS, confusion and memory difficulties that are supposedly caused by *Candida*."

"Antiyeast drugs are of considerable value in the holistic plan of action to restore a battered bowel ecosystem."

"How often and for how long do you use them?" Choua asked.

"Usually for no more than two to three weeks at a time, and on no more than three or four occasions during the first year of case management. I don't agree with those who use such drugs for months—sometimes for years—to root out *Candida* species."

"Why not? If *Candida* is the cause of the problem, why not eradicate it completely the way you clear strep throat with antibiotics?" Choua argued.

"Because it doesn't work that way. The issue is not *Candida*. The issue is the integrity of the bowel ecosystem. There are many other types of yeast, pathogenic bacteria, viruses and parasites. There are also the issues of the chemical environment of the bowel, transit time and digestive-absorptive dysfunctions."

"Do you think the *Journal* knows anything about your ideas of the battered bowel ecosystem?"

"Probably not. I've never seen an article in it that addresses the global issues of the bowel ecosystem—how it is battered by the inappropriate use of antibiotics, hormones and other drugs."

"And yet, it is forever ready to discredit ideas that it knows nothing about. And the better stuff is yet to come. Listen to this:

Proponents...urge that the avoidance of foods containing yeast or mold and the reduction of dietary carbohydrates are essential components of therapy...One possible criticism of our study relates to our focus on only one aspect of therapy—the efficacy of the antifungal drug nystatin. Our study design did not address other therapeutic approaches that have been advocated, including special diets, measures to control environment, or immunotherapy.

N Eng J Med 323:1722; 1990

Didn't I tell you the better stuff was yet to come?"

"So the authors of the report *knew* before beginning the study that they were going to include only one part of the therapy plan and would end up declaring the whole plan ineffective. Amazing!" I shook my head.

"Those are the miracles of double-blind research." Choua stretched his back and walked over to the window. "*Science has not failed medicine,*" he mumbled. "*The Prince Chaullahs of N^2D^2 medicine...*" He turned sharply to face me and then walked out without completing his sentence.

Those Rascal Faith Healers:
They Bad-mouth Chemotherapy

"Chemotherapy drug makers also play the numbers game well," Choua continued.

"How do they do that?" I asked.

"They talk great games, but the results! Well, that's a different matter, isn't it?"

"Chemotherapy does work for some cancers. Hodgkin's disease and multiple myeloma are good examples," I challenged Choua.

"Would you undergo chemotherapy if you had cancer of the pancreas?"

"No!"

"Why not?"

"Because it doesn't work."

"Do oncologists agree with you on this?"

"I think most of them would."

"Have you seen persons who were given chemotherapy for pancreatic cancer?"

"Yes, that's not uncommon at all."

"Why do oncologists prescribe chemotherapy for cancer of the pancreas when they know drugs do not work for this type of tumor?"

"Well, they have to..."

"Have to?" Choua erupted. "No! They don't *have to*! Nobody *has to* administer poisons that do not control cancer. The oncologists don't *have to* destroy their patients' immune defenses with drugs that do not work. They don't *have to* damage people

just because they feel compelled to do something. Why can't they
support those patients with natural, nondrug therapies that
enhance their antioxidant and immune defenses?" Choua lashed
out.

"They don't always work."

"At least they don't destroy whatever immune defenses a
patient has left. Tell me, Mr. Chemotherapy Defender, do
oncologists ever offer their patients any nonchemotherapy
options?" Choua's insolence seemed to grow by the minute.
"What happened to the patients' bill of rights? What happened to
the physicians' hippocratic oath?"

"Oh shush, Choua!" I rebuked him angrily.

STATISTICAL POWER FOR MODEST RESULTS

"Would you take chemotherapy if you had cancer?" Choua
finally broke the silence, still gazing through the window.

"Yes! Well, depending on the type of cancer," I answered
without looking up from my microscope.

"But you would do that only for a handful of cancers,
right?"

"Right. But it is hard to know what my real feelings
would be if I actually faced that choice. There are some studies
that create room for hope."

"What studies?" Choua stiffened and turned to face me
squarely.

"The meta-analysis study published in the January 4, 1992
issue of the *Lancet*. Didn't that study show appreciable benefits
of chemotherapy for breast cancer?" I demanded.

Choua gazed into my eyes for a few moments and then

walked out without saying a word. He returned several minutes later.

"Here, I want to read something. This is the February 26, 1994 issue of *Clinical Insights:*

The meta-analysis homogenized patients for the sake of statistical power in order to detect modest differences.

Now this is a cancer specialist from the Dana Farber Cancer Institute commenting on that *Lancet* study," Choua said after reading the quote.

"Meta-analysis does help sometimes. It combines the results of a large number of studies and brings out what may not be apparent from smaller studies," I commented.

"I should add that *Clinical Insight* is published by the maker of Nolvadex—tamoxifen used for breast cancer," Choua ignored my comment. "Don't you see even they have to admit they massaged the data to increase the statistical power in order to detect modest differences. That's the issue—*modest differences.*"

"But there were differences," I asserted.

"Look, I have no difficulty if some people insist on using poisons to kill cancer. Perhaps it does work for a small number of people. The real issue is this: What did the chemotherapy cats sacrifice in banning all nontoxic herbal, bioelectric and electromagnetic therapies? What did they give up when they totally ignored the potential of therapies that normalize the abnormal surface charge of tumor cells and so cause their regression? Or when they contemptuously dismiss the potential of salves that have been clearly shown to literally pull out the tumors? Or when they ignored David Seigal's work, which clearly showed that meditation and other nondrug supportive approaches helped women with breast cancer longer than those who were drugged? But why am I talking about cancer cats sacrificing anything? They never sacrificed anything. It is the poor folks with cancer whose lives were sacrificed," Choua ended his words with evident bitterness, and then picked up a journal. "Let's see what those who know about such things say about cancer treatment in the U.S."

The main conclusion we draw is that some 35 years of intense effort focused largely on improving treatment must be judged a qualified failure.

N Eng J Med 314:1226; 1986

MODEST RESULTS AT WHAT COST

"What is the true cost of those modest results for the patient?" Choua resumed after a while.

"Chemotherapy has its problems," I replied.

"Has its problems!" Choua repeated after me. "Such as: bone marrow suppression, progressive fatigue, weight loss, loss of hair, nausea and vomiting, liver and kidney toxicity, skin eruptions, and infections with opportunistic organisms."

"Yes."

"There are yet worse things."

"What?"

"The patient's knowledge that his immune system is being systematically destroyed. And that beyond the immediate toxicity of chemotherapy, there are late consequences of a damaged immune system."

"You mean tumors? A higher incidence of leukemia, lymphomas and other cancers that is encountered in persons administered chemotherapy?"

"And the ultimate price! Here, listen to this:

An oncologist colleague lately returned from an autopsy conference at my hospital and proudly announced that his patient, who had had widespread cancer, had died "cancer-free." The patient had succumbed instead to chemotherapy-induced lung disease. It is precisely this sort of thinking and practice, where our zeal to eliminate the cancer sometimes eliminates the patient as well.

Lancet 343:494; 1994

Eliminates the patient as well! Do they figure deaths caused by chemotherapy when they conduct their meta-analyses to detect modest differences?" Choua asked scornfully.

"Cancer is a tough disease. It requires tough therapies that sometimes prove fatal," I explained.

"I know *that*!" Choua groused. "The real issue is this: How do those chemotherapy cats justify their banning of all other nontoxic, nonkiller alternative therapies for cancer? What gives them the right to kill people by the thousand with chemotherapy, *then* revoke licenses of holistic physicians who seek nonpoisonous therapies for their patients suffering from cancer?"

"You exaggerate," I countered. "Chemotherapy works for many people and it is not nearly as toxic as you think."

"Exaggerate!" Choua pouted. "I will give you the statistics for a twenty-year study of chemotherapy for node-positive breast cancer. It was reported in the April 6, 1995, issue of the *New England Journal of Medicine*. Twenty-three of 207 patients (eleven percent) were alive without recurrent cancer in the chemotherapy group while eighteen of 179 (ten percent) had no cancer in the control group of women who were spared chemotherapy. That's a difference of *one* percent!"

"Hard to believe! Are you sure those numbers are correct?" I asked.

"That's not where it ends," Choua ignored my question. "Four (2.2%) women in the control group developed a second cancer in the opposite breast while 7 (3.4%) in the treated group developed cancer in the second breast. That more than wipes out the benefits of chemotherapy, doesn't it?"

"I didn't realize the data for disease-free survival with chemotherapy were that dismal," I replied. "But were there not more overall survivors in the treated group in that study?"

"Yes, there were, but since there was no real difference between the disease-free rates among the treated and untreated groups, one has to conclude that chemotherapy wasn't of much value. Some other factors must have been responsible for differences in other areas."

"What other factors?" I asked, confused.

"Perhaps because women given chemotherapy were

expected to get sick and were watched very closely while those in the control groups were simply ignored," Chous smiled impishly, then walked out.

IF THE TUMOR IS ALL GONE, HE MUST BE DYING OF TREATMENT

What the *Lancet* laments, of course, is not uncommon at all. Frank Schauberg, M.D., an internist at our hospital, told me about a dying patient who had been treated for cancer of the throat. He sent the patient to see his oncologist, then followed up with a call. Frank asked the oncologist if he knew why his patient was dying. The oncologist insisted that he had cured the cancer, and there was no evidence of any residual cancer. Frank finished the conversation by saying, "Well, the patient is dying. If cancer is not killing him, he must be dying of the treatment."

I recall instances when a patient died after chemotherapy and his oncologist appeared in the autopsy room asking the pathologist to sample all lymph nodes—and some tissues that clearly were not lymph nodes—to prove there was no residual cancer at death. The cause of death entered on the death certificate in such cases was never chemotherapy—though it clearly was. The pathologists write off the death as due to pneumonia or other infections. Even when such deaths are discussed in mortality conferences, no one ever delves into the issues of battered host defenses, or enumerates the many ways in which chemotherapy devastates the antioxidant and immune defenses, and kills. This is not a politically-correct subject to broach!

IMMUNE SUPPRESSION IN ASTHMA
WITH STEROIDS

Asthma affects more than 5 percent of the population in industrialized countries, yet it is underdiagnosed and undertreated. There is evidence that the prevalence and severity of asthma are rising. The number of deaths from asthma may also be rising contrary to the trend for other common treatable conditions. These alarming increases are occurring despite a marked increase in prescribed asthma therapy, which suggests that currently available therapy is inadequate or is not being used optimally.

N Eng J Med 321:1517;1989.

This is the beginning," Choua finished reading.

"I agree with the *Journal* there. The recent reports show an alarming increase in the number of people who die of asthma. The worst thing about it is that asthmatics who take asthma drugs die from the disease more often than asthmatics who do not. Frightening! Isn't it?"

"Why do you think that is?"

"Growing pollution and stress."

"How about allergy?"

"Well, everyone knows that mold and food allergies set the stage for asthma attacks."

"So, would you say treatment of asthma should focus on those issues?"

"Yes. Plus self-regulation and certain breathing techniques that are very useful."

"Do you think the *Journal* knows about those things?"

"Of course. That's basic stuff."

"Basic stuff! Choua looked at me askance. "Let's see what the Journal knows about the cause of asthma and what it preaches for treatment:

> ### *We conclude that asthma is almost always associated with some type of IgE-mediated (allergy) reaction.*
>
> *N Eng J Med* 320:271; 1989
> (Parenthesis added)

How many pulmonary specialists who treat asthma understand the relationship between mold and food allergies and asthma?" Choua asked.

"Probably most," I replied.

"How many of them do you think actively manage mold and food allergy for their asthma patients?"

"Probably few. Actually, I don't know of any, but, they probably refer their asthma patients to allergists."

"Well, I don't see how anyone can truly understand mold and food allergy *well* if he has never actively managed such cases,"

Choua rubbed it in.

"Well! You..."

"There is no well." Choua interrupted me sharply. "Let's us see what therapy the *Journal* recommends for asthmatics:

> *Asthma is a chronic inflammatory condition. The previous emphasis on bronchodilator therapy, which does not treat the underlying inflammation, may be misplaced. Earlier introduction of anti-inflammatory agents, such as corticosteroids or cromolyn sodium, is strongly recommended.*

N Eng J Med 321: 1525; 1989

Pushing steroids! Isn't that it?" Choua sneered.

"Steroids save lives in brittle asthma," I explained.

"Not one word about environment. Not one word about allergy. Not one word about nutrition. Load them up with cortisone, that is the great advice that the *Journal* has," Choua said angrily.

"They want to treat the underlying inflammation," I said calmly.

"What causes the underlying inflammation?" he groused.

"Mold and food allergy and chemical sensitivity," I acquiesced.

"So, why not treat the underlying cause? Why simply suppress the symptoms? And the steroids that also suppress the immune system, leaving them vulnerable to all kinds of infection, raising blood sugar and causing all kinds of metabolic problems. And there are yet other complications of steroids use. You don't often hear about such complications as psychosis in adults and cataracts in children. Is there any part of human biology that is immune to injury due to long-term steroid use?"

"None," I confessed.

"Science has not failed medicine, the Prince Chaullahs..." Choua broke out in laughter.

VITAMIN C IS A PREMIUM LIFE SPAN MOLECULE

"Vitamin C is a premium life span molecule. It matters little what the great *Journal* does or does not say about it," Choua said in an irate tone.

"The Journal has to say what the researchers found, whether it pleases you or not," I replied firmly.

"What kind of research is this? From one side of their mouths these researchers declare vitamin C to be valuable, and from the other side, they declare it useless. And all that in the name of science," Choua said bitterly.

"I don't think you understand science in medicine," I returned his anger.

"Science in medicine! Huh! No, these folks are not interested in science. The science of vitamin C is for anyone to see. Tell me, does it work? Is vitamin C good for the common cold?"

"Yes, it is" I nodded.

"Do you know anyone in nutritional medicine who accepts the *Journal's* pronouncement about vitamin C?"

"No."

"Yet, no one who ever tries vitamin C for the common cold will ever speak against its value. Only those professors who know nothing about nondrug therapies—and practice drug medicine—write for the *Journal* and denigrate nutrients."

"Why? Why do you think they write such things?" I Asked.

"Because drug companies pay them only to sing the drug songs."

"That's a mean thing to say," I reproached Choua.

"Mean thing to say, eh! Why don't you look at what vitamin C does? Isn't it the most efficient water-phase antioxidant in the body? Don't viruses cause disease by oxidant injury? Isn't vitamin C safe and cheap?"

"Yes, that's true, but the *Journal* has to report what is observed—that vitamin C didn't seem to make any difference," I stood by the *Journal*.

"Do you ever prescribe vitamin C as the only therapy for anyone?"

"No."

"Well, these brilliant drug doctors did! Why do you write about holistic molecular relatedness in human biology?"

"Because no nutrient molecule in the body works alone."

"So, multiple nutrients must be used to complement each other's roles."

"Yes."

"So when drug doctors conduct research with single nutrients at a time, it is fundamentally a flawed method. It's not valid scientific research, is it?"

"How else do you define the metabolic functions of individual nutrients?" I asked.

"That's different!" Choua screamed. "We are talking about the efficacy of nutrients for clinical disorders."

"If it isn't a scientific method, then what is it?" I needled him.

"Fraud! Total fraud!" Choua slammed his fist on the table, looked at me sternly and walked out.

THE NUTRITION SCIENCE OF DRUG DOCTORS, THE NUTRITION SCIENCE OF NUTRITIONISTS

"We have two nutrition sciences today," Choua returned the following day.

"I thought you believed science to be mere observation. Are you saying that nutrition can be observed in two ways?" I chided Choua.

"There is the true science of nutritionist-physicians who use nutritional therapies," Choua ignored my question. "They observe the clinical results, and so determine what works and what doesn't."

"And the other?" I asked, though I knew what his answer would be.

"Then, there is the phony nutrition science of drug doctors who search for the name of the disease so that they can suppress its symptoms with their *drug of choice*. They know nothing about nondrug therapies, make much noise about scientific medicine and declare nutritionists to be quacks."

"Give me a specific example," I demanded.

"Let's look at the vitamin E study published in the *Journal*. It proves my point effectively. The authors write:

> *After controlling for age and several*
> *coronary risk factors, we observed a lower*
> *risk of coronary disease among men with*
> *higher intakes of vitamin E...Public policy*
> *recommendations with regard to the use of*
> *vitamin E should await the results of*
> *additional studies.*

N Eng J Med 328:1450; 1993

This is good news for practitioners of nutritional medicine, isn't it?" Choua asked, after he finished quoting the *Journal*.

"Yes, it is," I replied.

"It further validates the use of this antioxidant vitamin for the prevention of heart disease and other degenerative disorders. Then the authors of the study conclude their paper with an entirely unexpected statement: *Public policy recommendations with regard to the use of vitamin E supplements should await the results of additional studies.*"

"It is a good study, Choua," I responded. "It adds to our understanding of the protective role of vitamin E".

"Vitamin E is the principal lipid-phase antioxidant in human biology. That's old knowledge. That's not where the problem is."

"Then, where is the problem?"

"The problem arises from their conclusion that people continue to limit the use of this vitamin until further study. The Recommended Daily Allowance for vitamin E is 30 IU. I don't know how the Prince Chaullahs of N^2D^2 medicine arrived at that number. You prescribe from 200 to 600 IU of this vitamin for most of your patients. Why is that?"

"I arrived at that number based on vitamin E's known antioxidant roles and my empirical clinical observations."

"Vitamin E is the principal fat-phase antioxidant. That means it's the first molecular defense against oxidation and denaturation of fat molecules in the body. Right?"

"Right!"

"Oxidized fat molecules are dead fat molecules that clog the wheels of fat metabolism. Such denatured fats sit on cell membranes like candy wrappers on mountain trails, forever and ever. These damaged fat molecules fill the cellulite cells, those mortuaries of dead fats."

""I agree," I added.

"Oxidized fat molecules disrupt the normal production of most hormones. Oxidized cholesterol molecules begin the initial injury that results in plaque formation in the arteries of the heart, brain, kidneys, legs and other body organs, leading to heart attacks, strokes, leg cramps, kidney failure and other vascular disorders."

"That too!"

"Oxidized fat molecules are promiscuous molecules that mate with and destroy any molecule that crosses them. Oxidized fat molecules and their denatured toxic cyclic fat compounds injure DNA molecules and turn into cancer cells. Vitamin E is expected to prevent the birth of such molecular mutants," Choua stopped and looked for my agreement.

"Go on, Choua, I responded.

"There are yet other protective roles of vitamin E. It is a natural antithrombin—it prevents clot formation in diseased blood vessels, but not in healthy vessels, unless they have been traumatized. It prevents excessive scar formation. It is a dilator of blood vessels and so improves circulation. It prevents conversion of nitrites in deli foods into cancer-causing nitrosamine compounds. Tell me, why do you prescribe ten to twenty times of the RDA amounts of this vitamin for your patients?"

"For all the reasons you just mentioned."

"Do you think the *Journal* knows all that?" Choua asked churlishly.

"I'm sure it does. This is all established knowledge. There is nothing speculative about this."

"So, tell me, why does the *Journal* insist on yet more studies before recommending higher doses of the premium fat-soluble antioxidant?"

"Because the *Journal* is very conservative."

"It is conservative when it comes to nutrients but liberal when it comes to drugs. It pushes hard for the use of drugs and mechanical gadgets, doesn't it?"

"You're entitled to your opinion," I answered.

"Why do you stop at six-hundred units of vitamin E. Why don't you prescribe more of this good stuff?"

"Because my colleagues and I know from experience that such doses are safe over long periods of time. If and when we learn that larger doses than these also do not create any long-term adverse effects, my colleagues and I will increase the amount."

"So you are an empiricist."

"Why can't the *Journal* see the empirical value in nutritional medicine?"

"I don't know. Go ask the *Journal*," I answered with irritation.

"Science has not failed..."

"Not that again," I moaned.

"I'M AFRAID QUACKS ARE BEING VINDICATED."

A colleague spoke those words and winked when he ran into me in a hospital corridor the week the *Journal* published the vitamin E paper. I didn't think I needed to tell him that nutritionists who prescribe antioxidants had been vindicated a thousand times before that *Journal* study. A large body of clinical reports documents the efficacy of this vitamin for a host of autoimmune, degenerative, and vascular disorders. Indeed, every week my copies of *Nature* and *Science* report how oxidizing molecules injure living organisms and how antioxidants protect them from such damage—reports that further lend weight to my theory that all diseases are caused by accelerated oxidant injury.

My colleague's comment brought back to me Choua's words about two nutrition sciences—the clinically-relevant nutrition science of nutritionists and the clinically-irrelevant nutrition science of drug doctors. How much validation of the clinical efficacy of nutrients do the disease doctors of drug medicine require?

COFFEE IS AN AGING-OXIDANT DRINK

"Coffee is bad for the heart," Choua resumed. "Coffee is good for the heart."
"So which one is it?" I asked.

"Both!"

"Both? How do you mean?" I asked, surprised.

"Do you forget the two studies of the *New England Journal of Medicine* I cited some days ago?"

"I remember," I nodded.

"Coffee is an aging-oxidant drink.   Plain and simple. Remember, that's your terminology! Do you think the *Journal* understands that?" Choua asked.

"Choua, you really do have a problem, don't you? The *Journal* publishes what its researchers find. It is not the *Journal's* responsibility to dig into such inconsistencies," I scolded him.

"Oh no!   So what is the *Journal's* responsibility? Publishing meaningless data to keep the waters muddy about clinical nutrition? Is that it?"

"You are impossible today, Choua! You have a one-track mind."

"Science has not failed medicine..."

"I know! I know! The Prince Chaullahs of N^2D^2 medicine have failed science," I said impatiently.

CURING DISEASE WITH SNIPPETS OF DNA

"Here is something interesting," Choua picked up a magazine and read:

Someday, says Anderson, physicians will simply treat patients by injecting snippets of DNA and send them home cured.

Time Magazine page 48 January 17, 1994

"Let's see what the record shows. Have the geneticists cured any genetic disorder yet?

"They are very hopeful."

"I know they are, but that's not what I asked. Have they cured any genetic diseases yet?"

"I don't know, I'm not up on that."

"Do you think it might work out that way? That fellow Anderson wants to inject snippets of DNA and send his patients home. Funny stuff! isn't it?"

"I would never underestimate what science and technology can do."

"The human body is designed somewhat differently than a Ford. You can't simply remove some genes and replace them with others."

"It might happen one day, Choua, I wouldn't put it past genetic engineering."

"It's not the engineering part I doubt," Choua countered. "It's the biologic consequences of such engineering that concern me. There are millions of genes that interface with each other to produce what we call health. What do you think the chances are that one can find and replace a damaged gene and have the patient live happily ever after?"

"No one lives happily ever after," I countered.

"You're right there," Choua spoke softly. "I just wonder how grotesque the outcome of such engineering would be. You go to the hospital ICU often. Don't you see the damage that is done there in the name of good science? Don't you see what passes for heroic efforts to prolong life in so many instances is nothing more than mutilation of tissues that only prolongs the dying process? Don't you see all that Stars War technology that pumps oxygen into the listless bodies of people who should be allowed to make their last journeys in silence and dignity? But you cannot do that? Can you? You claim to be scientists in medicine. What is science in medicine except when it is subordinated to higher demands of the human spirit?" Choua fell silent for a while, then picked up a magazine and read:

HOPE IN THE WAR AGAINST CANCER

It begins as a single cell and grows into a merciless disease that claims more than half a million Americans a year. But scientists are steadily unlocking its mysteries, and the fight against it may now have reached a turning point. New discoveries promise better therapies and hope in the war against cancer.

Time Magazine
April 25, 1994

Time sees much hope in the war against cancer. Do you?" Choua asked.

"We have to keep trying," I replied.

"Let's see if the *New England Journal of Medicine* shares the hopes of *Time Magazine*.

WE ARE LOSING THE WAR AGAINST CANCER

We assessed the overall progress against

cancer during the years 1950 to 1982. In the United States, these years were associated with increases in the number of deaths from cancer, in the crude cancer-related mortality rate, in the age-adjusted mortality rate, and in both the crude and the age-adjusted incidence rates...we are losing the war against cancer...

N Eng J Med 314:1226; 1986

The *Journal* is right on target," Choua said after he finished the quote. "The rate at which human genes are oxidatively damaged will far exceed the rate with which such damage can be detected, let alone repaired. *Time* will learn this some day. *Cancer is reversible*—but not with chemotherapy drugs."

ATTRACTIVENESS OF GLOOM

Because life expectancy is constantly going up, and we may well cure cancer and heart disease in the near future, doesn't all else matter little if we are increasingly healthy?

Science 55:265; 1992

"Science is out to dispel gloom," Choua resumed. "It entitled the editorial from which the above excerpt is drawn *Attractiveness of Gloom*. It doesn't leave much reason for gloom on the present scene. It has infinite faith in its capacity for solving all mankind's problems through the miracles of synthetic chemistry."

"Curing heart disease! Wow!" I exclaimed.

"How does science propose to cure heart disease?" Choua frowned. "With coronary bypass surgery? With angioplasty? With drugs? On what basis does *Science* make its pronouncement? Does *Science* have any data that support its conclusions? If so, why does it hide them from us?"

"I think the *Science* editorial addresses the issue in a humorous dialogue with one Mr. Noitall," I explained. "You say science has not failed medicine. I agree with that. The problem of heart disease, indeed, can be addressed effectively.

"*Heart disease is reversible*," Choua continued. "It is a correctable oxidative-metabolic disorder—and not a mere plumbing problem as your cardiac surgeons and 'angioplasterers' insist. Science has given us molecules such as EDTA, vitamin C, taurine, glutathione and N-acetyl cysteine that can reverse coronary artery disease. But if we were to pursue this matter seriously, we would face some serious obstacle, won't we?" Choua smirked.

"What?" I asked.

"The RDA stupidity! The N^2D^2 dollars! The drug medicine's abominable notion of the irreversibility of heart disease!"

DRUGS FOR MORAL JUDGEMENT

"Soon we will drugs to improve moral conduct," Choua

continued.

"What?" I asked, puzzled. "Drugs for moral conduct?"

"We use drugs to solve all other problems. Why not solve the problem of immortality in society with drugs? Why single out morality as a problem beyond the reach of drugs? Why not enforce morality on the recalcitrant with *morality-restoring* drugs?"

"That's a preposterous idea?" I protested vehemently.

"Not really. At least *Time Magazine* doesn't think there is anything wrong with it," Choua laughed. "Listen to this:

> *If moral judgement can be broken, surely the next step is to fix it. 'If the abnormality is in a discrete part of the brain that uses a specific neurotransmitter, we can develop a drug treatment,' suggests Dr. Synder.*

> *Time Magazine* July 11, 1994

Long live synthetic chemistry! Long live our drugs! " Choua chanted.

BLINDED FRONTIERS

"What is science?" Choua asked.

"Didn't we go over that before?" I asked.

"Science is the search for truth," Choua continued.

"Science is observation. Science is self-correcting," I

added, remembering how we had left the subject the previous time.

"Progress in science is based on two core elements: observation and the search for meanings of that observation," Choua seemed not to take note of my comment. "Theories based on previous observations set the framework for making new observations that lead to new theoretical constructs. Theories that cannot be validated with new observations are discarded."

"What happens when observations clash?" I reminded him of his previous comment.

"The great advances in medical science of this century have occurred in a similar fashion," Choua went on, again ignoring my question. "Observations of physical phenomena in disease led to new concepts of disease treatment philosophies. Advances in surgery, anesthesia, immunology, enzymology, and hormone and receptor chemistry took place when physical observations were supported by an understanding of the meanings of those observations. Now, progress in knowledge of the human genome is taking place in the same model."

"New meanings paved the way for new observations, and so on," I added. "Where do we go from here?" I asked, amused by Choua's flow of ideas.

"Back to basics! Back to the basic study of human energy dynamics."

"Isn't that what we are doing?" I asked, puzzled now.

ELECTRON TRANSFER MEDICINE

"In 1897, J.J. Thompson, professor of natural philosophy at Cambridge, discovered electrons," Choua continued. "That discovery opened new frontiers into the nature of matter. Progress in physics in this century has followed the same basic scientific model: observation-theory-new observation—modified theory, rejecting along the way all theories that were not validated by newer observations."

"Why do you think we physicians have not followed the lead of the physicists?" I asked.

"Because you chose to be blinded," Choua deadpanned, and then smiled. "And when that wasn't enough, you got yourself double-blinded."

"You know why the double-blinding was deemed necessary, don't you?"

"I don't care why it was deemed necessary. What is important is that it is unnecessary! No, it is actually pernicious and destructive," Choua answered angrily, then asked, "Isn't the human frame composed of matter? Doesn't the matter of human flesh follow the principles of physics? Aren't electron transfer events in human metabolism of significance? Don't your enzymes work by transferring electrons? Aren't the fats and proteins in the body built up and broken down with electron transfer events?"

"Yes! Yes!" I shouted impatiently. "I know *that*. But, it's different with sick people. We don't have the luxury of theoretical physics when the sick require immediate attention."

"Are you saying that you physicians are above the laws of physics?" Choua pouted. "Don't you need to understand the essential electron transfer events in health and disease? Don't you need such knowledge to plan scientifically valid therapies? Or is it that you physicians do not have the intelligence to understand what science is and how it progresses?" Choua howled.

"Don't talk down to me like that," I responded angrily.

"Physicists build on the body of old observations and theories based on those observations," Choua ignored my protest. "Then they proceed with new observations and base new theories on new observations. Why can't you do the same?"

"Electron transfer studies in clinical medicine?" I asked in disbilief. "You are crazy, Choua!"

"The physics of health and healing! That's the issue."

"What's physics of health and healing?"

"Injured tissues don't heal with drugs. They heal with the physics of health—with energy of minerals, vitamins, fats, proteins and carbohydrates. Why can't you see something that simple? Why can't you learn the physics of health and healing, and pattern your restorative therapies on that knowledge?" Choua was unrelenting. "Why do you always push drugs? Why do you..."

"Because drugs work," I cut him off in utter exasperation.

"Why do you think people consult physicians?" Choua suddenly softened his voice and asked.

"To have their illnesses treated and health restored," I recovered.

"Do sick people ever consult you so that you can celebrate your double-blind cross-over medical science?"

"No, I don't think so."

"The sick hope you will prescribe remedies that are safe and that work, don't they?"

"Yes, that's true."

"So you agree people want what works and what is safe?"

"Of course, I do."

"Do you think people prefer disease or health?"

"That's a silly question. Of course, health."

"So what does the *Journal* do to promote health?" Choua asked.

"It seeks to promote effective treatment for disease," I offered.

"There is a big difference between treating diseases and promoting health, Dr, Innocent," Choua shot back sarcastically. "Health has something to do with the quality of an individual's sleep. All the Prince Chaullahs of N^2D^2 medicine know is how to insert those awful machines up the nostrils of gullible people. They now claim that one in four American males need these gadgets.

"Health has something to do with visceral stillness—tranquillity of the whole being. All Prince Chaullahs of N^2D^2 medicine do is encourage people to take drugs for their abraded nerves. They pronounce that forty-four percent of Americans should take anxiety drugs.

"Health has something to do with human antioxidant and immune defenses. The Prince Chaullahs of N^2D^2 medicine publish all those expensive studies funded by public money showing that antioxidants such as vitamin C and E lower the incidence of heart disease. But then they advise their readers not to use the vitamins in excess of RDA. Do they ever realize how ludicrous their advice is?

"Health has to do with nutrition. And nutrition is about right choices in the kitchen. Do the Prince Chaullahs ever try to teach their patients differences between living foods, and oxidized, denatured and dead foods? Do they understand these differences themselves? When was the last time you read an article about optimal food choices published by the Prince Chaullahs of N^2D^2 medicine?

"Health has something to do with toxic pollutants. How often do the Prince Chaullahs educate their patients about their home and work environment? They recognize dioxin to be 'probably the most potent' carcinogen in rats, and then turn around to tell their readers that dioxin does not pose any definable risk to the general public exposed to it.

"Health has something to do with hope and spirituality. The Prince Chaullahs of N^2D^2 medicine disdainfully dismiss those subjects as matters of religion. They think hope and spirituality do not measure up to their scientific standards. When was the last time you read an article published by the Prince Chaullahs of N^2D^2 medicine about the role of hope and spirituality in healing?"

Choua finished his diatribe and looked at me with piercing eyes. I sat motionless. Minutes later, I got up for a drink of water. When I returned, he was gone.

Perfection of means and confusion of goals seem—in my opinion—to characterize our age.

Albert Einstein

Few things are as discouraging as the attitude of the practitioners of drug medicine toward preventive medicine. Among themselves, they do not believe preventive medicine has any role in their professional work. Yes, they do advise their patients to reduce stress by "relaxing", instruct them to quit smoking, drink less and lose weight. Some very enlightened practitioners even tell their patients to take a multivitamin tablet daily to prevent deficiency diseases. This is where it all ends. The practitioners of drug medicine know that none of this ever works. Hence, their belief that preventive medicine has no role in their clinical work.

Taken from
The Ghoraa and Limbic Exercise

Chapter 10

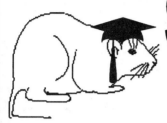

SEVENTH INSIGHT

Given an informed choice,
a vast majority of people prefer
nondrug therapy based on
Physics of Health
rather than drug regimens
based on
Chemistry of Disease.

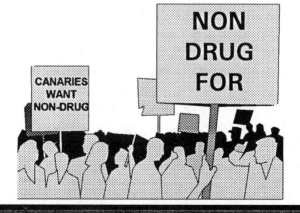

The Fifth Medicine

Choua returned after a few days, and as he often does, picked up a journal from my desk and buried his face into it without greeting me. I looked at him and wondered whether he was going to return to his favorite subjects of Prince Chaullah and N^2D^2 medicine, or whether he was going to broach a new issue. I waited for a while. Choua seemed lost in the journal. As far as he was concerned I wasn't in the room. I returned to my microscope.

"Medicine of physics," Choua muttered after a while.

"Physics?" I looked up from my scope.

"Yes, medicine of physics," Choua said without looking back at me. "That's the only way out of this mess."

"What mess?"

"Hundreds of millions of people drugged out of their wits by N^2D^2 docs all over the world. That mess!"

"I thought the subject might be different today," I teased. "But, first will you tell me what the medicine of physics is?"

"Folks have to learn to think more of the physics of health and less of the chemistry of disease," Choua replied, his eyes still fixed on the journal pages.

"Tall order! Isn't that? People can't get their vitamins and minerals straight, and you want them to think about the physics of health?"

"There is no alternative. The chemistry of disease has utterly failed people with chronic degenerative, ecologic, nutritional and immune disorders. Chemicals cannot reverse those disorders. People must seek answers in the physics of health."

"Crazy! Only someone like you could have thought this one up, Choua. How do you propose that people with chronic disorders should move from the chemistry of disease to the physics of health? The problem is that sick people need relief. At least drugs make that possible."

"Do you have any drugs that can reverse degenerative disease?" Choua abruptly looked up from the journal and challenged.

"Haven't we already covered that?" I protested.

"It has to be the fifth medicine based on physics of health." Choua ignored my question.

"Fifth medicine?" I asked, confused.

"The fifth medicine based on the physics of health."

"What are the other four medicines?"

"The first medicine was a medicine of the spirits."

"Do you mean the medicine of primitive man—of rituals, dances and trances?"

"The second medicine was the medicine of gross pathology," again Choua ignored my question. "It was based on the naked-eye study of dead or dying tissues."

"And the third medicine! Was that the medicine of the microscope?" I ventured a guess.

"Yes, Leeuwenhoek invented the microscope in 1719 and ushered in the era of the third medicine. The microscope became the arbiter of what disease was and what it wasn't," Choua chugged along.

"And the fourth medicine? What was that? A medicine of scalpels and X-rays?"

"The fourth medicine was—and continues to be—a medicine of blockage. It is based on the chemistry of disease. In this medicine, synthetic chemicals are used to block healing processes and suppress the symptoms that are associated with the healing responses. In this medicine, drug makers make drugs to block cellular enzymes, cell membrane channels, cell receptors, mediators of repair response, neurotransmitters and anything else that they might manage to block," Choua spoke solemnly.

"And then drug makers persuade physicians to use those drugs, is that the idea?" I asked.

"Now people must ask for—no, they must insist on—nondrug therapies of the fifth medicine based on the physics of health," Choua proceeded in a matter of fact way.

"And just what are the therapies of the fifth medicine based on physics of health?" I asked, my curiosity piqued.

"In prehistoric times, the tribal priest doubled as the tribal healer," Choua went on. "He proclaimed disease a punishment from angry spirits and sought to heal his flock by appeasing the offended spirits. To this end, he devised elaborate rituals for making offerings to wrathful spirits. Sometimes, when he realized the spirits were too furious to be calmed by animal sacrifices, he offered human sacrifices. He chose handsome young men and the prettiest damsels and devised perverse ways of taking their lives. On the side, he experimented with the medicinal effects of plants and crystals. Sometimes his plant potions and rock sorcery seemed to work. Or, more likely, the sick got better in spite of his therapies—just as the sick often get better in spite of drug therapies of N^2D^2 docs today. Since..."

"Venom! Choua's venom again!" I shook my head.

"Since mankind didn't become extinct," Choua ignored my protest, "we have to assume that the healing responses that Nature built in human beings worked."

"When do we get to the fifth medicine therapies? I'm still waiting for medicine based on the physics of health," I reminded Choua.

"The second medicine of gross pathology evolved very slowly," Choua ignored my reminder. "Dissection of dead bodies by the curious few among physicians rankled their peers in mainstream medicine in ancient and medieval times—just as innovations in nutritional medicine and clinical ecology irk disease doctors of drug medicine today."

"You can't help yourself, can you? Why do you have to give us the rub at each step?" I pretended to be offended by his remark.

"The gods of medieval medicine ridiculed the dissenters in medicine—as much as the gods of modern medicine deride ecologists and nutritionists today," Choua went on. "Still, the anatomists persisted in their dissections of human parts, often risking their lives at the hands of their peers in the *straight* medicine of their times."

"Straight medicine?" I suppressed a smile.

"Straight medicine—the status quo medicine—has always hated innovators. Mostly, it is a simple matter of protecting their positions and income. Sometimes, it is resentment with nondrug therapies that work. Now, that's not good for drug medicine, is it?" Choua sneered.

"The fifth medicine, Choua! I still await the fifth medicine," I asked impatiently.

"Leeuwenhoek invented the microscope primarily to satisfy his curiosity about the microbes that were believed to live in the bowel and expelled with the stools. Folks were interested in the happenings in the bowel even then, though I don't think they ever heard of *your* bowel ecosystem," Choua winked and continued. "I wonder if Leeuwenhoek ever had any inkling how he was to change medicine single-handedly and forever. Rudolph Virchow, the German physician-pathologist-statesman published *Cellular Pathology* in 1858, and that book earned him the title of the father of pathology. To this day, you physicians are incarcerated in the Virchownian thinking, and all your therapies are based on ideas of disease founded on the microscopic study of injured tissues."

"Physicians generally are conservative. They don't change their methods or opinions easily."

"Don't I know *that?*" Choua blurted. "They stay with what brings them riches and prestige. Innovation is hard work and it is risky. Why rock the boat! Except, of course, when it comes to new drugs and surgical procedures."

"Oh, shush, Choua!" I rebuked him. "What is the fifth medicine?"

"By itself, the fourth medicine is not bad. You do need potent, albeit toxic, drugs for acute, life-threatening illnesses."

"So what's bad about the fourth medicine?" I asked, puzzled.

"Synthetic chemistry is the science of turning and twisting natural molecules to invent new ones. It provides the foundation of modern pharmacology—the science of drugs that save lives in Star Wars medicine. Drugs are used to inhibit, inactivate, block, mimic and manipulate molecules in the body. The synthetic chemicals give you the tools of your trade for the acutely ill. The problem begins when you fail to see the difference between the needs of the acutely sick to interrupt destructive processes and the requirements of the chronically ill to restore damaged enzyme systems. All..."

"Let's move on to the fifth medicine," I pressed.

"All drug therapies for degenerative, ecologic and nutritional disorders are bound to fail in the long run. The champions of the fourth medicine do not understand this simple fact."

DISEASES ARE NOT
DRUG-DEFICIENCY DISORDERS

"Diseases are not drug-deficiency disorders," Choua continued.

"We need drugs for acute illness and for pain relief, anxiety and sleep," I remembered the tirade of the past few days, but still provoked him.

"Americans know that chronic illnesses are not caused by chemical deficiencies that can be healed by supplying the missing chemical as a drug. It is self-evident—even to those who need drugs for mere symptom suppression. The true answers to our global health problems are in our understanding of what health is, what disease is and the difference between the two. The issue is not that Americans do not see this and do not want nondrug therapies or that they reject the health benefits of effective methods of self-regulation."

"What, then, is the issue?" I asked, flustered.

"The issue is that they generally do not have access to professionals who are willing and able to provide the necessary support with care, compassion, and persistence."

"I am an optimist. I believe this will change. I see an ever-increasing number of physicians who want to learn about nondrug therapies."

"Absence of disease is not always presence of health," Choua threw my own words at me. "Between the states of health and disease is a transitional state of absence of health. Absence of health—the physics of health under stress—is a state that precedes disease. This simple fact is crucial for a genuine understanding of the fifth medicine of physics. But, you physicians cannot understand that, can you?" Choua asked sarcastically.

"The tide is turning in favor of nondrug therapies," I replied.

"Yes, the tide is turning, but not because of anything you doctors have accomplished. It is turning because people are beginning to realize that diseases do not arrive from Mount Olympus. Rather, chronic illnesses are related to environmental, nutritional and stress-related factors."

The New England Journal of Medicine
MAKES AN IMPORTANT DISCOVERY

"On January 28, 1993, the readers of the *New England Journal of Medicine* made a great discovery," Choua chortled.

"What?" I asked.

"They found out what common folks have known for decades: Americans prefer unconventional therapies—no, make that nontoxic, nondrug remedies—to toxic drugs. Listen to this:

The frequency of use of unconventional therapy in the United States is far higher than previously reported...Extrapolation to the U.S. population suggests that in 1990 Americans made an estimated 425 million visits to providers of unconventional therapy. This number exceeds the number of visits to all U.S. primary care physicians.

New England Journal of Medicine
328:246; 1993

Note the words *extrapolation to the U.S. population* in the above quote."
"Yes?"
"In a democratic society, a majority opinion determines what must be regarded as the dominant thought, right?"
"Right!"
"If we accept the data published by the *Journal*, it follows that Americans have clearly demonstrated, by their true-to-life actions, that they consider nondrug therapies *conventional* and drug therapies, unconventional."
"That's a twist!" I mused.
"Most drug doctors believe that people who accept nondrug therapies are ill-informed. They believe people take vitamins and herbs because of superstitious beliefs and irrational fears of synthetic chemicals. In reality, the opposite is true. Several studies

show that people who seek out nondrug therapies are in a higher socioeconomic strata. They are more educated and have greater financial resources so they can afford nondrug therapies."

"That's surprising!"

"Why should it surprise you?" Choua posited. "Educated folks understand that injured tissues heal with nutrients, not drugs. So they try nondrug therapies, and when they find out that they work, they simply continue to use them. Poor people cannot afford to pay for their health care twice: once in the form of health insurance premiums and a second time when they pay for nondrug therapies that are not covered by the insurance industry."

UNNECESSARY DRUGS

"How often are drugs used unnecessarily?" Choua resumed.

"Not uncommonly, but I don't have any precise statistics," I replied.

"Here, I'll read something:

...that 1.8 million older people had prescriptions for dipyridamole, a blood thinner that, the researchers say, is useless for all except people with artificial heart valves. Yet, only 36,000 Americans, half of them over 65, had heart valves put in.

The New York Times, July 27, 1994

"Explain that to me, please," Choua continued, putting the

paper down. "Tell me, how does that happen? Almost two million people are given a drug that only eighteen-thousand need—that comes to nine-hundred and ninety-nine persons taking the drug needlessly for every one who needs it."

"Why?" I asked.

"Because drug doctors have to give their patients something, and drugs are all they've got to offer. If they believed in nutrition, environment and self-regulation, they could have used many other therapies."

"That can't be the whole story, Choua," I disputed. "People insist that their physicians prescribe drugs."

"Nonsense!" Choua's voice suddenly rose. "People want their physicians to give them something, but that something doesn't have to be drugs. It could be nutrients! Herbs! Training in *your* limbic breathing."

"Very few patients are ready for that sort of stuff," I persisted.

"Not true! Not true!" Choua croaked. "People are ready for that stuff. Even the *New England Journal of Medicine* knows that. It's the N^2D^2 doctors who are not ready."

INAPPROPRIATE USE OF DRUGS

Close to a quarter of all Americans 65 or older were given prescriptions for drugs that they should almost never take, a study found.

The New York Times, July 27, 1994

"Why do you think that happens?" Choua asked.
"Why?" I asked.

"Doctors prescribe what the salesmen tell them to prescribe," Choua chuckled.

"That's ludicrous!" I said in disgust.

"Why don't you ask your hospital pharmacists how drug use changes after the drug speakers hired by the pharmaceutical industry leave the hospital?"

"That is a problem, I admit, but it is nowhere as bad as you make it," I protested.

"Isn't that how an ordinary drug becomes the drug-of-the-month? Isn't that how an inexpensive old drug is replaced by an expensive new drug that works no better? Isn't that how drug salesmen make their living? Isn't that how drug doctors who speak for drug makers earn their consultations? Look at the drug abuse:

SEVEN WRONGLY PRESCRIBED DRUGS FOR THE ELDERLY		
Drug	Percent Receiving	# of Prescriptions
Propranolol	6.27	4,995,358
Dipyridamole*	6.44	4,832,889
Methyldopa	4.52	3,663,512
Propoxyphene	4.83	2,412,308
Diazepam	2.82	1,547,111
Indomethacin	2.64	1,300,212
Chlorthiazide	1.95	1,135,497
Total	29.47	19,886,887

Source: 1987 National Medical Expenditure Survey conducted by the Federal Agency for Health Care Policy and Research.

DRUG INTERACTIONS

"The *New York Times* is concerned that older people are not properly informed about the risk of drug therapies," Choua said, picking up a copy of the paper.

"That continues to be a problem. What's your take on that?" I asked in jest.

"Don't you remember the older patients you saw in the emergency departments? Didn't they pull one drug bottle after another from their bags until no one could figure out what drug was being used for what purpose?"

"How does that happen?" I asked.

"You know how," Choua grinned. "They go to their family practitioners who prescribe drugs for sleep, anxiety and aches and pains. When these drugs stop working, the family doctor refers them to a rheumatologist who then prescribes potent anti-inflammatory drugs that cause gastritis and stomach ulcers. That takes them to gastroenterologists who prescribes yet other drugs to heal gastritis and stomach ulcers. Their drugs, in turn, ruin the normal acid secretion in the stomach without which food cannot be digested. The patients get indigestion, abdominal bloating and digestive-absorptive problems—eventually leading to serious disruptions of the bowel ecosystem. Now they get antibiotics that further damage bowel ecology. Stress, sleep and pain problems worsen, and if they didn't suffer from high blood pressure and heart palpitations before, they add those to reasons for seeing yet other doctors—the cardiologists. Isn't that how it happens?"

"To some extent," I replied.

"To some extent! Here, I'll read another piece:

Dr. "X" suggested that older people take lists of their medications to their doctors and ask about interactions and side effects. There are things that older people can do to help themselves and I think they should do them...

"This doctor, speaking for the *Times,* omitted one simple detail," Choua said, putting the paper down.

"What?"

"Genuine and reliable information about drug interactions *simply* does not exist."

"Now, that's not really true," I challenged Choua. "Pharmacists now have computerized files of drug interactions."

"Don't be silly!" Choua said tartly. "Has any drug company ever conducted a double-blind, cross-over study of any of its drugs used concurrently with a drug made by its competitor? Has anyone ever done double-blind cross-over studies of concurrent use of three, four or seven drugs?" Choua countered.

"I don't know."

"So, tell me where do pharmacists get their data about drug interactions from?"

"From reported cases."

"Aha! From reported cases of serious drug interactions. How often do you think doctors report toxic interactions of different drugs? Wouldn't they be setting themselves up for medical liability actions? The *New England Journal of Medicine* says thirty-six percent of hospitalized patients suffer from disorders caused by doctors. But, then aren't they talking about serious disorders that require hospitalization? How about all those reactions that go unrecognized and unreported? Reactions that are dismissed as inconsequential by drug doctors but that are very consequential for the patients! And how about mind-altering drugs that cause older people to trip, fall and break their bones? How often does that happen? How often is that reported?"

TEAM EFFORT: THE MORE THE MERRIER

"Drug doctors like the idea of team effort, don't they?" Choua asked.

"Don't tell me you have a problem with that," I replied.

"What do you get out of it?"

"It makes a lot of sense—shared responsibility, access to experienced opinions, less margin for error. Do you have a problem with it?" I asked, surprised.

"The more the merrier. Everyone contributes," Choua sneered.

"You can be so obstinate, Choua." I shook my head. "Yes! It's good to be safe, and consultants help minimize the margin of error."

"Team effort!" Choua mumbled softly. "Everyone does his thing. Everyone shares responsibility. Everyone prescribes."

"Oh! You are such a cynic!" I sighed.

"You physicians often lament drug abuse," Choua retorted. "Yet, you merrily prescribe drugs for sheer symptom suppression —fully recognizing that other physicians on the case are prescribing additional drugs just as merrily for the same patient. Tell me that's *not* the case!" Choua dared me.

A Friendly Challenge

"What philosophy of medicine will work better for chronic disorders?" Choua asked a few days later. "Drug medicine or nondrug holistic medicine?"

"I'm not sure I understand the question," I said.

"The question is simple. Who will get better results for chronically ill patients, Betty Best Internist, M.D., or Avita Average Holistic, M.D.?"

"It depends. I don't know how good a diagnostician Dr. Betty Best is or how competent Dr. Avita Average is."

"Suppose we design a clinical outcome study to test the idea?"

"Only you could have conceived a notion like that, Choua," I said, holding back a smile. "How can you draw valid conclusions by comparing the results of just two physicians?"

"We will pick seven university-trained Betty Bests with more than ten years of experience each with drug therapies. Next, we will ask seven Avita Averages, experienced in nondrug therapies, to participate in the study."

"Who will select the patients?"

"No one! There will be no patient selection. We will take seven-hundred consecutive patients with chronic degenerative, immune, ecologic, nutritional and stress-related disorders. We will divide them into two groups of three-hundred and fifty subjects, each matched for age, sex and the general disease category. We will then ask each of those fourteen physicians to manage one subgroup of fifty patients each for seven years."

"For seven years? You're not serious, are you?" I was flabbergasted by Choua's proposition.

"We'll give them full freedom to use any and all therapies they wish for a period of seven years," Choua ignored my question.

"Do you really believe such a study can ever be undertaken?"

"Why not? University internists spend hundreds of millions of dollars of public money on their drug research. Why can't they find two-hundred dollars for such a study?"

"Go on! Dream, Choua, dream," I exhorted him. "One hundred thousand dollars for holistic doctors? On second thought, maybe the Office of Alternative Medicine will fund such a study."

"Ah, the Office of Alternative Medicine! No, they are wolves in sheep's clothing."

"Oh! You don't like them either?" I expressed surprise. "That's really odd. I thought that was a great step ahead."

"Why don't you review the list of research grants they approved?" Choua scowled. "They are all single-issue-single-therapy protocols—and if they are silly enough to persist with their frivolous notions of medical research—the outcomes are entirely predictable."

"How so?"

"Either there will be no success or they will fudge the results."

"Now you are being silly! How can you be so sure of that?" I asked in frustration.

"The essence of empirical medicine is slow, sustained restoration of the normal energetic-molecular pathways of human biology. Natural therapies work best when they are integrated with a valid philosophy of healing. Can the Office of Alternative Medicine ever design a study to conduct a true test of a lifelong philosophic approach to health and healing? My friend, I'm not being silly. The folks who dole out tax money at the Office of Alternative Medicine are incarcerated in N^2D^2 notions. They have no understanding of the core philosophy of empirical medicine."

"So what's the answer?" I asked with resignation.

"Long-term outcome studies in which practitioners of both systems are given free reign to apply their philosophic principles for some years and then the sick are asked to evaluate the results. The NIH will never get any place as long as they are stuck with their infantile N^2D^2 notions of health and healing."

"Oh, God!" I moaned. "Let's get back to the study protocol."

"Fine! Fine!" Choua grinned. "We will carefully record the symptoms as defined by the patients at the time of initial consultation, and we will ask the physicians to meticulously record their physical findings."

"And you really think you will find seven university internists who will have nothing else to do except play this game with you?" I mused.

"It will not be a *game*," Choua snapped acidly. "It will be a serious test of the two medical philosophies—a type of definitive study that has never been undertaken before."

"And you believe holistic physicians will win, don't you?" I laughed at Choua's innocence.

"I don't believe they will win. I *know* so," he dead-panned.

"Seven Betty Best Internist, M.D.s! And seven Avita Average Holistics! An interesting proposition, Choua. I have to hand it to you," I laughed.

WILL ANY BETTY BESTS FROM BAYLOR OR BROWN TAKE THE CHALLENGE?

"It seems like a crazy idea to me, Choua. Do you think anyone will take it seriously?"

"It's not a crazy idea, and those who talk the loudest about science in medicine should have the courage to accept the challenge."

"That's not my question. Will any Betty Bests from Baylor or Brown take the idea seriously enough to consider it?"

"Why do you keep saying it is not a serious idea?" Choua snapped. "What could be more serious than testing the two philosophies of medicine with true-to-life case histories? I'm talking about a seven-year outcome study. That should take a lot of variables out of the picture."

"But who would want to get involved in such a study for seven years? So much work!"

"Now, that's a silly argument," Choua spoke sharply. "University doctors do drug studies that last for years and years, don't they? How long did the Framingham studies last? How long did the Harvard aspirin and the Lipid Research group studies last? How many millions of dollars of public money were spent on those studies? And what did the people get in return? Some bloated numbers to promote drug use when the real data were abysmally poor—pushing cholesterol-lowering drugs with concocted risk reduction of forty-four percent when the real reduction in the rate of heart attacks was only one percent. Why can't the NIH find a few hundred-thousand dollars to do a study to compare long-term clinical outcome with drug and nondrug therapies? Perhaps some drug companies will fund it. After all it *might* prove the superiority of their drugs," Choua said in a mocking tone.

"You're so sure of yourself, aren't you? You really *do* believe the Avita Averages will win, don't you?"

"Yes! Yes! I do," Choua yowled. "There is no chance of Avita Averages losing. None whatsoever. I don't doubt for a moment that they will beat Betty Bests hands down if such a study were ever undertaken."

"You shouldn't make dogmatic statements, Choua. You hurt your credibility. You are making a big claim for holistic physicians, and I don't see how you can be certain of the results."

"Let's see." Choua stared at me for a while and then continued, "I am absolutely certain Avita Averages with their nondrug therapies will come out way ahead of Betty Bests with their drug regimens for two sets of reasons."

"What?" I asked, my curiosity peeking.

"First, the therapies that Betty Bests will use and those that Avita Averages will employ. Betty Bests will prescribe seven years of blockade of normal healing responses. Avita Averages, by contrast, will offer seven years of supportive therapies. Injured tissues heal with nutrients, not drugs. Remember, those are your words."

"And the second set of reasons?" I asked, a trifle flustered.

A DIRTY TRICK

"We will play a dirty trick on Betty Best. We won't let her use her favorite gimmick," Choua grinned.

"What favorite gimmick?" I asked, surprised.

"Of excluding the patient from assessing the long-term

benefits of therapies! You see, that's where the problem begins. University doctors strenuously exclude the patients from the process of determining what therapies work and what do not. And we won't let them play that silly game in this study. Those who suffer will decide what works—those who push pills won't. Seven years is a fair time for people who suffer to evaluate what therapies offer them the most benefit and least toxicity."

"And you are sure Avita Averages will come out on the top if patients evaluate the results?" I expressed doubt.

"All you have to do is to randomly take some of your charts. How many doctors does an average patient see before he consults you?"

"Four, maybe five! Sometimes I see them after they have seen ten or more."

"How many drug regimens did they try before they saw you?"

"I may be looking at a very skewed patient population. Almost all patients now see me because they want to get off their drug therapies," I explained.

"Why? Why do they want to get off their drug regimens? Because the drugs don't work after a while and drugs cause side effects. And also because drugs cost a lot of money."

"To an extent, that's true," I agreed.

"Let's see how Betty Bests and Avita Averages will provide care for their assigned patients with chronic degenerative, immune, nutritional, ecologic and stress-related disorders."

"Go on, Choua, I'm listening. This stuff is getting more interesting."

"Degenerative disorders will include heart disease and arthritis. Immune disorders will include recurrent infections, skin disorders, collagen diseases such as lupus, and underactive or overactive thyroid glands. Environmental problems will include asthma and chemical sensitivity. Sugar roller coasters, hypoglycemia and adverse food reactions will be the common nutritional disorders. And stress-related disorders will, of course, include sleep difficulties, anxiety and panic attacks, high blood pressure and such problems as stomach ulcers."

"That's not a bad list of clinical problems. Betty Best Internist, M.D., and Avita Average Holistic, M.D., see such patients every day."

"Now let's see how patients with these chronic disorders will fare with their physicians?"

"Okay," I agreed.

SEVEN YEARS OF BLOCKADE MEDICINE, SEVEN YEARS OF SUPPORTIVE MEDICINE

"Let's assume that Betty Best will provide medical care according to the highest standards of excellence prevailing in university hospitals today. Of course, those standards of excellence are standards of drug regimens. Right?" Choua asked in a naughty tone.

"Right!" I acquiesced.

"Let's also assume Avita Average will also employ the prevailing nondrug therapies—choices in the kitchen, oral and injectable nutrients, herbs, allergy management, physical therapies and meditation. Agreed?"

"Agreed."

"As far as clinical problems such as sugar roller coasters, adverse food reactions, chemical sensitivities, yeast overgrowth and chronic fatigue are concerned, Betty Bests will dismiss them as all-in-the-head problems—to be treated, if at all, with antacids, antianxiety drugs or antidepressants. Right? I mean the university internists don't believe such problems exist because their existence has never been proven with their *blessed* double-blind cross-over studies."

"Well..."

"Well what?" Choua interrupted me sharply. "Betty Bests have been trained to dismiss those problems as hypochondria."

"But hypochondria *does* exist, doesn't it?" I objected.

"Fine, fine! So it exists. What interests me is this: Betty Bests obviously will not search for physical causes of what they believe is hypochondria or all-in-the-head problems. And, if they have to give those patients anything, they'll prescribe Valium, Ativan or antidepressants. Right or wrong?" Choua gawked.

"I'm afraid you're right," I responded.

"Of course I am!" Choua said forcefully. "The same will hold for ecologic disorders such as headache and fatigue caused by sensitivity to formaldehyde, solvents and other pollutants. Betty Bests don't believe in them and so will not address those issues or will prescribe mind-altering drugs. Do you agree?"

"Yes. Perhaps there will be some exceptions."

"Are you saying that there are some university internists who believe chemical sensitivities are real disorders?" Choua raised his eyebrows.

"Okay! Okay!" I yielded. "Go on."

"For sleep problems, Betty Best will prescribe more pills or order sleeping machines that patients can stick up their noses when they go to bed. That will also be the case with TMJ and other stress-related disorders—more of those awful contraptions to be stuck in people's mouths or noses."

"Some internists might prescribe biofeedback or meditation," I countered.

"How many university internists do you know who teach biofeedback or meditation to their patients?" Choua groused. "How many of them meditate themselves?"

"There is more to good medicine than just that," I rebutted.
"What?" he asked, surprised.
"Correct diagnoses."
"Oh that!" Choua seemed relieved. "Will Betty Bests make better diagnoses? Is that what you mean?" he asked.

SHARPER DIAGNOSES, AWKWARD CONCEPTS

"University internists will be much sharper than holistic doctors in making diagnoses. I don't think there can be any doubt about that," I replied.

"Sharper diagnostic labels!" Choua laughed scornfully. "Yes, I agree Betty Bests will be more glib with their diagnostic terminology. They are more adept at throwing around their tongue-twisting medical jargon—just like you pathologists do when you are not sure of what you are looking at. The longer the pathology report, the less its substance! Isn't that what you told me once?"

"You're a master of obfuscation! You turn and twist everything until it suits your purpose," I complained.

"Obfuscation? I don't know what that is," Choua softened a bit. "But don't forget how we designed this study. Participating physicians will be given full freedom of therapies for seven years and patients who suffer will rate the results. It wouldn't matter to patients how elegant or inelegant the diagnostic labels used for them might be. Diagnostic labels wear thin for the sick. What they want is good health—high energy level, deep sleep, freedom from pain and anger, normal bowel transit time with healthy bowel movements and ability to enjoy personal time. Betty Best hasn't got any drugs to offer for any of that, does she?"

"Go on," I replied.

"Avita Average may be laughed at for the awkwardness of her clinical concepts of health and disease but all her nondrug therapies are designed for restoration of energetic and physiologic dynamics of human health. Slow and sustained, her therapies will facilitate healing responses, won't they?"

"Yes."

"After seven years, only clinical outcome will count. The glow of Betty Best's dazzling diagnoses will be long forgotten when the time comes for patients to rate their physicians. What will be remembered instead are frequent infections, bloated bellies, aching heads, disturbed sleep, sugar roller coasters, anxiety, heart palpitations, cold hands and feet, persistent fatigue, skin rashes, hurting muscles, menstrual irregularities, PMS, thinning hair, swollen joints, enlarged neck glands, anger, hopelessness and..."

"Will the litany ever end?" I interrupted Choua.

"Stop to realize that we are pitting seven years' worth of drug toxicity against seven years' worth of optimal choices in the kitchen, nutrient and herbal support, allergy management and benefits of self-regulation, *Ti Chi*, yoga and massage. Now, you tell me, is there a comparison?"

DRUGS BY THE BUCKET FOR BETTY BEST

"Let's look at the buckets of drugs Betty Best will use for her patients and then consider what approach Avita Average will adopt," Choua said, standing at my office door next day.

"Didn't we cover that yesterday?" I asked.

"I made up a list of the nutrients and herbs Avita Average will use and I'll give you a list showing the ranking of new, refill and the total number of prescriptions that drug doctors used in

1994. That will help me make my case for Avita Average and against Betty Best."

"Amazing! It's amazing how sure you are that holistic doctors are going to win over university internists," I laughed.

"Just glance at the lists first," Choua pressed. "First, the drug list published in the February 28, 1994 issue of *American Druggist*, then a list of nutrients and herbs that I prepared:

DRUG PRESCRIPTIONS IN 1994			
RANK	**REFILL Rx**	**TOTAL**	**NEW Rx**
1	Premarin	Premarin	Amoxil
2	Procardia	Zantac	Trimox
3	Synthyroid	Amoxil	Ceclor
4	Zantac	Synthyroid	Xanax
5	Lanoxin	Procardia	Augmentin
6	Vasotec	Lanoxin	Premarin
7	Cardizem	Xanax	Zantac
8	Xanax	Trimox	Amoxicillin
9	Ortho-novum	Vasotec	Cipro
10	Mevacor	Cardizem	Synthyroid
11	Proventil	Ceclor	Naprosyn
12	Provera	Augmentin	Lanoxin
13	Capoten	Proventil	Procardia
14	Lopressor	Naprosyn	Acetaminophen
15	Calan	Provera	Seldane
16	Micronase	Prozac	Vasotec
17	Coumadin	Mevacor	SMX-TMP
18	Prozac	Seldane	Propoxyphen
19	Dilantin	Orthonovum	Prozac
20	Ventolin	Capoten	Zoloft

20 COMMONLY USED NUTRIENTS	
RANK	**NUTRIENT**
1	Vitamins C, E and A
2	Magnesium
3	Taurine
4	Pantothenic Acid
5	Protein Formulas
6	Vitamin B complex
7	Pyridoxine
8	Bowel ecology protocols
9	Gastric Ecology Protocol
10	Herbs for blood ecosystem
11	Herbs for liver ecosystem
12	Herbs for parasites
13	Herbs for sleep and stress
14	Essential fatty acids
15	Essential amino acids
16	Zinc and molybdenum
17	Other minerals
18	Plant progesterones
19	Folic acid and DHEA
20	Herbal teas

Avita Average will use vitamins C, E and A along with minerals such as zinc and selenium to give her patients essential long-term antioxidant support and protect their cell membranes from oxidant injury. She will use vitamin B complex members to streamline the energy and detoxification systems of the body. Taurine will be used as one of the most effective cell membrane protectors. When oxidant stress pokes holes in the cell membrane, what's inside the cell hemorrhages out and what is outside floods the cell innards. That explains why Avita Average will use large amounts of magnesium and potassium with sparing quantities of calcium and other minerals. Molybdenum is a mineral co-factor for sulfite oxidase enzyme system that is so important in detoxification pathways.

"Avita Average will use essential oils to stabilize cell membranes and protein formulas composed of eighty-five to ninety-five percent partially hydrolyzed and digested plant- or animal-derived proteins to provide amino acids for producing hormones, enzymes, neurotransmitters and structural proteins, and..."

"And for providing slow, sustained energy to offset sugar roller coasters," I completed his sentence. "We know all that."

"Sugar roller coasters that trigger insulin roller coasters that, in turn, bring on adrenaline roller coasters are some of the most common problems. But, of course, Betty Best will dismiss all that as hypochondria."

"Not all of them," I challenged him.

"Drug doctors are not into metabolic nutritional problems. Drugs are the tools of their trade," Choua shrugged. "Another important area that Betty Best will ignore completely will be the damaged bowel ecosystem. Avita Average, on the other hand, will use plenty of herbs to restore the damaged bowel ecosystem: echinacea, astragalus, pau D'arco, burdock root, golden seal, alfalfa, licorice, ginger root and garlic. She will use vitamin C, magnesium, potassium, taurine, psyllium and cascara to normalize the bowel transit time that is often prolonged in patients with chronic nutritional, immune and ecologic disorders. And for the liver ecosystem, they will..."

"I know! I know!" I interrupted Choua. "She will use milk thistle, turmeric, red clover, dandelion root, fennel seed, fenugreek, Jerusalem artichoke and black radish."

"Also, she will use lipotropic factors—methionine, inositol, and choline."

"Some mainstream physicians are beginning to use lipotropic factors to prevent liver injury after viral hepatitis," I offered.

"Meanwhile, Avita Average will search for intestinal parasites," Choua went on, "not the way Betty Best will do this by sending a stool specimen to the laboratory. Avita will perform an anoscopy and take swabs of the rectal mucus where parasites hide. And then she will stain the slides with specific antibodies against parasites."

"Is this lecture going to end?" I asked, frustrated.

"And they will use herbs such as artemisia, pringamoza, gossypol and others that have been tested and found efficacious for centuries, not like the drugs that have been tested on mice and medical students for weeks or months in your blessed double-blind cross-over studies."

"You can't help yourself, Choua," I said in anger and rubbed my temples with both hands.

"Do you have a headache?" Choua asked, lowering his voice in concern. "I thought you cured your migraine years ago with your limbic stuff."

"No, I don't have a headache," I nearly screamed. "Your words are boring holes in my temples."

"Oh, that!" Choua blinked. "Incidentally, Avita Average

will teach her patients something about breathing for stress control, and something about anger and hostility."

"Betty Best will also do that," I injected.

"Yes! But physicians who practice nondrug, empirical medicine are much more inclined to focus on those issues than are N^2D^2 docs. I often wonder if it is holistic medicine that makes physicians more compassionate and sensitive or if holistic physicians are more humanistic to start with, and so are drawn to natural methods of caring for the sick? Certainly, holistic practitioners address anger, hostility, stress and sleep more readily than drug doctors. Isn't that so?" Choua asked.

"I don't know," I answered, wondering whether there was indeed something to Choua's observation.

DRUGS FOR DISCIPLINE

"How will Betty Best treat children with hyperactivity and attention deficit disorders?"

"With psychological counseling and, if necessary, with Ritalin, amphetamines or related drugs."

"Does psychological counseling really help problems caused by sugar roller coasters, food allergy and stress?"

"Not really," I confessed.

"So, ultimately the only thing Betty Best will offer to her little patients is drugs. Isn't that true? I mean it will be drug prescriptions once the formality of psychological counseling is done with and talk therapy found useless for such disorders."

"I'm afraid, you have a strong case."

"How bad is this problem? How fast is this epidemic spreading? Here, I'll read something:

The results reveal a consistent doubling of the rate of medication treatment for hyperactive/inattentive students every four to seven years such that in 1987, 5.96% of all public elementary school students (in Baltimore county) were receiving such treatment.

JAMA 260:2256; 1988

How will Avita Average address those problems?" Choua asked after reading the journal excerpt.

"With nutritional and ecologic approaches. By eliminating orange juice, candies, colas and cakes, and by looking into food sensitivities and mold allergy."

"And?"

"And by paying attention to the bowel ecosystem."

"I certainly agree all human antioxidant and immune defenses are plants rooted in the soil of the bowel contents. All essential antioxidant and immune battles are waged—and won or lost—in the bowel. Even when holistic physicians talk about the essential detoxification role of the liver, they often neglect the guardian angel of the liver ecosystem. It's the bowel ecosystem that protects the liver ecosystem from the onslaught of toxins. Without the bowel barriers, the liver would be so inundated with undigested foods, macromolecules and toxins that it could never function. As good as the liver is in breaking down toxins, it has a finite capacity. Without the bowel protection, it would go under within a few hours."

ANTIBIOTICS FOR LITTLE JANES AND JOHNNIES

"How will Betty Best manage ear infections in little Janes and Johnnies?" Choua resumed.

"With antibiotics and with ear tubes," I replied.

"How well do antibiotics work for recurrent ear infections in children?"

"Antibiotics do not always give satisfactory results."

"So, what do you do for your little Janes and Johnnies?"

"Actually, Choua, they do extremely well if you can identify the reasons why they catch ear infections frequently in the first place. I have never yet seen a child with ear infections who does not have food sensitivities, and most of them have mold allergy as well."

"So, an underlying allergy causes the edema that blocks the tubes connecting the throat with the middle ear."

"Yes."

"Why doesn't Betty Best see that? Why doesn't she manage allergy right so little Janes and Johnnies don't develop recurring ear infections?"

"I suppose because she doesn't believe that such an allergy exists, or at the very least that it has anything to do with ear infections."

"Do they think ear infections come from Mount Olympus?"

"No, infections are caused by microbes."

"But why only in some children? Why not in everyone? Betty Best will never ask that question."

"Oh, shush, Choua!" I laughed.

"You said antibiotics do not always give satisfactory

results. How often does that happen?" Choua laughed too.

"I don't know the statistics."

"Well, I do!" Choua reached for a copy of a journal, "Here is a quote about the efficacy of antibiotics for ear infections:

> *... the effect is limited (six patients need to be treated to improve the outcome in one) and is of relatively short duration.*
>
> *JAMA* 271:1349; 1993

The effect is limited! Now, you see how it works, don't you?" Choua rubbed his hands.

"That's a gross misrepresentation! You can prove anything that way—just take things out of context, quoting bits and pieces from articles to make your point," I protested.

"Taking bits and pieces, eh!" Choua groused and shuffled the pages of the *Journal* rapidly, and then read:

No significant differences were shown between placebo and antibiotics in the eight studies of long-term outcome of OME (otitis media with effusion).

JAMA 270:1344; 1993

No significant differences! This is a meta-analysis of *eight* studies. It was conducted to resolve the brouhaha over treatment of ear infections in children with long-term broad-spectrum antibiotic therapies. That's not taking bits and pieces from literature," Choua frowned.

"There are other studies that show antibiotics do work," I persisted.

"I know! I know! There is that study published in the *New England Journal of Medicine* that drug doctors are fond of quoting."

"But that is a good study and it shows that antibiotics work for about half the children with ear infections."

"Yeah! Yeah!" Choua grimaced, picked up a copy of another journal and said, "This is the truth behind that famous *New England Journal of Medicine* study:

...a 4-year study which found that children who took amoxicillin for a middle ear infection were twice as likely to be cured as those who took a placebo, or inactive substance. The team's work was published in the Feb. 19, 1987 New England Journal of Medicine...However, one of the Pittsburgh researchers disagreed with that conclusion. He submitted a separate paper to the **New England Journal of Medicine,** *citing no appreciable differences between the antibiotic and the placebo. Charges flew back and forth, and it took until Dec 18, 1991, for the second paper to be published, in the* **Journal of the American Medical Association (JAMA).**

Science News 146:332; 1994

Charges flew back and forth! So much for the *rigorous* science of the *Journal.* It publishes the side of the story that says antibiotics worked for half of the children but refused to publish the other side that showed antibiotics to be useless. See the magic of medical statistics! The same data is reported as a clear proof of antibiotic efficacy and again as a clear proof of their ineffectiveness."

"So, how do you know which interpretation is right?" I asked.

"The second! I *know* antibiotics cannot work for ear infections over the long haul," Choua snapped and picked up the copy of the *JAMA* issue again. "Listen to this:

The pathogenesis of OME involves eustachian tube dysfunction as well as, in some cases, the presence in the middle ear of pathogenic bacteria. It is perhaps unreasonable to expect that a brief course of antibiotics will produce lasting benefits for this condition, given the continued role of the eustachian tube dysfunction.

JAMA 270:1350; 1993

Unreasonable to expect lasting effects! How can anyone reasonably expect long-term benefits of therapies that do not address the underlying food and mold allergies? Do you know what is the most remarkable thing about this article?" Choua asked as he looked up from the page of the *Journal.*

"What?" I asked back.

"The Betty Bests from Case Western Reserve University School of Medicine who wrote the article did not mention one word about the allergy that causes eustachian tube dysfunction and subsequent fluid in the ear."

"A bad mistake!" I agreed.

"How many children do you see who live on antibiotics for ear infections and have ear tubes inserted repeatedly?"

"It's not uncommon."

"How often do these little Janes and Johnnies show all negative test results for food and mold allergy?"

"Not often."

"Not often? Does it ever happen?" Choua's eyes narrowed.

"You're right, Choua," I yielded. "I have never seen that in my practice. Our children with ear infections almost always show evidence of food sensitivities as well as mold allergy."

"Here is another interesting item:

The group collected nasal mucus at regular intervals between age 1 month and 24 months from 216 infants in Buffalo who had never taken antibiotics before. They found that 96 percent of M (Moraxella) catarrhalis bacteria did not respond to penicillin, 90 percent were unaffected by ampicillin and 19 percent did not respond to trimethoprim-sulfamethaxozole, all antibiotics commonly used to fight otitis media...We have learned that some commonly used drugs are no longer valuable..."

Science News 146:333; 1994

Some commonly used drugs are no longer valuable! What do you think little Jane's chances are of escaping such a course of antibiotics when her mother takes her to Betty Best?" Choua asked.

"Not every university pediatrician rushes to prescribe antibiotics for kids with otitis media," I replied.

"When university pediatricians do not give antibiotics, what else do they do? Do they ever prescribe herbs and nutritional therapies for otitis media?"

"I don't think so."

"So their choices are limited to prescribing antibiotics or doing nothing at all. They will insert ear tubes or do nothing. Since they don't believe in food allergy or mold sensitivity, they obviously aren't going to look to right choices in the kitchen or immunotherapy for answers. Right?"

"Right!" I moaned. "Let's go on to the next subject, shall we?"

EAR TUBES ARE TWO-WAY CHANNELS

"When pediatricians recommend ear tubes for little Janes and Johnnies, do they ever tell the parents that ear tubes are going to expose to the outside what nature meant to be kept closed?" Choua asked.

"The middle ear chamber is not a closed chamber," I corrected Choua. "It is at all times in communication with the back of the throat which, of course, is part of the oral cavity. So, insertion of an ear tube in a child is not all that bad."

"I would think a pathologist would have more sense than to give that kind of silly explanation," Choua frowned.

"What's the difference?" I asked, angry at his insolence.

"Which way do the secretions travel? From the throat to the middle ear chamber, or from the middle ear to the throat?" Choua asked, tersely. "Which way do the cilia in the eustachian tubes direct the flow?"

"From the ear to the throat," I confessed, embarrassed at my obvious error.

"Is there any structure in the external ear that prevents entry of microbes into the middle ear via the ear tube?"

"No."

"You're a pathologist. You write about ecorelationships. You can't bypass nature's barriers and not pay a price. Why don't you write about that?" Choua exhorted. "Aren't there studies that show the downside of ear tubes?"

"I thought you didn't believe in medical statistics," I pointed out. "So, it is okay to use medical statistics when they support your contentions and it isn't acceptable when they refute your positions. Is that it?"

DRUGS TO DROWN SENSES

"Let's move on to drugs for drowning the senses," Choua suggested, without commenting on my remarks—that was so much like him, never acknowledging when he lost an argument.

"Drowning the senses? Whose senses?" I asked.

"Drugging people to calm them!" Choua continued. "Because when they are offended, they scream. Now, we can't have people screaming in the workplace, can we?"

"Oh! You mean anxiety problems and panic attacks."

"And sleep disorders and jitteryness and heart palpitations."

"What about them?"

"How will Betty Best treat anxiety attacks and sleep problems. Let's talk about that."

"No!" I said emphatically. "You have wailed against them

enough."

"Then, we will talk about what Betty Best will do for the poor and downtrodden—those who live Valium-deprived lives."

"No!" I repeated firmly. "You had your day with that as well."

"Shall we take up the matter of drugs that Betty Best will administer to those who stay awake at night?"

"Not that either!" I declined equally firmly.

"How about breathing machines Betty Best will stick up the noses of their patients after they diagnose one of their seventy-one sleep disorders?"

"Choua, haven't we covered all that enough?" I asked, irritated by his persistence.

"Poor Betty Best! You won't let her practice her craft. How will she ever make a living?"

"Oh shush, Choua!" I scolded him.

DRUGS FOR DEPRESSION: THE DEMISE OF AN AMINO ACID

"What will Betty Best do for depression?" Choua continued.

"Depression is a tough problem. You have to use antidepressants often."

"How will Avita Average manage depression?"

"Not well, I'm afraid!"

"What do you do for depression?"

"I think the only true long-term answer to that problem is self-regulation and meditation, but that takes months or years for patients to learn well enough to be effective—and self-regulation is so much harder for people who are depressed."

"So what do you do for depression while you teach them autoregulation?"

"They suffer."

"What else do you do?"

"Eliminating metabolic roller coasters helps. Teach limbic exercise. That helps! Instill hope! Spirituality! Anything that helps. Of course, it's true that creating hope is easy, sustaining it for a depressed patient takes every ounce of a physician's energy."

"What about tryptophane?"

"Ah, tryptophane! That used to be quite valuable when used with tyrosine. Tryptophane at night to support serotonin—the major night neurotransmitter—and tyrosine in the morning to support epinephrine—the principal day neurotransmitter! That helped almost all depressed patients, though not sufficiently to avoid drugs in all cases."

"So, why aren't those amino acids used now?"

"You know why, Choua! The FDA banned them a few years ago."

"Why did the FDA ban the use of an essential amino acid that is present in milk, meats and other foods?"

"Because some batches of tryptophane were thought to be contaminated."

"Thought to be?"

"There were a few patients who suffered from eosinophilic myalgic syndrome, but I'm not sure that was a valid entity. I don't know if there ever was any valid proof that tryptophane ever hurt anyone."

"How many hundreds of thousands of people are made sicker by antidepressants? Are there any antidepressants that never cause serious side effects?"

"None!"

"So, why doesn't the FDA ban all antidepressants? What

is it about nutrients that irks them so? A few people come down with a reversible disorder due to a chemical contaminant and they ban the amino acid. Millions of people suffer from drug toxicity yet that is acceptable. How do they justify that?"

"Ask the FDA that question," I responded.

SEVEN YEARS OF BETA AND CALCIUM CHANNEL BLOCKADE

"What will the beta blockers do? Of course, block the beta receptors. So for a while they control heart palpitations or lower blood pressure. Do beta blockers ever reverse heart disease? Do they ever dissipate the stress that causes high blood pressure? Or eliminate the risk factors that cause heart attacks or high blood pressure? If Betty Best doesn't already know this at the beginning of this study, she will certainly find it out by the end. Seven years is a long time to block someone's beta receptors. Tell me, why do you need to block anyone's beta receptors in the first place?" Choua stopped to breathe.

"I guess because overactivity of beta receptors causes heart palpitations and high blood pressure. So it makes sense to block the overactive receptors," I said evenly.

"For seven years? For twenty-one years? Or would it be the remaining life span of the patient? Don't you see the absurdity in your logic? If the beta receptors are overactive, it means they are being overstimulated by something in the internal or external environment. Why not take the time to find out what those factors might be and address them?"

"Get real, Choua!" I said angrily. "You live in a world of your own. Those problems are real and heart palpitations can quickly get out of hand and prove dangerous."

"All the more reason to identify and remove the irritants! Limbic walks! Limbic breathing! Gratitude! Meditation! Spirituality. Aren't those the things you talk and write about and teach your patients?"

"University internists are not set up to do such stuff," I explained.

"That's the point! Betty Best cannot do what people with overactive beta receptors really need. She only knows how to prescribe drugs and drugs cannot solve the underlying problems, Mr. Pathologist!" Choua howled.

"You know, you can drive anyone crazy with your logic," I recoiled. "Most people simply are not ready for that stuff."

"How many people do you know who are not ready for that stuff?"

"My practice is different," I confessed.

"What does Betty Best use calcium channel blockers for?" Choua was unrelenting.

"For heart disease and high blood pressure."

"How do channel blockers work?"

"By blocking the channels! How else?"

"Do you think nature made channels in cell membranes so they can be blocked for decades without bad effects?"

"No, we need drugs for angina," I countered.

"Do calcium channel blockers reverse heart disease?"

"Of course, not!"

"Do they remove the factors that cause decreased blood vessel tone that results in hypertension?"

"I don't think so.

"Does Betty Best know all that when she prescribes those drugs for young people? Does she tell her patient the drugs are forever because they do not remove the basic cause of illness?"

DRUGS FOR BRONCHIAL TUBES IN PROTEST

"What is asthma?" he resumed after several moments.

"Attacks of wheezing that interfere with breathing. Tight bronchial tubes that do not let air in," I replied.

"Why do bronchial tubes tighten up during an asthma attack?"

"Because that's all they know. I mean I don't think they know how to write poems or computer software," I jested.

"Good! Good! I like that. Bronchial tubes don't write poetry when they protest the air they breathe or the immune reactions that occur within them. How do asthma drugs work?"

"They loosen up the bronchial tubes in spasm," I replied.

"And also shock the heart every time, don't they?" Choua scowled. "Isn't that the reason asthmatics who use inhalers regularly die earlier than those who don't? Wasn't that the gist of the British and Canadian studies?"

"Yes," I capitulated.

"So asthma drugs do not cure asthma, do they?"

"I don't know if anything cures asthma."

"Yes, that's true. But when you properly diagnose and treat mold allergy, and when you test for food sensitivities and eliminate or reduce the intake of foods that trigger bronchial spasm, you take away the reason for the bronchial tubes to rebel and go into spasm. Isn't that true? You presented the results of your asthma outcome studies at the Academy meetings. Isn't that what you showed?"

"Can we talk about something else, Choua?" I pleaded.

"If Betty Best isn't already aware of such things, she will

be after seven years," Choua spoke with a gentle smile.

KILLER OF IMMUNE CELLS, SAFE FOR OTHER TISSUES

"What does Avita Average do for patients with autoimmune disorders?"

"Supportive therapies! All the things that we have talked about several times," I replied flatly.

"Food and mold allergies, kitchen choices, herbal and nutrient therapies, minimizing exposure to pollutants and meditation. Right?"

"Right, but why do I suffer such a litany every time?" I protested.

"Just to make a point that all of Avita Average's therapies for immune disorders are supportive in nature. Now, let's move to Betty Best. She loves to suppress the immune system, doesn't she?" Choua asked impishly.

"Your cyclopean eye sees things in crooked ways," I teased.

"My cyclopean eye sees it clearly." Choua wasn't miffed. "What does Betty Best prescribe for rheumatoid arthritis, juvenile arthritis, lupus, psoriasis, temporal arteritis? Isn't it steroids? And when steroids don't work, she prescribes toxic chemotherapy drugs, doesn't she?"

"Choua, you don't understand!" I answered, frustrated. "Patients suffer and their suffering has to be relieved."

"How many times have you put a patient on long-term steroid therapy?" Choua sneered.

"I don't remember ever doing that because..."

"Because you manage your difficult problems with aggressive nondrug therapies and intramuscular or intravenous nutrient therapies," Choua cut me off rudely.

"It would be nice if you let me make my points myself," I said bitterly.

"Let me read a quote:

This drug has been found to cause the death of lymphocytes by apoptosis and to have relatively low toxicity toward other tissues.

Remarkable statement, isn't it?"

"It's not remarkable. It's astoundingly stupid," I answered with disbelief.

"Why? Why is it stupid?" Choua asked.

"Because the lymphocyte is an essential cell of the immune defense system," I explained. "How can any drug kill immune cells and be declared relatively safe. This is an absurd statement if I ever heard one!"

"I'm glad you said that! I didn't. This is a direct quote from page nine of the July 2, 1994 issue of the prestigious *Lancet.*"

"I don't believe the *Lancet* could have printed such an utterly stupid statement. The lymphocyte is the quarterback immune cell of the body. Killing lymphocytes is tantamount to total destruction of the immune system. No one can live for any length of time after his immune cells have been killed. No matter what the short-term advantages of lymphocyte killer drugs may be, such drugs cannot *not* damage all other body organs. Isn't that what we learned from chemotherapy drugs?"

"Well said! Well said!" Choua spoke condescendingly. "This article was written by the Betty Bests who are touting cladribine for multiple sclerosis. Cladribine, as you know, is a drug used in chemotherapy of lymphomas and leukemias when other drugs fail because it is such an efficient killer of helper T-lymphocytes. You will recall this was the article in which Betty Bests played that dirtying-up-the-placebo trick to make the placebo effect look so bad that the drug effect looked good by contrast."

"That's awful!" I felt angry.

"Now, you watch how Betty Best will carry this game further. She will tout this immune-killing drug for other autoimmune disorders. I hear there are studies going on to test this drug for hepatitis and lupus. It's sickening. They'll destroy whatever little immune defenses those poor patients are left with."

"How does Betty Best justify this?" I asked, a lump in my throat. "How do they convince the patients to enter such studies? What happened to informed consent?"

"Ah! Informed consent!" Choua moaned. "You don't think Betty Best is foolish enough to tell the patient the whole truth—that the drug is an immune cell killer, a lymphocyte destroyer. And that no matter what the short-term benefits of the drug may be, it is bound to get the patient for good. Do you think any patient will be gullible enough to fall for that? No sir! The way to entrap the unsuspecting sick is to first dazzle them with marble edifices of Star Wars medicine, mesmerize them with Star Wars medical technology, subdue them with white coats and dangling stethoscopes, and then pull out the consent forms showing how much public tax money has been allocated to the research protocol. Then the poor patient is ready for the kill! Then Betty Best can destroy whatever helper T immune cells he has left in his body."

"You don't need to be so graphic, Choua," I said, feeling sick.

"Here, I've a suggestion for you. You like to write. Why don't you ask the U.S. Congress to allocate some funds to study the long-term dire consequences of immunosuppressant drugs for chronic immune disorders? Evidently, Betty Best will not expose her dirty linen. Why don't you? On second thought, don't bother. Congress never allocates any money except when Betty Best decides who gets the money. There is no point to all this."

Of Maggots, Magnetism
and Medicine Men

"Enough about Avita Average and Betty Best!" I said with irritation. "Tell me, what is your medicine of physics?"

"What do maggots know about magnets that men of medicine in your medical schools do not?" Choua asked back.

"What do maggots have to do with physics in medicine?" I asked, exasperated.

"Maggots know things about health and sickness that your university internists do not," Choua replied churlishly.

"Will you for once give me a straight answer?" I asked, my temper rising.

"Do you know what happens if maggots are put in a cardboard box and a magnet is put close to the box?" Choua asked.

"What?" I asked, my anger melting as my curiosity took over.

"Maggots will move away from the side of the cardboard box closer to the north pole of the magnet."

"Is that really true?" I asked.

"Because they know the north pole is not good for them. They know if they do not move away from it, the magnetic influence of the north pole will kill them."

"Wow! Who told you that?" I couldn't contain myself.

"I think it was Albert Roy Davis who first wrote about such effects. There have been many others who studied the effects of magnetism on biologic systems."

"What do the maggots do if the box is small and they can't move away from the north pole?"

"Clever rascals, those maggots! They bore their way out of the cardboard box." Choua grinned.

"What happens if you put the south pole of the magnet close to the box?"

"They luxuriate!"

"Fascinating stuff! You are not making it up, are you?" I asked, uncertain of his demeanor.

"No," Choua grinned broadly this time. "Why does that surprise you. Don't you do your limbic run every morning facing east? Why not face west? Remember what you wrote in *Ghoraa*!"

"What?" I tried to see the link between my morning run and the maggots boring their way out of the cardboard box to escape the north pole of the magnet.

"You forget what you wrote. Facing east means the right side of your brain—the limbic side as you fondly term it—is under the calming influence of the south pole of the planet Earth—and sheltered from the excitatory influence of the north pole. See, maggots know what the ancients knew! Fascinating, isn't it? The ancients wrote about the benefit of facing east for morning meditation. Didn't they?" Choua chortled.

"Amazing! And funny!" I exclaimed.

"Do you think Betty Best knows how maggots react to the physical effects of electromagnetic forces on biology?"

"Oh, so that's what you mean by the physics of health!" I said, amused by Choua's circuitous way of answering my earlier question about the medicine of physics. "But, Choua, this is good for fun and games. Surely, you don't mean we treat serious problems with magnets. I mean, we have had enough problems with snake oils."

"You amaze me," Choua suddenly turned somber.

"What did I do?" I asked with bewilderment.

"You are a sharp pathologist but kind of slow when it comes to common sense," he grimaced.

"Why do you insult me at each step?" I nearly screamed.

"You practice empirical medicine every day and you write quite a bit about it," Choua was unaffected by my outburst. "But then you say things that reveal your ignorance about the *core* philosophy of empirical medicine."

"What core philosophy of empirical medicine?" I asked.

"Empirical medicine is about doing as many nontoxic things as you can to comfort the sick and reverse his illness," Choua replied softly. "When you use magnets for therapy, that's not all you do. In empirical medicine, you try *everything* that is nontoxic and likely to facilitate healing. Can't you understand something that elementary? You don't use magnetic field as the only therapy. I know it has a weak effect. You use it along with other weak but safe therapies based on the physics of health." His tone abruptly turned harsh again.

"Okay! Okay! You made your point," I groaned.

"The north pole kills bacteria; the south pole stimulates their growth."

"Then how is it that bacteria live at all? Why doesn't the north pole kill them all?" I saw the obvious weakness in Choua's statement and challenged him.

Choua seemed baffled for a few moments. I felt good at his discomfort. It isn't often that I see Choua speechless. Then he scratched his temple, looked around my office, pulled out a journal from a pile on the rug and read:

"Magnetosomes are intracellular, iron-rich, membrane-enclosed magnetic particles that allow magnetotactic bacteria to orient in

the earth's geomagnetic field as they swim.

Science 259: 803; 1993

Do you see, Mr. Innocent, that magnetic effects exist to guide living beings and not to kill them! But you can't see such simple things, can you? The north pole of a magnet kills bacteria when held close to them because its magnetic field is very strong due to close proximity. The geomagnetic fields are much weaker so they simply provide guiding influence to bacteria in their swim. Do you see what N^2D^2 medicine has done to your thinking faculty, Mr. Pathologist?"

"You are so obnoxious and..." I fumed and stopped myself in mid-sentence.

"The same physical effect occurs in human tissues," Choua continued, completely indifferent to my anger. "When holistic physicians use magnetic therapies, it is only to facilitate the healing response, recognizing that the magnetic effects may be mild. Many magnetic field researchers have reported beneficial effects of magnetic fields in a host of clinical disorders, including inflammatory and degenerative diseases. You have seen a few patients who report some benefits, haven't you?" he asked calmly.

"Yes, but how I could be sure of the value of magnetic therapies?" I calmed down. "There were so many other variables."

"You don't understand the core philosophy of empirical medicine, do you?" Choua shook his head. "*Variables are not important in chronic disease. Reversal of disease is!* Why is that so hard for you to understand? In empirical medicine, you use what is safe and works—for years, for the whole life span, not just for a few weeks or months. We are not talking about the three-months-mice-or-medical-student research which Prince Chaullahs of N^2D^2 medicine are so fond of."

PULLING ELECTRONS OUT, PUSHING ELECTRONS AWAY

"How does a cancer cell differ from a noncancer cell?" Choua asked me the next day.

"A cancer cell continues to multiply mindlessly while a noncancer cell replicates only when needed for the healing response," I answered.

"How does a cancer cell differ from a noncancer cell in a physical sense?"

"A cancer cell has a much stronger negative charge on its cell membrane. Noncancer cells usually have -2 to -3 millivolts surface charge and a cancer cell may be as high as -200 to -300 millivolts."

"What does that mean?"

"A cancer cell has a whole lot of electrons on its membrane."

"How does that happen?"

"I wish I knew. It probably has something to do with the mode of metabolism in a cancer cell—the mode in which sugars are burned up without utilizing oxygen—and also perhaps with the way a cancer cell produces hydrogen peroxide in quantities much larger than those seen in a noncancer cell. Electrons accumulate at the cell membrane to compensate for excessive positive charges within the cell. But, why do you ask me these questions?"

"Because there is a wonderful opportunity here to treat cancer using the physics of health rather than the chemistry of disease," Choua spoke seriously and then chuckled suddenly, "but it won't happen!"

"Why?" I asked, bewildered by the abrupt changes in Choua's tone.

"A simple machine required to remove the excessive charge will take about two-hundred dollars to build but it will take four-hundred million dollars to get FDA approval. So no one will be foolish enough to try that."

THERAPIES BASED ON PHYSICS OF HEALTH

"Do you know why they revoked Dr. David Saunder's license?" Choua asked when he returned after some hours.

"I heard it had something to do with magnetic therapies, but I'm not sure," I replied.

"You heard right!" Choua said in a terse tone and walked to the window. "Why are drug doctors adamantly opposed to magnetic therapies?" he asked without looking at me.

"Because they have not been proven effective with valid scientific studies," I offered the usual explanation.

"Valid scientific studies, my foot!" Choua erupted. "It's disgusting how such things work. All drug doctors use MRI scans these days. Don't they see what MRI stands for: magnetic resonance imaging."

"What does that have to do with magnetic therapies?" I asked, confused about Choua's reference to MRI scans in a discussion of magnetic therapies.

"Everything! Drug doctors accept electromagnetic technology as valid only if it leads to drug therapies or surgery. When energy technologies are used to promote health by physical, nondrug approaches, they balk and declare them unscientific and those who practice them quacks and charlatans."

"Well..."

"All ancient Chinese therapies based on the concept of *Chi* energy are dismissed as ineffective and wasteful. All Indian yoga energy methods are rejected as witchcraft. Effective massage therapies are looked down upon as perversions of the obsessed. Homeopathy is effective for hundreds of millions of people all over the world. Almost one-third of Europeans regularly use such remedies. Yet, the drug doctors insist homeopathy is a fraud. Why? Because they cannot understand the physical principles upon which it is based!"

"Because modern science wants *hard* proof for the efficacy of therapies," I interjected.

"Hard proof, my foot," Choua shrieked. "Haven't I shown you the deception of the *hard* proof of the beloved drug therapies of disease doctors? Do you want more proof of that? Do you?" Choua fumed.

"No! No!" I recoiled. "I don't need any more of your discourses on drug therapies."

"When you're stuck with poor results, how do you diagnose food sensitivity?" Choua howled.

"With electrodermal conductance technology," I replied.

"That's what I mean by the medicine of physics! When you teach your patients self-regulation, what technologies do you use?"

"Electrodermal conductance and electromyography."

"That's what I mean by the medicine of physics! How do you assess oxidative stress on blood proteins and blood cells?"

"By high-resolution microscopy."

"That's what I mean by the medicine of physics!" Choua bellowed.

Dysregulated Money Metabolism

"Money metabolism in medicine in the U.S. is dysregulated," Choua spoke after a while.

"How so?" I asked.

"Medicine in the United States metabolizes money in ways that no one can understand. Certainly, it baffles your economists more than any other group. It was not so many years ago that people were dismayed at medicine because it spent nearly five-billion dollars of public funds. There was a general sense then that the cost of sickness in the U.S. was exorbitant. More troubling than that was the fact that it was not clear what that money was buying for our citizens."

"Technology costs money."

"In 1995, things are quite different," Choua went on. "Now you take in stride an annual bill of one trillion dollars and glibly dismiss any talk about what this money is or isn't buying for you. The Clinton Administration and Congress now share a common pursuit: how to finance the projected increases in health care by taxing cigarettes and liquor. Now, isn't that a riot?"

"I do not have any grasp of numbers that reach in hundreds of millions, let alone in trillions," I replied.

"You doctors thought the cost of care didn't matter. Well, it does! Do you know what I think will do you doctors in?"

"What?"

"Star Wars technology. You thought it was too much of a bother to listen to a patient when he complained of a headache. You thought it was easier to send him for an MRI. Well, the chickens are coming home to roost. Now, the insurance company pays you fifty-dollars for your consultation and twelve-hundred dollars to the fellow who owns the MRI machine. Do you see the problem?"

"I'm afraid it will get worse," I agreed.

"You gave up high-touch medicine for no-touch high-tech. And now that is killing you. The irony is you keep looking for answers in more technology. You drug doctors have a death wish."

THE MORE MONEY BETTY BEST SPENDS, THE SICKER HER PATIENTS GET

"The incidence of breast, prostate and many other cancers is increasing. The incidence of asthma and other chronic lung disorders is increasing. The incidence of arthritis in our young, including children, is increasing and so is the incidence of other ecologic and immune disorders.

"Hyperactivity and attention disorders among our children used to be uncommon problems. By 1987, one of every sixteen children in the public elementary schools in Baltimore county were on drugs for discipline in school (*JAMA* 260:2256;1988). A more frightening part of this survey was what the researchers described as 'consistent doubling of the rate of medication for hyperactive/ inattentive students every four to seven years.' I know of some communities in the U.S. where—thanks to some aggressive school psychiatrists and obliging pediatricians—up to ten percent of school children are drugged for discipline. I wonder if such care givers have ever heard of sugar-insulin-adrenaline roller coasters that are driving many children into hyperactivity and inattentiveness.

"Chronic fatigue is a spreading pandemic. After dismissing tired young people as overprivileged, underworked yuppies, N^2D^2 docs are reporting chronic fatigue as the presenting complaint in twenty-one to twenty-five percent of their patients *(JAMA* 257:2303; 1987 and 260:929; 1988).

"You proudly claim that health care in the U.S. is the best in the world—a pretty safe statement as long as we make it out of the earshot of Western Europeans and the Japanese. What we don't say—largely because we have no compelling reason to show others our dirty laundry—is that we are really very good for *people near death.* We do not quite understand what health is—when was the last time the *New England Journal of Medicine* published an article defining what health is and how one might go about teaching people how to preserve it?

"You proudly claim that we must be the best in the world or foreigners wouldn't choose to come here over any other place for heart surgery. Actually, they do, but somehow they neither seek our clearance before surgery nor inform us after it. I wonder what we can do about that! Cardiac surgery—as those who successfully reverse heart disease with chelation therapy know—is not a hot item anyway.

"For acute, life threatening illnesses, intensive medical and surgical care is expensive but clearly essential. Indeed, for such care, the U.S. is peerless. The case for management of chronic ecologic, immune, nutritional and stress-related disorders, however, is quite different. You know from personal experience that nondrug therapies widely used in Europe, China, India and other countries offer superior clinical outcomes at a fraction of the cost that we Americans pay. The only physicians who question this statement are those who have had no direct experience with such therapies.

"Let me show how the cost of care stacks up in different countries:

HEALTH CARE SPENDING PER CITIZEN, 1991, U.S. DOLLARS	
United States	$2,868
Canada	$1,915
Germany	$1,659
France	$1,650
Sweden	$1,443
Italy	$1,408
Japan	$1,307
Great Britain	$1,043
Spain	$ 848

Source: *Organization for Economic Cooperation and Development*

"The Canadians always look to the U.S. for enlightenment, don't they?" Choua asked.

"Who told you that?" I asked.

"I know they don't like to admit that, but that's the reality. Don't they pattern their health care after the U.S.?"

"No, not really. Look at their health care system. It's quite distinct from our."

"There may be a slight difference here and there in the reimbursement plan, but I'm talking about the philosophy of medicine. The Canadian N^2D^2 docs loathe the holistic physicians in Canada with as much zest as they do here in the U.S., don't they?"

"In that sense, you're right," I confessed.

"Here is an interesting quote about Canadian medicine:

Canadians are proud of a system that generally provides good care...But spending in recent years has grown nearly as fast as in the United States, and is outstripping the ability of the public sector to pay...

German hospitals have fewer pieces of high-technology equipment than most big urban hospitals in the United States. Still, with a mounting demand for medical services, costs have been soaring here too, putting the insurance funds billions of dollars in the red last year.

The New York Times November 14, 1993

See, common sense in medicine is as uncommon in Canada as it is in the U.S."

"How does Betty Best fare in Canada?" I asked.

"Just as poorly as she does in the U.S. She is infatuated

with drugs just as much her American sister."

HOLISTIC MOLECULAR RELATEDNESS IN HUMAN BIOLOGY

"In *The Butterfly and Life Span Nutrition,* you wrote about the principle of holistic molecular relatedness in biology. What does that mean?"

"Just what it says—that no molecule in human biology works in a vacuum, each is related to every other no matter how different or distinct it might appear."

"Do you think Betty Best knows about that principle?"

"It's a simple principle. I don't see any reason why she wouldn't."

"How could she prescribe drugs for single symptoms and still profess to practice in accord with the principle of holistic molecular relatedness?" Choua sneered.

"That is a problem," I confessed. "University internists really cannot use that principle. It doesn't fit into the practice of drug medicine."

THERE ARE NO BIG FINISHES IN CHRONIC DISEASE

"Betty Best will do a lot of tests and then make elegant diagnoses. Next, she will pull out her prescription pad. For a while, her patients will feel better. Drugs do suppress symptoms."

"Drugs *do* work and we *do* need them," I said emphatically.

"Betty Best has a big problem."

"What's that?" I asked.

"Betty Best hasn't yet found out that there are no big finishes in chronic disease," Choua murmured softly and looked out the window.

"How do you mean? What big finishes?"

"There are no big finishes in chronic disease," Choua repeated, without turning to face me. "Months later, the glory of the diagnosis dissipates. Drug efficacy diminishes. Toxic effects of drugs accumulate. The oxidative coals of chronic disease simmer."

"So?"

"Years later, chronic disease persists—usually gets worse. Betty Best will have to keep changing her drugs, substituting newer, more potent and toxic drugs for the older drugs that won't work anymore. At the end of the seven-year-blockade, Betty Best will be left with sicker patients who require increasing doses of drugs."

"As usual you exaggerate," I admonished Choua.

"Exaggerate?" Choua shifted uneasily. "Name one drug that will be as effective after seven years of regular use as it was when first prescribed."

"There are millions of people who regularly take drugs with good results," I offered a defense for the safe use of medications.

"I know. And there are just as many millions who hate the daily ritual of taking drugs," Choua snapped. "I sometimes wish the older Betty Bests would have the courage to reflect on their work. Reflect on the fate of children who were given radiotherapy for tonsillitis or enlarged thymuses and who now have underactive thyroid glands and cold sensitivity! Consider the outcome of rearing children on antibiotics, who now suffer from chronic fatigue states! See the hideous obesity of people given steroid therapy! Think about the misery of young women with cancer of the cervix caused by DES hormone given to their mothers during their pregnancies! Recognize the destruction of immune defenses by chemotherapy drugs administered to patients with injured immune systems! Sense the disappointment of men made impotent by their high blood pressure drugs! Know the anger of people who had coronary bypass surgery only to be told a year later that they needed to have their chests cut open again!

"I sat with Jim the other day while he had a chelation drip. He had a bypass operation in 1984. He was told he needed a second operation in 1987. He was taking five cardiac drugs and suffered daily chest pains and heart palpitations. That's when he started chelation therapy. I saw a progress note you wrote in November, 1994. He didn't take a single pill after January, 1994. He walks three to four miles a day. As far as an occasional episode of chest tightness is concerned, he simply breathes it away with limbic breaths. When you first saw him, his wife insisted on therapy but he simply talked about leaving this world with dignity. Now he looks at his heart disease as a past event—a bad nightmare. Oh, how I wish Betty Best could sit with him and listen to his story! How I wish she could see him swell up with anger at the mere mention of heart surgery!" Choua heaved as he finished the last sentence and then slowly left the room.

Courageous or Reckless

The efficacy of nutrients and herbs in the management of chronic disorders has been well-known to hundreds of thousands of physicians who use such therapies and to hundreds of millions of people all over the world who have received such therapies. The only doctors who do not know about them are those who have never tried them.

Several years ago, I presented a paper about nutrient therapies for ecologic disorders at the meeting of the American Academy of Environmental Medicine. During the break, a physician in his late seventies came over, warmly shook my hand and said,

"Dr. Ali, you are a courageous man!"

"Thank you," I replied courteously.

"You are a very courageous man," he repeated.

"Thank you again," I repeated, wondering what it might be that seemed to have impressed him.

"No, really, you are a courageous man. Quite extraordinary!" he went on.

"That's awfully nice of you, but tell me what did I do to be regarded as courageous?" I asked, curious about his exuberance. "What did I say that was so extraordinary?"

"Nothing! It wasn't anything that you said," he smiled.

"Oh! Was it the way I said it?" I asked, quite curious about his comment now.

"No, it wasn't that either."

"So, then what was it?"

"What you said was true. I know that."

"How do you know it was true?" I asked, my curiosity piqued.

"What you said about nutrient therapies is true. I know that because I have used them for over fifty years now."

"So then what is it that makes me extraordinary?"

"Your courage."

"Courage? What is courageous about saying nutrients work?"

"Dr. Ali, I have been going to medical meetings for decades. I have never seen a man of your credentials stick his neck out and talk about treating his patients with vitamins and herbs. University doctors talk a lot about vitamins and minerals but they never have the courage to put their research findings into practice. They talk much about nutrients but never prescribe them for their patients. Those of us who practice nutritional medicine have talked about vitamin therapies for decades, but always in hushed tones and only behind closed doors. Never out in the open the way you are doing it. It takes a lot of guts to do that. You are a courageous man, an extraordinary man."

Courageous or reckless! I murmured to myself. *Extraordinary or foolhardy.* Who knows?

No shrine is holier than the human frame,
for it houses the human spirit.

Caring for this shrine is a scared trust, sacred for the patient and sacred for the physician. It is this trust which sets medicine apart from other professions.

The Cortical Monkey and Healing

Molecular medicine is not an easy way out for the poorly informed physician. It is not an exemption from the labor of learning and knowing. Knowledge of the molecules of physiology of fitness, of pharmacology of nutrients, of chemistry of environment, of immunology of allergy, of pathology of autoimmunity and biology of self-regulation—these are the essentials for the practitioner who takes this less travelled road.

The Cortical Monkey and Healing

Chapter 11

Betty Best in Seven-Board Wonderland

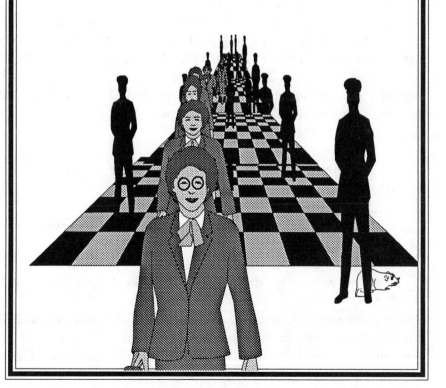

Rats
and Food and Nutrition Board

A tall, slender intern in a white coat entered my office and politely asked if I had time to review the lung biopsy of her patient. I pulled the biopsy slides from a pile of trays, then invited her to sit across my double-headed microscope and study the lesion with me. Pleased with my offer, she sat down on a high stool by the microscope, removed her glasses, and peered through the eyepieces of the scope. She spoke as she looked, giving clinical information about the case. The slides showed an epidermoid cancer—a common type of lung malignancy among smokers. With the microscope pointer, I demonstrated the microscopic features of that cancer type. She asked a few questions about the biologic behavior of various types of lung cancer, talked a little about the treatment options, thanked me profusely for taking time to go over the case with her and left.

"A caring and a compassionate young doctor!" Choua remarked.
"Yes." I replied.
"Soft-spoken and knowledgeable! She has a nice way about her. She will do well."
"I think so."
"She will make an excellent Betty Best Internist, M.D., won't she?"
"Oh shush, Choua!" I said, annoyed at Choua's uncalled for comment. "You can't help yourself, can you? You see a young woman at the threshold of her medical career. She looks good. She

speaks well. She obviously knows her stuff. But all your cyclopean eye can see in her is a Betty Best. Shame on you!" I scolded Choua.

"That's the point," Choua retorted. "Why aren't nice young physicians like her drawn into your natural ways of facilitating the healing response? Why are they always pulled by drug medicine? Why are they not persuaded to pursue the kind of medicine that saves people from surgery rather than the one that uses scalpels on them? Why can't nice women like her do the right things?"

"Oh shut up, will you?" I screamed at him. "Get off her case. Poor thing! All she came here was to look at the biopsy of her patient. And you can't help but make your ugly comments."

Choua seemed shaken by my harsh words. He opened his mouth to say something but changed his mind and looked down instead. My anger melted as I saw him look around timidly then pick up a tenth edition of the *Daily Recommended Allowances* that lay on my desk. Next, he buried his face into the opened pages of the book and started reading. I went back to my microscope.

"What do you think of RDAs?" I asked after several moments, a trifle uneasy for scolding him.

"Rubbish!" Choua mumbled, without looking up from the book.

"And government RDA experts?" I prodded.

"Pseudoscientists peddling petty pseudoscience," he muttered, his face still buried in the open book.

"No, seriously, Choua, what do you think of the experts who sit on the Food and Nutrition Board and establish RDA amounts for nutrients?" I pressed.

"RDA! That's rats stuff!" Choua looked up, still looking unnerved, then went back to the book, "Pretty stupid, isn't it? That ratty RDA stuff!"

"Strong words! Be polite, Choua" I said gently. "The members of the Board are eminent professors from prestigious medical schools."

"I didn't say they were not eminent professors from prestigious medical schools," Choua said, somewhat apologetically, looking squarely at me now. "I said they are pseudoscientists peddling petty pseudoscience. Talking about things they know nothing about."

"You're cranky today. Or, shall I say, in a ratty disposition?" I humored him.

"Rubbish!" Choua grimaced. "I mean that RDA stuff is for the rats, guinea pigs and the like. It is the ratty nutrition of N^2D^2 docs. It has nothing to do with real people. It's the pseudoscience rubbish of the pseudoscientists of N^2D^2 medicine!" Choua continued petulantly.

"C'mon Choua, RDAs must have some value. I mean, why else would physicians everywhere in the world accept them?" I pressed.

"Physicians everywhere?" Choua frowned. "You don't buy that rats nonsense. Do you?"

"Well! I don't, but the majority of physicians do." I answered haltingly.

"Do they?" Choua's eyes narrowed. "Do they really?"

"I think, they..."

"How many docs take one, two or more thousand milligrams of vitamin C? Isn't that mega-dose vitamin therapy? Far in excess of the ludicrous ratty RDA amounts?" Choua interrupted me. "That RDA stuff is for intellectual dissertations at medical conferences and patients! It isn't for the physicians or their families."

"Some do," I agreed.

"Some? That's not what I hear. Most of N^2D^2 docs take vitamin pills themselves and give some to their family members as well," Choua said testily.

"That's true," I conceded. "So?"

"So what?" Choua looked perplexed.

"So, what do you think of RDA?" I reiterated my question.

"What do I think of RDA?" Choua repeated after me, articulating each word slowly. "I think RDA is a perverse notion."

"A perverse notion?" Choua took me by surprise.

"Yes! A perverse notion! A pernicious idea! A misbegotten creed of pseudoscientists," Choua groused. "A stupid and silly concept—an utterly unscientific notion that denies hundreds of millions of sick people the nutrients that can help them recover from illness. It's a pernicious idea because it slanders nutrient therapies and pimps drug therapies."

"Now that's absurd," I contradicted him. "Explain to me how the concept of RDA pimps drugs?"

"It prevents hundreds of thousands of physicians from prescribing effective nutrient therapies for degenerative, ecologic, immune and nutritional disorders. Since it blinds N^2D^2 docs to safe, nontoxic alternatives to drugs, they have no choice but to use toxic drug therapies. It is the most calamitous invention of N^2D^2 doctors. And..."

Choua stopped in mid-sentence and began to shuffle pages of the RDA book. Choua usually has strong opinions, and he does not mince words when expressing them. Like most of my colleagues in nutritional medicine, I consider the idea of RDA obsolete and irrelevant to my clinical practice. Choua is right about mainstream physicians as well. Most of them think RDA values are too conservative. But, RDAs—a perverse notion? A pernicious idea? I thought Choua had gone too far. Still, Choua's choice of words jolted me a bit. I looked at Choua in silence for some moments. His eyes were glued to the pages of the book. Choua has a remarkable ability to say highly inflammatory things

about a subject one moment, and then be totally engrossed in
another the next moment. I regarded him with amusement for
some more moments, then decided to provoke him.

"Perverse notion. Bah, humbug!" I teased. "Tell me,
Choua, why do government experts hang on to RDAs if the idea
is so pernicious? What's in it for them?"

"Experts, my foot!" Choua responded with irritation.

"C'mon, Choua, be reasonable. Why do government
experts hold RDA so sacred?" I persisted.

"How do these government experts become experts in
human nutrition?" Choua frowned again.

"I guess because they specialize in these matters, that's
why?"

"Specialize in *what*?" he asked, his voice turning shrill at
the last word.

"Nutrition. Recommended Daily Allowances." I answered
evenly.

"You read a lot about nutrition. Don't you?" Choua asked,
his voice calm now.

"Some." I answered.

"You have read the names of the people who sit on the
Food and Nutrition Board—the folks who establish RDA values.
Haven't you?"

"Yes, I have."

"Do any of them actually practice nutritional medicine?"

"I don't know. Well...No. Not to my knowledge." I
admitted.

"You travel extensively for medical conferences. Don't
you?"

"Some."

"And you often lecture about treating diseases with
nutrients?"

"Yes, that's correct."

"Have you ever heard any of the Board members lecture on the treatment of diseases with nutrients?"

"I don't recall!"

"You see a lot of patients treated by other doctors. Have you ever seen a patient who was managed nutritionally by any of the Board members?"

"I don't think so."

"You publish clinical outcome studies of nutrient therapies. Have you ever seen any article by any of the Board members reporting success or failure with nutrient therapies for chronic diseases?"

"They publish epidemiologic studies about the efficacy of various nutrients," I posited.

"That's not what I mean!" Choua snapped. "I mean nutrient therapies for real people with real illnesses!"

"Well..."

"Well, then tell me, what makes members of the Food and Nutrition Board experts on human nutrition?" Choua asked belligerently. "They don't practice nutritional medicine. They practice drug medicine. They don't prescribe nutritional therapies. They pimp pharmaceuticals. They don't conduct research in the clinical uses of nutrients. They perform double-blind cross-over drug studies. They don't lecture at clinical nutrition conferences. They speak at drug conferences."

"But, Choua," I protested, "basic research has to precede clinical use of nutrients."

"Rats research?" Choua pouted. "Yes, I agree they are experts of rat research? Experts in feeding this vitamin or that mineral to mice or medical students for weeks or months? Yes, that too! Experts of double-blind and cross-over statistics? Yes, why not? But experts of clinical nutrition for humans? That they are not. It's amazing how *you* cannot see something *that* simple.

"You can't help but distort things," I observed acidly.

"For several years, you have conducted seminars in nutritional medicine," Choua ignored the irritation in my voice. "You have done so at the Instruction Courses of the American Academy of Environmental Medicine and the American Academy of Otolaryngic Allergy. Did you ever see any member of the blessed Food and Nutrition Board at those seminars?" Choua asked.

"I don't recall," I replied.

"You presented the results of your clinical studies about the efficacy of nutrient protocols at the conferences of the these two academies as well as at the meetings of the American College for Advancement in Medicine. Did you ever see a member of the Food and Nutrition Board at any of those conferences?"

"I don't think so."

"You conduct postgraduate training seminars in nutritional medicine at the Institute of Preventive Medicine in Denville, New Jersey. Did any member of the Food and Nutrition Board ever express an interest in reviewing your clinical results?"

"No!"

"Don't your clinical research and lectures bring you in contact with almost all members of the rather small community of nutritionist-physicians in the United States? Did any of those physicians ever tell you anything about clinical nutrition they might have learned from members of the Food and Nutrition Board?" Choua pressed.

"No," I yielded.

"Those RDA experts have no true-to-life clinical experience with nutrient therapies, do they?"

"Well..."

"Well what?" Choua interrupted me sharply. "The notion of RDA is a pernicious notion—and you know that! Those Food and Nutrition Board members are not scientists. They're pseudoscientists. Science, as you say, is observation. It is the search for truth. And true science in medicine is the science of empiricism. What is effective and safe and saves human lives is worthy of use, and what is toxic and hurts the sick, over the long haul, is unworthy. Do you agree?" Choua asked, his piercing eyes fixed on my face.

"Yes. No!" I blurted. "Science is not ignoring accumulated scientific knowledge about the structure and function of molecules in the body. You simply take things to an absurd degree. You can't turn your back on all the body of scientific knowledge about nutrition, can you?"

"You don't understand, do you?" Choua shook his head contemptuously. "Those who don't care for the sick with nutrients have no business talking about science in clinical nutrition. You and your RDA experts! *The double-blinded disciples of Aesculapius leading gullible Betty Best.*"

Rats
and Medical Curriculum Boards

"Do you know how N^2D^2 medicine makes N^2D^2 docs?" Choua asked me the next day.

"How?" I prepared for another onslaught.

"Medical students are intelligent and inquisitive young people. It isn't easy to sanitize their minds and divest them of those innate characteristics," Choua said impishly.

"Venom! Choua's venom again!" I suppressed a smile. "Pray, tell me Choua, how do medical schools sanitize the minds of medical students?"

"It is a grand plan—a carefully-crafted well-orchestrated strategy for actions. Slowly, persistently and inexorably, medical education strips them of common sense in matters of nutrition, health and disease," Choua winked.

"Go on," I prodded.

"How many practicing doctors do you think are affiliated with the medical school in Newark, New Jersey?" he asked.

"I don't know. Probably several hundred," I replied.

"Listen to this:

It is preferable to get antioxidants from foods like vegetables and fruits, because you are getting other nutrients and trace elements along with them.

This is a Ph.D.—not a medical doctor—writing in the winter 1994 issue of *HealthState*, the Magazine of UMDNJ New Jersey University of the Health Sciences."

"So?" I replied. "That's not bad advice."

"Not bad advice? Eh!" Choua grimaced. "Do you think this Ph.D. practices clinical medicine?"

"I don't think so. I mean Ph.Ds are not licensed to practice clinical medicine."

"So when this great magazine wishes to educate medical students about nutrition, the only person it can find to write about nutrients is a Ph.D. who is not allowed by law to practice clinical medicine. Why do you think...?"

"That's absurd!" I interrupted Choua. "Physicians do not have a monopoly on nutritional science. There are many people who earn their doctorate in nutrition and become very knowledgeable in nutrition science."

"I'm not talking about the ratty RDA nutrition of N^2D^2 docs," Choua retorted. "I'm talking about the clinical use of nutrients to manage sick people. The magazine couldn't find a single internist to write about his own clinical experience with nutrients! It couldn't find a single family practitioner to do that! Not a single pediatrician to do it. They had to pick a Ph.D., who has no real sense of what nutrition is all about, or how nutrients can be used to reverse chronic disorders. And he goes on to pronounce that people do not need antioxidant supplements."

"You know how it is in our medical schools. Nutritional medicine is considered quackery," I explained.

"Here is another illuminating quote," Choua continued. "Listen to this:

He does not take large doses of antioxidant supplements nor does he recommend it to others, though he does take a multivitamin occasionally. Instead, he makes a conscious effort to eat plenty of fresh fruits and vegetables. 'My first recommendation is to eat a balanced diet,' he advises.

A multivitamin occasionally!" Choua sneered. "Such foolish advice we can do without. I wonder why he takes an occasional multivitamin pill? What good can an occasional multivitamin pill do for him anyway? Why bother at all?" Choua snarled.

"Don't you think you are taking it too far?" I asked.

"What credentials does he have to advise people about nutrition any way?" Choua grunted. "He is not a clinician. He does not see sick people. He has never tried nutrient therapies. He has never evaluated the clinical efficacy of nutrients administered by others. What, on God's green earth, gives him the right to feed such nonsense to impressionable Betty Best?"

"Ease off the poor guy, Choua." I tried to calm him down. "You are reading too much into the piece. Probably all the editor of the magazine wanted to do was to carry an article about nutrition."

"So the editors can claim that they are enlightened and recognize the need for good nutrition?"

"I mean, I don't know if there is anyone at the medical school who practices clinical nutritional medicine. Besides..."

"That's the point!" Choua was now plainly agitated. "They

interviewed this poor Ph.D., who knows nothing about clinical nutritional medicine, because the practicing doctors there know nothing about nutrition there. And yet, they hail him as a nutrition expert who talks about a balanced diet. What, may I ask, is a balanced diet?" Choua frowned.

"Balanced diet! Oh, well..."

"What would someone like him know about balanced diet anyway? I bet all he knows about a balanced diet is what the dairy and orange industries and cholesterol cats have told him about it. It's pathetic, the way the magazine celebrates its nutrition experts. One silly statement follows another. Here, listen to this:

If you decide to supplement your diet, what's the right amount of antioxidant to take? According to Dr. XYZ, it's anybody's guess. Scientist have been unable to come up with an exact recommendation. Dr. XYZ suggests: 200-800 units of vitamin E; 1,000 to 2,000 milligrams of vitamin C; and 30 milligrams of beta-carotene daily. He says these amounts are based on continuing studies.

The RDA value of vitamin C is a mere 60 milligrams, and here he is advocating 1,000 to 2,000 milligrams of vitamin C! That's more than thirty 30 times the RDA value. Isn't someone prescribing mega-doses of vitamins a quack? Doesn't this make Dr. XYZ a quack? Aha! A quack on a medical school faculty?" Choua leered.

"Physicians are beginning to see the need for large doses

of micronutrients," I replied.

"How do you think those poor medical students cope with that? One expert tells them not to take any vitamin supplements while the other recommends thirty times the RDA amount of vitamin C!"

WHOSE SCIENCE?

"There are two sciences in medicine today," Choua snickered. "First, there is a ratty nutrition science of N^2D^2 docs who push drugs and put down nutrient therapies. Second there is the nutrition science of nutritionist-physicians who seek to reverse chronic disease with nutrients. Poor Betty Best! She has a large problem. She had a teenager's idealism to help the sick. In high school, the Food and Nutrition Board got to her with its stupid notions of RDA, and then in medical school, the Ph.D.s are out to get her with their erudite but phony dissertations about the clinical efficacy of nutrients. What chance does poor Betty Best have?"

"I think things are changing."

"Waiting for Godot, eh!" Choua blurted. "The gullible Betty Best! She is taught nutritional medicine by those who know nothing about it—have no true-to-life experience with it. Medical curriculum boards are populated by N^2D^2 docs whose knowledge of nutritional science is limited to the use of vitamin C for the prevention of scurvy, thiamine for beriberi, niacin for pellagra, vitamin B_{12} for pernicious anemia. The only clinical nutrition she will learn in medical schools is that nutrients are of no value in the care of the sick."

"At least they now talk about Vitamin C in doses of 1,000 to 2,000 milligrams daily," I sounded a note of hope.

"Poor Betty Best! She lives in a wonderland," Choua spoke with biting sarcasm. Her teachers teach her things of which they know nothing. She has no chance of using common sense—no chance of helping her patients with nutrient therapies when she leaves medical school. She looks up to her teachers. Alas! They are incarcerated in N^2D^2 medicine. She is destined to drug her patients for every symptom, every infirmity!" Choua replied with biting words. "*The double-blinded disciples of Aesculapius leading gullible Betty Best.*"

Rats,
and Hospital Medical Boards

Choua looked at me with impassive eyes for several moments, rubbed the back of his neck with both hands, picked a copy of a journal from my desk and started reading something. I went back to my surgical pathology cases.

"Are nutrient IV drips beneficial?" Choua asked me, without looking up from the pages of the journal.

"You know my answer to that question. Why would I use intravenous nutrient infusions if they were not very beneficial?" I replied. "What do nutrient IV drips have to do with that intern any way?"

"How do nutrient IVs help?" Choua ignored my question.

"We can manage many viral infections with nutrient IV drips and avoid unnecessary antibiotics. We often control severe asthma attacks, or at least markedly reduce the drugs required to control wheezing, with magnesium, molybdenum and vitamin B_{12} drips. My associates and I obtain good clinical responses for our patients with severe, disabling chronic fatigue. When given preoperatively and postoperatively, nutrient IV drips promote wound recovery and reduce the incidence of infections. Of course, EDTA infusions are very effective for solving problems caused by poor circulation such as leg cramps or intermittent claudication. There are many other good indications for IV infusion therapies."

"So, nutrient IV drips are useful. Why don't doctors in hospitals use them?"

"Because nutritional medicine is not practiced in hospitals. Mainstream physicians believe that micronutrients given in excess of the RDA amounts are of no clinical value."

"The RDA amounts! That rats stuff again! Why do N^2D^2 docs think nutrient IVs cannot help?" Choua pressed.

"Because hospitals are for very sick patients."

"Huh! You mean very sick people in the hospitals don't need nutrient IV drips while the not-very-sick people in your office do?" Choua winked.

"No! It's not that," I answered, flustered by his reasoning. "Didn't I tell you that physicians in hospitals do not believe in nutrient therapies. Also, nutrient IV drips may not work in acutely ill hospitalized patients."

"Have nutrient IV drips ever been tried in hospitals? If not, how can any one say that they are not useful in speeding up recovery from acute illnesses?"

"You have a point. But..."

"But what?" Choua cut me off rudely. "Nutrient IV drips can promote the healing responses in doctors' offices, but not in hospital wards. Is that it?"

"In a way that's true," I said. "Acutely ill patients require potent, rapid-acting drugs and nutrients don't work rapidly."

"Are you saying that nutrient drips promote the healing response but cannot be used as supplementary therapies for acutely ill hospitalized patients?"

"I didn't say that," I protested.

"So why don't N^2D^2 docs ever use nutrient drips in the hospitals?" Choua returned to his earlier question.

"Because nutritional medicine just isn't practiced in the hospitals—physicians there do not believe in it. It's that simple!" I replied, exasperated.

Choua laughed lightly but said nothing. We remained silent

for a while. I felt relieved by the break in his relentless interrogation. Then Choua broke the silence and resumed,

"What would happen if Betty Best, that young intern, were to administer a nutrient IV drip to one of her patients in a hospital?"

"She will be probably be censored."

"By whom? By her supervising resident? By her attending physician? Or would it be some N^2D^2 doc sitting on the hospital medical board? And why would she be censored?" Choua fired a volley of questions.

"Because there are established standards of care in the hospitals and physicians abide by them. And those standards do not include nutrient IV infusions. Besides, interns in hospitals are not allowed to use unconventional therapies. She will have better sense than to order a nutrient IV drip," I shot back angrily.

"Oh yes! The hospital standards of care!" Choua mocked. "Standards of drug therapies, yes! Standards of nutrient therapies, no! Makes sense, doesn't it? Tell me, how much do N^2D^2 docs on hospital boards know about nutritional medicine?"

"You see things differently with your cyclopean eye," I said sarcastically."

"Will they censor the intern because they know nutrient IV drips do not work or because they have been programmed not to think beyond their rats stuff?" Choua asked scornfully. "Do they think vitamin C is only for scurvy? And what about magnesium? Since there is no known named deficiency syndrome for this mineral, when will they ever use it? Or it is because they are totally and utterly committed to drugs? Is this about caring for the sick or about protecting their turf?"

"Well..."

"Do these fellows who sit on hospital medical boards practice nutritional medicine?" Choua cut me off rudely.

"Why do you ask me questions if you do not have the patience to wait for my answer?" I retorted angrily.

"Do hospital medical boards ever discuss nutrition for hospitalized patients?" Choua ignored my question.

"Yes, they do!" I sighed.

"Is that RDA nutrition—the rats stuff of N^2D^2 docs—or is that the real thing?"

"What's the point of all this?" I asked, growing weary of Choua's unending questions.

"Who supervises the work of hospital dieticians?" Choua sidestepped my question.

"Usually one of the gastroenterologists serves as the chairman of the hospital dietary committee." I answered.

"Do gastroenterologists practice real nutritional medicine? Or are they also committed to that ratty RDA nutrition?"

"They do recommend different types of diets for various gastrointestinal disorders."

"That's not my question," Choua snapped. "Do they practice nutritional medicine? Do they use nutrients to reverse any disorders? Do they look at adverse food reactions and food allergies the way you do? Do they teach patients how to avoid sugar-insulin-adrenaline roller coasters? Do they think of the bowel as a delicate bowel ecosystem or do they see it a dark, gurgling tunnel that sometimes grows polyps?"

"I don't think gastroenterologist think ecologically," I confessed. "At least not those I know."

"So what is it that they supervise?" Choua taunted.

"Policies and procedures," I replied firmly.

"Aha! Policies! And procedures!" Choua drawled with mock surprise. "Policies and procedures for what? And based on what? The stupid rats notion of vitamins and minerals! Nutrients given in silly RDA amounts to treat deficiency diseases? Tell me, when was the last time you saw a case of scurvy treated with vitamin C? Or one of beri beri cured by vitamin B_1? Or one of pellagra cured with nicotinic acid?"

"I don't remember," I replied curtly.

"Do N^2D^2 docs on hospital boards ever realize foods might have something to do with disease?" Choua remained unaffected by my irritation. "Do they ever wonder if nutrients might facilitate the recovery process after an acute illness? Or after a surgical procedure? They do not know anything about nutrient therapies, yet they are so ready to censor physician-nutritionists."

"As usual you are exaggerating, Choua," I said acidly.

"Exaggerating! Am I?" Choua groused.

"Who told you that physicians in hospitals do not believe in food sensitivities?" I countered. "But hospitals are for acute medicine, and not for diagnosing food sensitivities."

"Do you think it doesn't matter if you feed acutely ill patients food they are sensitive to? Or is it that food-sensitive patients leave their food sensitivities at home when they check into hospitals?"

"Funny! Very funny stuff, Choua!" I replied with growing irritation. "There are more pressing clinical problems in hospitals than worrying about food reactions."

"How clumsy of me?" Choua rubbed his head in sarcasm. "How silly of me not to realize that it is okay to feed patients in hospitals foods that they are allergic to? I'm puzzled by one thing though: Since N^2D^2 docs on hospital boards don't use nutrients to treat diseases and since they also don't think that food sensitivities are relevant to care in the hospital, why do they go through the trouble of writing policies and procedures for nutrition?" Choua scowled.

"There are other things," I felt uneasy advancing an argument I didn't believe in. "There are issues like special diabetic diets, salt intake and the amount of proteins," I explained.

"Counting! So that's it! Counting calories and milligrams

of sodium? Is that it?" Choua gored. "Is that the depth and the breadth of nutrition science practiced in hospitals?"

"Choua, I don't think you understand the workings of a hospital dietary department," I held my ground. "There are other issues."

"What other issues?" Choua shot back. "Whether to serve patients Classic Coke or Pepsi? Whether to serve Maxwell House coffee or Folgers? Or is it about using aspartame or saccharin in desserts? Or perhaps those policies and procedures are to determine whether the napkins are Far Eastern yellow-green or patriotic red, blue and white? Or, maybe it's all about more substantive issues—whether the meals are served before the night shifts leaves or after the morning staff arrives?"

"Don't be silly, Choua," I replied curtly. "Serving hundreds of sick people with different nutritional requirements is not a mean task. It takes much planning and schedules that..."

"Aha! The schedules!" Choua cut me off rudely. "How awkward of me not to understand something that elementary? Isn't that what dietary policies and procedures are about? Schedules for receiving food deliveries, schedules for stocking shelves with canned foods, schedules for ovens and schedules for dishwashers?" Choua was unrelenting.

"Those *are* important considerations," I nearly yelled at him.

"Important for the administrative staff, yes!" Choua raised his voice too. "But, for N^2D^2 docs, no! Don't you see the difference between the two? Physicians should be interested in the metabolic nutritional needs of the sick, in subjects of *your* oxidative storms, how nutrients can be used to put them out, in how human energy pathways disrupted by disease can be restored. Don't you see physicians in hospitals need a broader perspective of health, disease and nutrition?"

"Hospitals don't make money teaching people nutritional

science. Nutritional medicine has no constituency in hospitals. Understand that for God's sake," I closed my eyes and rubbed my eyes for relief. "That's not my choice. I'm just telling you the way things are."

"Surely, the managers in the dietary department know more about food deliveries and dishwater schedules than N^2D^2 docs who supervise them," Choua spoke softly now. "So then the bottom line is that those who establish dietary policies and procedures in the hospitals know less than those who follow them," Choua chuckled.

"Hospitals are for acutely ill," I repeated.

"How many years have you served on the Medical Executive Committee of your hospital? Eighteen years? Or is more than that? Did the committee ever invite a practicing physician-nutritionist to advise them about their dietary policies and procedures during those years?"

"Don't be ridiculous," I replied sternly. "Why would a hospital board invite a practicing physician-nutritionist to advise it? Practicing nutritionists are not welcome in our hospitals."

"I thought so!" Choua said solemnly, ignoring the harshness in my tone. "Did the committee ever invite experts in any other discipline in medicine to address the committee?"

"Yes, it did—several times."

"Experts in what?"

"Infectious diseases."

"To tell you about cheaper antibiotics to save money? Or, was it to teach you how to avoid antibiotics?"

"That's ludicrous, Choua. Patients in hospitals need their antibiotics," I said angrily.

"Drug experts, yes! Physician-nutritionists, no! Why? Because nutrition is not important, is that it?" Choua shook his head.

I decided not to answer. Choua stared at me for a few moments, then walked to the window and looked out. We were quiet for several moments. Conversation with Choua can be unnerving. I was driven to the limit of my patience, and welcomed a respite, brief as I knew it would be. Then Choua turned to look at me and broke the silence,

"Do hospital boards ever discipline any physicians—punish them for mismanaging patients, for professional misconduct?"

"Of course, they do! But only when discipline is really necessary," I replied.

"What would happen if Betty Best ordered a nutrient IV drip for her patient with lung cancer?"

"Didn't I tell you before she would be reprimanded."

"Why?"

"Because nutrient IV drips are not considered good science."

"Only drugs make good science. Is that it?" Choua said sharply and continued, "When conducting their inquisitions, do medical boards ever consult other specialists as experts in the field?" Choua asked.

"Yes, they do!" I replied.

"Did a board ever ask a pediatrician to sit in judgment of the work of a psychiatrist?"

"No! That wouldn't be very smart, would it?" I replied tersely.

"Did a board ever ask an orthopedist to sit in judgment of the work of an ophthalmologist?"

"Why would any board do so? Why do you pester me with such silly questions?" I protested.

"Did a board ever ask a radiologist to sit in judgment of the work of a pathologist?"

"No! No! No!" I replied, exasperated.

"So, who would the board consult if they were to hold disciplinary hearings against a physician-nutritionist accused of *criminal* misconduct of administering an EDTA IV drip? You just told me it would not allow a physician-nutritionist to appear as an expert in defense. What other specialist would it invite as an expert witness? A jaw surgeon? Or would it be a Betty Best who performs coronary bypass surgery? The heart surgeons hate chelation therapy, don't they? Chelation is bad for their plumbing business! Right?" Choua said churlishly.

"Get off her case, will you?" I replied angrily. "In the U.S., therapies are accepted only if they meet the double-blind cross-over criteria of efficacy."

"Oh, silly me!" Choua pouted. "How could I forget about your *blessed* double-blind cross-over? Everyone knows physician-nutritionists are quacks, utterly unfamiliar with modern, scientific drug medicine. How can a hospital board accept them as experts when they use nutrients rather than drugs? It wouldn't be real, would it? What *is* real is that they will ask some university professor who has never practiced nutritional medicine to give an expert opinion on a matter that he knows nothing about. Now that would be real! Wouldn't it? *The double-blinded disciples of Aesculapius leading the blind.*" Choua sneered and disappeared into the hallway.

Rats
and Insurance Medical Boards

"Poor Betty Best! If she survives brainwashing by the first three rats boards, surely the fourth board will get her," Choua announced himself next day.

"What are you whimpering about now?" I asked.

"If Betty Best resists the Food and Nutrition, medical curriculum and hospital medical boards, she now faces the fourth board of insurance companies," Choua elaborated.

"You are an equal opportunity abuser, Choua. I was wondering when you were going to get to the insurance boards," I jested.

"Why don't the insurance companies see the obvious?" Choua asked.

"What's that?" I asked back.

"That nutritional medicine is far safer and less expensive than drug medicine."

"Because the medical boards of insurance companies do not believe in nutritional medicine."

"Catch 22! Isn't it? They don't believe in it so they don't try it. Because they don't try it, they don't find out it works."

"This is a serious problem," I agreed, "both for the professional as well as the patient."

"The insurance companies will happily pay $60,000 for coronary bypass surgery that will do nothing to reverse coronary heart disease, but they deny a patient $4,000 for EDTA chelation therapy that will dramatically improve circulation to the heart and prevent heart attacks. They will pay for expensive drug therapies and refuse to cover much less expensive nutrient therapies. Why don't they see the obvious cost savings for everyone? Their medical boards don't like Avita Average, do they? There must be some Olympian wisdom in that which escapes us mortals," Choua laughed.

One day Aubrey Worrell, M.D., a good friend and past president of the American Academy of Environmental Medicine, expressed his frustration with the way a major insurance company in his state refused to pay for the nutritional and environmental therapies that he prescribed for his patients. He collected several case histories of patients who suffered from nutrient deficiencies that were documented with the appropriate laboratory analysis. Then he met with a doctor from the medical board of that insurance company. This is how their conversation went after reviewing the clinical and laboratory data together:

"I have these case histories of people who are sick, and their laboratory test results show clear-cut evidence of nutrient deficiencies. They required nutrient therapies that I prescribed. Then you declined reimbursement. What shall I do for them?"

"We do not pay for nutrient therapies," the insurance doctor asserted. "We recognize only controlled scientific studies—double-blind cross-over proof of efficacy. We go by the RDA guidelines."

"But this *is* scientific data," Dr. Worrell protested.

"We need published scientific studies," the insurance doctor intoned, calmly but firmly. "What you are showing me are anecdotal items. We require properly conducted double-blind cross-over studies."

"But I'm a clinician. I don't conduct double-blind cross-over studies. My patients may be anecdotes for you but they are real people and so are their health disorders."

"Please be reasonable," the insurance doctor retorted. "Case histories of individual patients do not constitute controlled studies. We need hard data obtained with double-blinded studies."

"If not with nutrients, how else can I treat nutritional disorders?"

"We only recognize scientific, double-blind, cross-over studies." The insurance doctor repeated.

"Do you think I can morally treat nutrient deficiencies with the drugs you pay for."

"It's not a morality issue. At our company, we don't recognize nutritional medicine. We only follow established science. We insist on blinded, controlled studies."

"And you think it is good science to use drugs for people who need nutrients instead."

"We don't do medical research in our insurance company. We follow the RDA guidelines here.

"Don't you think I am medically liable to my patients if I do not treat documented nutrient deficiency states with appropriate nutrient therapies?"

"Dr. Worrell, please understand that we can only go by double-blind, cross-over studies. I'll be happy to see such studies if you have any."

DRUGS FOR NUTRIENT DEFICIENCIES

"Tell me what imbecile would insist on using drugs for documented nutrient deficiencies? What idiot would ask for double-blind, cross-over studies after nutrient deficiencies have been established with appropriate laboratory tests?" Choua fumed.

"Choua, be polite when you disagree with others," I

counseled.

"Does he tell the same thing to N^2D^2 docs? Does he ever talk about double-blind, cross-over nonsense when they use a drug for a disease when the use of that drug has not been validated with his *blessed* double-blind cross-over studies? You know that goes on all the time, don't you?"

"Yes," I agreed. "Tell me, why do you think insurance companies promote drug medicine but oppose nutritional medicine?"

"That's no secret. Insurance companies have big stakes in drug companies. Everyone knows that."

"But that doesn't explain why physicians who work for insurance companies should oppose nutritional medicine."

"Why should this be a mystery. The N^2D^2 docs, sitting on insurance medical boards, are just as ignorant of nutritional medicine as are the N^2D^2 docs who sit on the first three boards—the Food and Nutrition Board, the curriculum boards and the hospital boards. Poor Betty Best lives in a seven-board wonderland. N^2D^2 docs who take jobs with insurance companies usually do so when they are ready to retire or when they are plainly disgusted with the clinical practice of drug medicine."

"If they are really disgusted with drug medicine, Choua, why don't they actively support nutritional medicine?"

"You can be so simple-minded." Choua seemed to grow weary. "N^2D^2 docs do not take jobs with insurance companies to battle for their beliefs. It's just a job for them—fewer hours, plenty of coffee and doughnuts, no sick people to care for, no clinical failures to cope with, no responsibilities. Why would they want to get into trouble with N^2D^2 docs? They worship at the altar of the rat gods of the double-blind, and the rat gods solve all their problems. *The double-blinded disciples of Aesculapiuys worshipping at the altar of the gods of the double-blind.*" Choua shrugged and walked out.

Rats
and State Licensing Boards

Linda, a 28-year-old manager in a New York City advertising firm, consulted me for depression, muscle aches, fatigue and multiple allergies. As a teenager, she had "as much energy as her girlfriends." In college, she came down with infectious mononucleosis causing malaise and fatigue that lasted about seven weeks and restricted her to bed. She received steroids and multiple courses of antibiotics for it. Intermittent fatigue persisted even after she returned to school. She received more antibiotics for episodes of sore throat and common colds.

About two years later, a common cold caused severe fatigue, joint pains, abdominal bloating and mental confusion. She saw her primary physician who referred her to the local medical school where she saw several physicians including two professors of medicine. They treated her with antiglobulins, Acyclovir (an antiviral drug), and antidepressants. After some initial improvement, she went into deep depression and was hospitalized for two weeks, during which time she received multiple drug therapies. It was a very traumatic experience for Linda, because "I knew they were pouring drugs into me without knowing what they were doing."

She continued to suffer from recurrent sore throats, malaise, irritability, muscle aches and fatigue. She consulted some other physicians who prescribed yet more drugs. Finally, she consulted a physician who worked at a nutrition center and who prescribed nondrug therapies including intravenous nutrient drips. With such therapies, she "felt better than she had since the time she came down with infectious mononucleosis." She remained well for several months and returned to work, then the original problem began to come back. After reviewing clinical details of her case, I asked why she had come to see me rather than the physicians and professors at the university whom she saw earlier.

"Because I don't want to be a guinea pig anymore," she replied.

"What do you mean?" I asked.

"Because I have read enough about steroids and antiglobulin serum and Acyclovir and antidepressants. I now know what their long-term toxicities are."

"Why didn't you go back to the nutrition center where they successfully treated you before?" I asked the next logical question.

"Because they are now closed."

"Closed?" I asked with surprise.

"Yes! They were put out of business by the state medical board."

After finishing a review of Linda's medical history, I asked the staff to take her to an examination room and began to write my notes.

"The system never fails to protect its own, does it?" Choua asked sarcastically after Linda left.

"What system are you ranting about?" I asked.

"The system that protects the turf of N^2D^2 docs and puts all competition out of business," Choua jeered. "Poor Avita Average! She has no chance of survival."

"Well, we really do not know why they closed that place, do we? They seemed to have done well for Linda, but we don't know what else they did that wasn't right. We don't know why the

Board found it necessary to put them out of business."

"You don't! I do," Choua snapped. "Licensing boards hate Avita Average's guts!"

"Your cyclopean eye sees things only one way," I teased. "When you see a problem, you immediately think there is a doctor's hand behind it."

"My cyclopean eye?" Choua asked belligerently. "How many teenagers have you seen who suffered from chronic fatigue and depression and were turned into zombies by antidepressants and anxiety drugs? Tell me, did a state licensing board ever close down the office of a N^2D^2 drug doctor who fed too many mind-altering drugs to teenagers?" Choua shot back.

"Choua, we just do not know the facts of this case." I wanted to disentangle myself from the conversation.

"When was the last time a state licensing board revoked the license of a drug doctor who put little boys and girls on Ritalin, amphetamines and other drugs without ever bothering to find out if those poor children might be reacting to foods, molds or sugar roller coasters?" Choua was unrelenting.

"What," I sighed, "is the point of all those questions?"

"The point, Dr. Innocent, is that Linda got sicker and sicker with scientific drug therapies prescribed by those who exult in double-blind drug research. And that includes two professors of medicine! The only relief she obtained was from some *quack* she saw at some nutrition center. When her illness returned, she wanted no part of the scientific drug medicine. She wanted empirical, nondrug therapies and nutrient IV drips which had worked earlier. But, she couldn't have access to them because some state licensing board, in its infinite wisdom, had shut the nutrition center down."

"I can't comment on the case because I don't have the facts. There *are* charlatans in medicine. And they *do* bad things to many gullible patients. The public trust has to be protected." I was reaching the limits of my patience.

"Public trust! Huh!" Choua retorted. "Did any state licensing board ever shut down an operating room because the surgery performed in it was unnecessary?" Choua ignored my comment.

"It isn't always clear when surgery is unnecessary."

"Oh! Is that so? Is that really so?" Choua scowled. "Even when those TMJ specialists perform their *look-and-leave* surgery? You know what kind of surgery that is, don't you?" Choua frowned.

"What kind of surgery is that?" I asked even though I knew what Choua referred to.

"The open-the-joint-look-in-and-get-out surgery—the kind TMJ specialists love to perform. They open the jaw joint, look in, leave the things the way they found them, then close the joint. That's what that anesthesiologist told you. Didn't she?"

LOOK-AND-LEAVE SURGERY

Choua referred to a conversation that we had with an anesthesiologist who told us about this novel concept of *look and leave* surgery. I asked her how such an operation helps the patient. She smiled and said, "If the procedure helps any, it must do so by relaxing the spastic jaw muscles with the anesthetic we use." I found the concept of *look-and-leave* surgery amusing, but the idea behind it was really not new. Many years earlier, during my surgical training in Mayo Hospital, Lahore, Pakistan, I saw patients who had their gall bladders removed only to have symptoms recur within months after the surgery. "At least we removed the gall bladder from the differential diagnosis of your bellyache," we would console the patient and look for some other cause of his pain, some other body organ to remove. That is how we were brought up to think.

"What is TMJ?' Choua's words brought me back from my thoughts.

"You know what it is—a painful dysfunction of the jaw —temporomandibular joint—caused by excessive clenching of teeth. Why do you ask?"

"TMJ occurs as a result of persistent spasms of jaw muscles caused by chronic stress. Right? Now, do you think the use of a surgical scalpel is ever justified for problems caused by chronic stress? Isn't it a reprehensible abuse of surgical privileges?" Choua frowned.

"The joint exploration does seem to help some people," I said lamely.

"The concept of *look-and-leave* surgery does not surprise you?" Choua shouted. "But, on second thought, why would it surprise *any* pathologists? The TMJ surgeons shave a bit of the joint cartilage and remove some of the synovial joint lining. Such tissue is usually normal. Unremitting pressure of clenched jaws may cause some tissue edema and thickening but those changes are the consequences and not the cause of TMJ. But you know all that. You examine the tissues removed at surgery."

"Yes, we do."

"Do you send such cases to the hospital tissue committee for review?"

"We did, but don't anymore," I replied.

"I know why!" Choua grinned wickedly. "The TMJ surgeons were asked to explain why they removed normal tissues from the jaw joints. The surgeons soon found a solution to the problem: They stopped sending samples to the pathologist, and turned their *shave-the-joint-lining* surgery into *look-and-leave* surgery. The pathologist stopped receiving tissue, so there were no more ugly questions for TMJ surgeons to answer. A brilliant solution to an awkward problem. Right?" Choua chirped.

"You can't help but exaggerate, Choua," I reprimanded him. "The jaw joints are sometimes badly damaged in accidents and the victims do benefit from TMJ surgery."

"How often?" Choua posited. "How often is TMJ surgery done for trauma to the jaw? One in ten? Or is it one in one hundred?"

"That's the Chouese view of things again," I teased him.

"What sufferers of TMJ need is someone to teach them how to keep their jaw muscles relaxed," Choua's face softened to acknowledge my feeble attempt at humor. "But we all know there is no money in teaching people how to relax their tight jaw muscles. The TMJ surgeons know that the big bucks are in surgical procedures. Tell me, has a state licensing board ever shut down a TMJ surgery center? Those centers continue to mint money by performing their *look-and-leave* surgery, don't they?"

"I don't know enough about those things," I shrugged in resignation.

"Don't just keep repeating that silly defense," Choua hissed with sudden anger. "The N^2D^2 doctors on licensing boards are smug in their ignorance of essential environmental and nutritional issues. Drug and scalpels are all that they know and can use. Ask them about nutrition and human metabolism and they look at you as if you are from Mars. Ask them a question about the impact of environment on human biology and they go berserk. And these people decide who is fit to practice medicine and who is not! *The double-blind disciples of Aesculapius dispensing their Olympian justice.*"

Choua can be abrasive without realizing it. I decided not to provoke him any more. We were silent for some time, then I got up to examine Linda. When I returned Choua was gone.

Choua joined me for lunch the following day.

"Tell me, what else do the state licensing boards do to save Americans from the quackery of nutritionist-physicians?" Choua broke the silence.

"You are so cynical, Choua. The state boards have a responsibility to safeguard the interests of their citizens.

"What responsibility? To make sure that no citizen can have access to nutritional medicine?" Choua grimaced.

"There is no arguing with you. No point to it at all!" I fidgeted with a fork and knife.

"Why do you defend state licensing boards? Why do holistic physicians get into trouble with state licensing boards for their philosophy of medicine? Why aren't N^2D^2 docs ever investigated for their medical philosophy?" Choua ranted.

"Why?" I asked calmly.

"Because N^2D^2 docs have no philosophy of medicine! That's why! For them, it is all so simple: Name the disease, then name the drug. There is no need for philosophy in N^2D^2 medicine. Poor Avita Average! Her license is revoked because she tries to protect her patients from drug toxicities and unneeded surgical procedures."

"I don't know if that ever happens. There are usually other reasons. But, you do have a valid point. Mainstream physicians are not investigated as long as they limit their work to the use of drugs and scalpels."

"Do the N^2D^2 docs who sit on licensing boards ever wonder if they are qualified to sit in judgment of nondrug therapies? Do they ever have the courage to disqualify themselves when they are required to judge matters that they are incapable of judging?"

"They should, but they don't," I confessed.

"Why did they close the nutrition center that helped Linda?"

"I don't know! I don't know!" I groaned. "I told you I don't know the facts of that case."

"You don't see the obvious." Choua shook his head. "In hospitals, Betty Bests punish Avita Averages without first consulting the experts in that field. And Betty Bests are just as eager to destroy Avita Averages when they sit on state licensing boards. They never think of asking for expert opinion from those who practice nutritional and environmental medicine. I bet they are never troubled by such concerns. Do N^2D^2 docs ever really try to understand the chemistry of nutrients? The metabolic roles of nutrients? Do they ever wonder why nutritionists insist on looking at nutrients for their metabolic roles?"

"I don't know." That seemed like a short answer.

"Do N^2D^2 docs ever think beyond their silly notions of deficiency diseases?" Choua was relentless. "Do N^2D^2 disease doctors ever think about the roles of nutrients in health preservation? Do they ever think of the roles of nutrients in the aging process? Do they ever think of the roles of nutrients in disease reversal?"

"I don't know."

"Quackery! Expensive urine! Fringe physicians! Sound familiar?" Choua dug deeper.

"I know! I know! But you have to..."

"Have to do what?" Choua interrupted me again. "Your government experts think that micro-nutrients are needed for the prevention of deficiency diseases only. It seems so silly to me. I'll ask you again, when did you last see a patient who suffered from scurvy because he was deficient in vitamin C?" he inquired.

"I don't really remember." I replied.

"Did you ever see one?"

"No." I admitted

"Do you ever expect to see one?"
"Not really."

I had to admit, in nearly four decades of studying medicine, I had never seen a case of scurvy. In fact I do not remember ever hearing a case of scurvy described in the hundreds of nutrition conferences in which I have participated. I never heard my colleagues talk about using vitamin C to treat a scurvy patient. And, it seems highly improbable that I will ever see such a case for the rest of my years in clinical medicine.

"Tell me what do you think is the most important water-soluble antioxidant in your system?" Choua resumed.
"Ascorbate! I mean vitamin C" I answered in a matter-of-fact way.
"Now, tell me what is the most important free radical scavenger in your system?"
"Vitamin C?" I answered tentatively.
"Which vitamin has been used by more physicians for acute and chronic viral infections?"
"Vitamin C! It's common knowledge among nutritionist-physicians."
"What do oxidant injury, free radical stress and viral infections have to do with scurvy?"
"Nothing! I mean I don't know," I answered, trying to recall if I had ever read anything linking these things.

What does scurvy have to do with viral infections? I wondered about what possible relationship might exist between the two. Then I wondered why Choua raised this question. Does he know something about it that I don't? Or, was he simply drifting?

"The clinical efficacy of micronutrients is suppressed in the

United States," Choua resumed. "There are effective nondrug, nutrient and herbal therapies for immune and degenerative disorders. But N^2D^2 docs are not interested in them. They thrive on suppressing all nondrug and nonscalpel therapies. They love to punish holistic physicians, don't they? Some of them spoil for kill everytime a nutritritionist-physician is hauled before them. Others join the killers like the French women who brought their knittings to executions and urged the executioners on. All this in the name of science in medicine! There are no double-blind, cross-over studies to support the use of nutrients and herbs, they declare. *The double-blinded...* "

"*Double-blinded disciples of Aesculapius defending the public trust!*" I completed Choua's sentence in good humor.

Rats and FDA

Choua has strong opinions on everything. Strangely, I have never heard him take on the Food and Drug Administration.

Choua is an equal opportunity abuser and rails against different hierarchies in medicine with equal zest. No one is immune to his vitriolic attacks—not the Food and Nutrition Board, not medical school curriculum boards, not hospital disciplinary and state licensing boards, and not insurance boards. But, for some reason, I never hear him criticize the FDA. That is strange, because almost everyone I know in environmental and nutritional medicine is disgusted with what they believe is the FDA's heavy-handedness. When the FDA banned tryptophan—an essential amino acid that nutritionists favor over all other nutrients for depression, anxiety and sleep disorders—there was a nationwide hue and cry. But the FDA didn't budge. Tryptophan remains banned to this day. Choua never said a word against the FDA fiat.

"What do you think of the FDA?" I asked him one day in jest.

"They do their job," Choua replied nonchalantly.

"That's quite amazing!" I expressed my surprise. "*You* don't wail against the FDA!"

"The FDA is a government agency trying to do its job as best it can. What's amazing about it?"

"What's amazing about it?" I said, surprised. "The holistic world is bitter at their heavy-handed persecution of physicians who use nondrug therapies. You know how the FDA invades the

holistic clinics, confiscates their vitamin supplies and brings severe
action against them. And you don't think there is anything amazing
about your indifferent attitude to the FDA?"

"They are government agents doing their jobs. That's all!"
Choua repeated indifferently.

"Why are you so FDA-friendly?" I pressed. "There has to
be a reason. Are you afraid of them?"

Choua afraid of someone? The thought amused me. He is
an iconoclast, living in his own cocoon, impervious to events that
trouble most of us who practice environmental and nutritional
medicine. The things that concern most people are of no interest
to him—about the only time he argues passionately is when he
speaks against what he believes to be the tyranny of drug medicine
and when he puts down mainstream medical philosophy. That, of
course, is a daily occurrence. In those areas, Choua is totally
uninhibited. So the thought of Choua being afraid of the FDA was
amusing.

"So, tell me, Choua, are you afraid of the FDA? Is that
why you never take them on?" I asked.

"What's there to be afraid of?" Choua shrugged. "I've got
nothing to protect—no turf battles to fight. I just don't think the
FDA has a role in this. They are simply government agents doing
their thing."

"Then what was all that stuff about Mount Fudge and the
Mount Fudge-Blind Association?" I prodded.

"Olympian matters are for gods to discern and fix. I'm just
a story-teller," Choua grinned.

"I still don't get it, Choua!" I pressed. "How can you see
all the mischief caused by the FDA and say nothing? I mean, it's
not that you ran out of things to say, is it?"

"Nah!" Choua smiled. "It's none of that. It is just that the

FDA is composed of government agents doing their thing."

"Stop repeating that silly sentence!" I said testily.

"Suppose you are on an interstate highway and there is no traffic. You take liberties with the 55-mph speed limit and drive at 65-mph," Choua replied calmly, completely ignoring my harsh tone. "A cop nails you for speeding and gives you a ticket. Is that wrong?"

"It's not wrong, but it isn't right either," I countered, recognizing the frivolousness of my assertion.

"It isn't right because you do not agree with the law," Choua replied evenly. "You think when the interstate is empty, you should be allowed to driver faster. You forget cops do not write laws. If there is a silly law, you should write to your lawmakers, not take it out on the poor cop. After all, he is just a government agent doing his job."

"So?" I didn't know what else to say.

"So you see the FDA is a government agency. The folks at the FDA have no opinions of their own. They are neither scientists nor clinicians. They do not conduct research studies nor care for the sick. The only reason people work there is because they have neither the discipline of the scientist nor the diligence of the clinician. They have no minds of their own. Do you think the physicians at the FDA, who banned the use of tryptophan, knew anything about it?"

"Now, that's a good example," I countered. "Tell me, wasn't it a travesty? Millions of people all over the world take this essential amino acid as a precursor for the neurotransmitter serotonin. Along with tyrosine, we used it as a substitute for antidepressants and a natural aid to sleep in anxiety states. How many people got hurt with a contaminated lot of tryptophan? Five? Fifteen? How many hundreds of thousands of people will be hurt by antidepressants because they won't have access to tryptophan? How many will walk like zombies from taking mind-numbing drugs? Does anyone at the FDA think of that? And you still exonerate the FDA?" I asked in total disbelief.

"Yes!" Choua replied emphatically. "You miss the point. The doctors at the FDA are incapable of making those value judgments. I told you they have no expertise in such matters. They have no opinions of their own. The problem is not the FDA."

"Then, what is the problem?" I asked with resignation.

"The editors of your prestigious medical journals," Choua dead-panned.

"Wh...t!" I choked.

"The tyranny of N^2D^2 medicine begins with the editorial boards. They are the real villains in this maddening seven-board wonderland of Betty Best. They publish papers that push drugs and demonize nutrients and herbs. The folks at the FDA are not clinicians, nor do they conduct any clinical research. They are not paid to *think*. They are beaurocrats. They simply read what the editors of medical journals publish and blindly follow. *The double-blinded disciples of Aesculapius...*"

"That's crazy!" I yelled.

Rats and Editorial Boards

"The evil lurks in the editorial board rooms," Choua spilled more venom. "It's the editors of your prestigious medical journals who will not allow publication of articles about nondrug therapies—nutrients, herbs and physical methods of facilitating the process of disease reversal. They publish only drug studies. So poor Betty Best only reads about drug medicine."

"You overstate your case," I challenged Choua.

"Poor Betty Best! All she reads are articles pushing pills for anxiety," Choua ignored my comment. "And articles that tell her she should attach sleep machines to her nose when stress keeps her awake at night. Drugs for aches and pains, drugs for food reactions, drugs for environmental sensitivities, drugs for sugar-insulin-adrenaline roller coasters, drugs for abdominal bloating, drugs for constipation and drugs for the diarrhea caused by them, drugs for confusion and drugs for the brain fog caused by them, drugs for..."

"Is this litany going to end somewhere?" I asked with irritation.

"Poor Betty Best! Where does she get information about natural, nondrug therapies for the same problems? The N^2D^2 editors of drug journals never publish papers about the ways to enhance the antioxidant, DNA enzyme repair and immune defenses. Why should they? There are no advertising dollars in that?"

"There is good nutrition literature out there if any Betty Best is really interested," I challenged him.

"When did you last see an article in the *New England*

journal of Medicine that defines health, or describes how health may be preserved with nutritional, environmental and self-regulatory approaches? When was the last time you read an article about nondrug approaches to disease reversal in the *Annals of Medicine*? Did you ever see any such article?"

"I know that problem exists, but you spoil your case by exaggerating it," I advised.

"Exaggerating my case, eh?" Choua frowned. "The FDA does not ban herbs. It doesn't disallow vitamin therapy. The FDA doesn't stop anyone from using EDTA chelation for reversing coronary heart disease. The FDA does not put scalpels in the hands of heart surgeons. It does not force them to perform coronary bypass surgery, which does nothing to reverse heart disease except make sure the patient will forever need multiple drugs—and with some luck, return for a second, possibly a third bypass. You know how it is, don't you? All successful businesses are built on return business," Choua smirked.

"You and your cyclopean eye. You only..."

"That's a problem," He replied.

"You are totally out of order," I said harshly.

"Professors who sit on the editorial boards are responsible for the mess American medicine is in, not the FDA," Choua shrieked.

"That's a new one for me, Choua. I have never heard that before. Folks in nutritional medicine fear the FDA, not professors in some medical school."

"It's *the* professors!" Choua was adamant.

"That's absurd! Ludicrous," I spoke with annoyance.

"The folks at the FDA are innocent."

"Innocent? That's crazy," I screamed. "Choua, you are the only living soul in the nutrition community that defends the FDA and accuses professors in medical schools. Our professors do not make the rules. They don't write regulations. They have neither enforcement authority nor..." I protested.

"That's not the point," Choua interrupted sharply.

"Then what's the point?" I asked in frustration.

Choua stared at me with quizzical eyes and fell silent. I held his gaze, though I was confused and irritated by his sudden withdrawal. Then he walked to the window and looked out. Choua has this annoying habit. In the heat of an argument, he suddenly withdraws. After some minutes, my irritation subsided and I returned to my microscope.

"It all starts with the editors of medical journals," Choua spoke softly, still looking out. "They neither practice nutritional medicine nor are they aware of the healing potential of nutrients. They do not see patients who get better with nutritional therapies, and are unwilling to listen to the clinical findings of nutritionist-physicians. Yet they are convinced that nutritional medicine is only for the treatment of diseases that do not exist. They make sure that only drugs and scalpels get space in their journals."

"Why are they so malicious about nutritional medicine?" I provoked him.

"I don't know if they are malicious. They may be simply stupid about it." Choua answered in a matter of fact way.

"Stupid!" I was taken aback. "No one ever calls them stupid, Choua." I recovered.

"Why are you so sensitive about the word stupid? All of us are clever about some things and stupid about others. The editors of medical journals, I'm sure, are very clever about research in drug therapies and the practice of drug medicine, but they are obviously quite stupid about the fundamental premise of empirical medicine." Choua spoke both gently and firmly.

"Pray, tell me, Choua, what might that fundamental premise of empirical medicine be?" I jeered.

"That empirical medicine can only be practiced in a broad, integrated way—with sound knowledge of human biology, right choices in the kitchen, proper diagnosis and management of food and mold allergies, ample oral supplements and judicious use of injectable nutrients, skillful use of herbs, optimal environmental controls, effective methods of self-regulation, and slow, sustained exercise. Now, that's good empirical medicine. Doing what is safe and works! Is that too hard to understand?" Choua asked.

"Not really, but..."

"But there is nothing that medical editors hate more than the word empirical, right? They like their drug data pure and pristine—one drug at a time, double-blinded and crossed-over. What essential physiologic processes drugs block is of little concern to them. How toxic will the drugs be in months and years to come? That question doesn't bother them. How long will the victims of their drug research papers suffer the damage caused by drugs? The editors are not interested in such questions."

"It's hard to know what works and what doesn't without controls," I advanced the usual argument made by editors.

"Nonsense!" Choua erupted. "Nonsense! Sheer nonsense!" Choua seemed to grow angrier each time he repeated himself. "Do you follow the abominable double-blind, cross-over method when you do clinical outcome studies?"

"No, I don't!" I replied.

"Why not?" Choua pressed and then changed the subject. "Do you sometimes change your nutrient therapies?"

"Yes."

"Why?"

"Because I don't want to keep using what doesn't work."

"Aha! What works! So you do find out what does and doesn't work, don't you? Tell me, has any journal ever sent you articles for peer review?"

"Yes."

"I'm not talking about holistic journals. I mean has any mainstream journal ever asked you to review an article written by a nutritionist? Who reviews the articles about nutrient therapies? Practitioners of drug medicine, right?"

"Right!" I agreed.

"Now, tell me how can N^2D^2 docs conduct peer reviews of articles written by nutritionist-physicians? What kind of peer review is that?"

EDITORIALS FOR SALE

"What do you think of editorials for sale?" Choua asked one day.

"Don't be silly. No one *sells* editorials," I replied.

"You always underestimate the ingenuity of the merchants of N^2D^2 medicine. N^2D^2 dollars have an enormous buying power."

"Who feeds you such nonsense?" I asked.

"*The New England Journal of Medicine,*" Choua deadpanned.

"Don't be ridiculous! The *Journal* would never do that. It is very careful about ethical issues."

"You know me. I don't make things up," Choua winked. "Listen to this:

The practice of buying editorials reflects the growing influence of the pharmaceutical industry on medical care.

N Eng J Med 331:674; 1994

Ghostwriting to sell drugs is quite popular in the drug industry. For the right price, N^2D^2 docs are easily persuaded to submit ghostwritten papers to the journal under their name. Easy money! Why not?"

"That's amazing!" I couldn't contain myself. "I didn't know the editorials that I've been reading for years were bought by drug companies. Incredible! I don't think too many physicians know that. I wonder how many times even the editors might be duped. Do the editors always know when they publish bought editorials?"

"You don't, Dr. Innocent! Everyone else does," Choua chimed.

"How can any journal ever justify that? I have never heard such a thing," I said, vexed by Choua's revelation. "That is outright fraud, isn't it?" I asked, troubled.

"I'm glad you said that, not me!" Choua smiled, then continued, "Here is another interesting quote:

The caller said that I would not really have to do much work on this project. I would discuss the matter with them, and they would then have a professional writer compose the editorial, which I could modify as I saw fit. I would earn $2,500 for what was estimated to be several hours of work.

N Eng J Med 331:673; 1994

Earn $2,500! Do you know how this professor of public health was going to earn this money?" Choua frowned.

"How?" I asked, trying to maintain my composure.

"Interesting! An interesting explanation!" Choua smirked. "Listen to this:

> *The editorial was to be about the potential legal liability incurred by physicians who prescribe drugs that may have sedative side effects, such as antihistamines.*

> *N Eng J Med* 331: 673; 1994

Aha! An editorial against the use of drugs that have sedative effects! *How noble*?" Choua waved his arm in mock admiration. "But wait! Why would they pay a couple of thousand dollars to advise doctors not to use drugs? That doesn't make sense, does it?"

"No, it doesn't," I agreed.

"The purpose of the editorial was not to persuade N^2D^2 docs to refrain from using drugs. It was to encourage them to use a competitor's drug, the one who was paying for the hired gun. Now do you see the scheme of things? Clever! Ain't it?" Choua grinned broadly.

"Hard to believe!"

"This Harvard professor was to be hired by a high-power New York medical public relations firm to do a hatchet job on a competitor's drug. What's hard to believe there?"

"Oh no!" I shuddered.

"There is still more to come," Choua chuckled. "This professor teaches at the Harvard School of Public Health. Now isn't that fascinating? A New York public relations firm hiring a Harvard professor of *public health* to push drugs! What could be more elegant than that? Promoting public health by pimping drugs?"

"But Choua, this professor obviously didn't take the offer. Otherwise he wouldn't have written the article."

"That's not what kills me," Choua erupted. "What is astounding here is that a New York public relations firm would dare to ask a Harvard professor of public health to pimp drugs. New York firms are not populated by the scatterbrained. They didn't approach this professor so that their clever marketing strategy can be exposed. They would never try such a thing unless they knew it could work. How many Harvard professors do you think fell for this trick, sold their name—and their souls—for money, before this one yelled cop?"

BETTY BEST
AND SEVEN-BOARD WONDERLAND

"Poor thing, Betty Best Internist, M.D.!" Choua continued somberly. "She doesn't have a chance in the seven-board wonderland. She had a teenager's dream to help the sick without hurting them—and good nutrition seemed to make sense to her. The first sharp blow to her teenage idealism was dealt by the Food and Nutrition Board. It planted the pernicious RDA notion in her head. Nutrients, she was told, were necessary only to prevent ten or twelve deficiency diseases. And that's all!

"She worked hard to get into a medical school. Some Ph.Ds., who know nothing about nutrient therapies, reinforced the perverse notion that only quacks use nondrug nutrient and herbal therapies. She is too overwhelmed by her daily quota of material to be crammed to ask the basic question: If the injured tissues do not heal with nutrients, with what do they heal?

"As an intern, she looked up to her attending physicians for counsel and knowledge. Their ignorant animus against natural therapies spilled out of their ears and noses. If any part of her natural inquisitiveness toward the role of nutrients and herbs survived years of assault by N^2D^2 hospital docs, and if she tried a nutrient injection, she was promptly censored by the hospital medical board.

"She enters clinical practice and is swamped by drug representatives peddling their newest and most efficient drugs, killer antibiotics guaranteed to decimate the patient's bowel ecosystem. If she bumps into an article about nondrug therapies and wants to help her patient naturally, she is in for a rude awakening. The N^2D^2 docs at the insurance medical boards are as committed to drugs as their hospital peers. They contemptuously deny her claims for reimbursement. (They were trained by geek N^2D^2 docs, who call themselves quack-busters, to view all nondrug therapies as health frauds.) Betty Best and her patient learn fast—both are denied payment. If she foolishly persists, the N^2D^2 docs at the insurance board report her professional misconduct to the N^2D^2 docs on her licensing board.

"By now, Betty Best has matured. She has forgotten her teenage resolve to care for the sick with best the possible therapies. She now shuns anyone who talks about alternative therapies. I can't bite the hands that feeds me, she tells herself as she thinks of referring physicians. By now, she has also learned what happens to miscreants who overstep the bounds of N^2D^2 medicine. They are hauled before disciplinary committees. And if they do not desist, their licenses are revoked.

"Betty Best knew the folks at the FDA were dragons. One doesn't awaken sleeping monsters. Betty Best was not *that* stupid! She didn't want any part of omega-6 oils, tryptophan and everything else that the FDA chose to focus on. The practice of medicine was hard—and getting harder by the day. Patients had to be seen. Children had to be played with, at least on weekends. Sometimes, her husband didn't quite understand the pressures on her. Why engage in frivolous things such as disagreeing with the FDA? she reasoned.

"Now, Betty Best Internist, M.D., lives in a seven-board wonderland. She has very little time for herself. She can ill-afford being out-of-touch with current advances in drug therapies. Certainly she cannot allow anyone to think that she is unfamiliar with the latest drug-of-choice. So many journals to read! How does she keep up? So many drug names to learn—and each with a long list of toxic side effects! She knows one drug increases the toxicity of the other. She looks around to see how others cope with the avalanche of new drugs, and the new and novel uses of scalpels. Poor Betty Best! She has to be among the best. Finally she figures it all out—just as everyone else figured it out before her. She chooses the *New England Journal of Medicine.* The thing about the *Journal* is that it is safe. What fool would dare to defy the *Journal?*"

Choua heaved as he spoke those last sentences, stopped, looked me in the eye for a few moments, then disappeared into the hallway.

I love doctors and hate their medicine.

Walt Whitman

*Perfection of means and confusion of goals
seem—in my opinion—to characterize our
age.*

Albert Einstein

In acute illness, our perfection of means is astounding. Advances in medical technology are breath-taking. Our surgical prowess is daunting, the potency of our drugs supreme.

In chronic nutritional, ecologic and stress-related disorders, our confusion of goals is equally astounding. We seem to think nutritional medicine is a hoax; clinical ecology is treatment of non-existent diseases; and self-regulation is a pursuit for the feeble-minded.

We seem to think that energetic-molecular events that initiate disease, and cell membrane dynamics that perpetuate it, are of little relevance to clinical medicine. We seem to think that to name a disease is to understand it, to classify is to conquer it and to suppress its symptoms with drugs is to cure it.

Our principal clinical strategy is this: disease *prevention* is a patient's responsibility. When someone is near death, we will pull him out of the jaws of death with our Star Wars medical technology.

How could we, the healing profession, be so utterly wrong?

Index

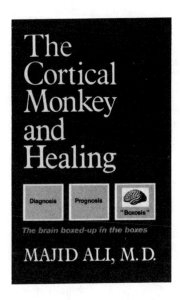

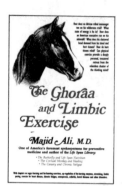
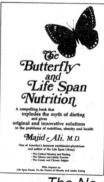

LIFE SPAN BOOKS

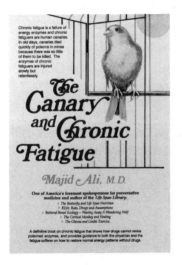

The definitive book on chronic fatigue.

Providing not only the clinical outlines for non-drug reversal of chronic fatigue, but also the rational and scientific basis of hope and optimism that is so sorely lacking in 'human canaries'.

Reversing chronic fatigue <u>without</u> drugs and <u>with</u> hope and non-drug therapies

The Canary and Chronic Fatigue

Majid Ali, M.D.

ISBN 1-879131-02-1

The Life Span Library of the Scientific Basis of Health

From the author of
The Canary and Chronic Fatigue
& RDA:Rats, Drugs, and Assumptions

WHAT DO LIONS KNOW ABOUT STRESS

MAJID ALI, M.D.

While we know what it means to be relaxed, we also know this knowledge does not always help us in our controlling stress.

The problem for many of us is not the absence of desire to control stress, it is knowing how to do it.

A practical approach to controlling stress without drugs

What Do Lions Know About Stress
Majid Ali, M.D.